Migraines and Beyond: Advances in the Pathogenesis and Treatment of Chronic Headache Disorders

Migraines and Beyond: Advances in the Pathogenesis and Treatment of Chronic Headache Disorders

Editor

Yasushi Shibata

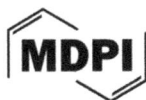

Basel • Beijing • Wuhan • Barcelona • Belgrade • Novi Sad • Cluj • Manchester

Editor
Yasushi Shibata
Faculty of Medicine
Mito Medical Center
University of Tsukuba
Tsukuba
Japan

Editorial Office
MDPI AG
Grosspeteranlage 5
4052 Basel, Switzerland

This is a reprint of articles from the Special Issue published online in the open access journal *Neurology International* (ISSN 2035-8377) (available at: https://www.mdpi.com/journal/neurolint/special_issues/4AO2CL3C12).

For citation purposes, cite each article independently as indicated on the article page online and as indicated below:

Lastname, A.A.; Lastname, B.B. Article Title. *Journal Name* **Year**, *Volume Number*, Page Range.

ISBN 978-3-7258-1809-9 (Hbk)
ISBN 978-3-7258-1810-5 (PDF)
doi.org/10.3390/books978-3-7258-1810-5

© 2024 by the authors. Articles in this book are Open Access and distributed under the Creative Commons Attribution (CC BY) license. The book as a whole is distributed by MDPI under the terms and conditions of the Creative Commons Attribution-NonCommercial-NoDerivs (CC BY-NC-ND) license.

Contents

About the Editor vii

Yasushi Shibata
Continuous Research of Headache and Migraine
Reprinted from: *Neurol. Int.* 2024, 16, 59, doi:10.3390/neurolint16040059 1

Horia Pleș, Ioan-Alexandru Florian, Teodora-Larisa Timis, Razvan-Adrian Covache-Busuioc, Luca-Andrei Glavan, David-Ioan Dumitrascu, et al.
Migraine: Advances in the Pathogenesis and Treatment
Reprinted from: *Neurol. Int.* 2023, 15, 67, doi:10.3390/neurolint15030067 2

Eleonóra Spekker and Gábor Nagy-Grócz
All Roads Lead to the Gut: The Importance of the Microbiota and Diet in Migraine
Reprinted from: *Neurol. Int.* 2023, 15, 73, doi:10.3390/neurolint15030073 56

Maria Papasavva, Michail Vikelis, Vasileios Siokas, Martha-Spyridoula Katsarou, Emmanouil V. Dermitzakis, Athanasios Raptis, et al.
Genetic Variability in Vitamin D Receptor and Migraine Susceptibility: A Southeastern European Case-Control Study
Reprinted from: *Neurol. Int.* 2023, 15, 69, doi:10.3390/neurolint15030069 73

Oliwia Szymanowicz, Izabela Korczowska-Łacka, Bartosz Słowikowski, Małgorzata Wiszniewska, Ada Piotrowska, Ulyana Goutor, et al.
Headache and *NOTCH3* Gene Variants in Patients with CADASIL
Reprinted from: *Neurol. Int.* 2023, 15, 78, doi:10.3390/neurolint15040078 85

Nicola Benedicter, Karl Messlinger, Birgit Vogler, Kimberly D. Mackenzie, Jennifer Stratton, Nadine Friedrich and Mária Dux
Semi-Automated Recording of Facial Sensitivity in Rat Demonstrates Antinociceptive Effects of the Anti-CGRP Antibody Fremanezumab
Reprinted from: *Neurol. Int.* 2023, 15, 39, doi:10.3390/neurolint15020039 100

Yasushi Shibata and Sumire Ishiyama
Neurite Damage in Patients with Migraine
Reprinted from: *Neurol. Int.* 2024, 16, 21, doi:10.3390/neurolint16020021 116

Leonidas Mantonakis, Ioanna Belesioti, Christina I. Deligianni, Vasilis Natsis, Euthimia Mitropoulou, Elina Kasioti, et al.
Depression and Anxiety Symptoms in Headache Disorders: An Observational, Cross-Sectional Study
Reprinted from: *Neurol. Int.* 2024, 16, 26, doi:10.3390/neurolint16020026 129

Paolo Manganotti, Manuela Deodato, Laura D'Acunto, Francesco Biaduzzini, Gabriele Garascia and Antonio Granato
Effects of Anti-CGRP Monoclonal Antibodies on Neurophysiological and Clinical Outcomes: A Combined Transcranial Magnetic Stimulation and Algometer Study
Reprinted from: *Neurol. Int.* 2024, 16, 51, doi:10.3390/neurolint16040051 143

Yasushi Shibata, Hiroshige Sato, Akiko Sato and Yoichi Harada
Efficacy of Lasmiditan as a Secondary Treatment for Migraine Attacks after Unsuccessful Treatment with a Triptan
Reprinted from: *Neurol. Int.* 2024, 16, 48, doi:10.3390/neurolint16030048 159

Reem Suliman, Vanessa Santos, Ibrahim Al Qaisi, Batool Aldaher, Ahmed Al Fardan, Hajir Al Barrawy, et al.
Effectiveness of Switching CGRP Monoclonal Antibodies in Non-Responder Patients in the UAE: A Retrospective Study
Reprinted from: *Neurol. Int.* **2024**, *16*, 19, doi:10.3390/neurolint16010019 . . . . **169**

Yan Tereshko, Enrico Belgrado, Christian Lettieri, Simone Dal Bello, Giovanni Merlino, Gian Luigi Gigli and Mariarosaria Valente
Pulsed Radiofrequency for Auriculotemporal Neuralgia: A Case Report
Reprinted from: *Neurol. Int.* **2024**, *16*, 25, doi:10.3390/neurolint16020025 . . . . **184**

About the Editor

Yasushi Shibata

Yasushi Shibata graduated from the School of Medicine, University of Tsukuba, Tsukuba, Japan. He received medical and surgical training at the University Tsukuba Hospital and affiliated hospitals. He conducted basic and clinical research at Harvard Medical School, Boston, the Beth Israel Deaconess Medical Center, Boston, and the Massachusetts Institute of Technology, Cambridge, MA, USA. His main research interests are headache, cerebrovascular diseases, head injury, neuroradiology and brain tumor. He published more than 130 research papers and more than 50 edited textbooks. He has received many research grants and awards. He is now a Full Professor and the Director of the Department of Neurosurgery, Mito Medical Center, University of Tsukuba. He is the on the board of the Japan Neurosurgical Society and the Japan Stroke Society, as well as on the executive board of the Japanese Society of Neuroradiology, the Japanese Headache Society, and the Japan neurosurgery English forum. He was accredited as Headache Master by the International Headache Society in 2013. He is also the member of many international academic societies. He has also worked as an Editor-in-chief or editorial member and reviewer for many international journals.

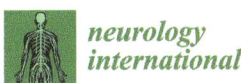

Editorial

Continuous Research of Headache and Migraine

Yasushi Shibata

Department of Neurosurgery, Mito Medical Center, University of Tsukuba, Mito Kyodo General Hospital, Miyamachi 3-2-1, Ibaraki 310-0015, Japan; yshibata@md.tsukuba.ac.jp

1. Introduction

Headache is a common disorder with high prevalence. Migraine is known to heavily disturb the daily life of patients. So, the direct social and indirect economic losses caused by absenteeism and presenteeism have been reported to be huge. Recent developments in new drug therapies are specific and effective for most patients with migraine. However, there are still some patients whose condition cannot be controlled using current therapies. We need continuous research to effectively use these new medications.

2. Discussion

This Special Issue includes a variety of basic, translational, and clinical research and case reports. A step-by-step understanding of migraine pathophysiology is crucial for clinical decision making and future research.

Because there are no clinically available diagnostic biomarkers of migraine, the diagnosis and evaluation of patients' headaches has solely depended on interviews regarding their clinical history and symptoms. Migraine biomarkers are a hot area of research. Some neuropeptides could be commercially available markers of migraine. Another biomarker may be imaging methods such as magnetic resonance imaging (MRI). Studies of these biomarkers could provide effective diagnostic tools and indicators of the effects of treatment.

We understand that genetics is also involved in the various forms of headache including migraine. Some specific genetic diseases are accompanied by clinical migraine. However, a single gene causative of migraine has not been demonstrated. Genetic studies of headache disorders will identify the causal mechanisms of those genes and clinical headache. These studies will provide fundamental therapy strategies for these headaches.

Clinical studies and clinical case reports provide insight for daily clinical practice. We can use many drugs and some interventions, such as neuro-stimulation. These therapies have been effective in some patients. In clinical practice, we must select these therapies according to each patient. These therapeutic strategies, including their ideal combinations, need more research.

3. Conclusions

I hope this Special Issue contributes to the current understanding of migraine and headache. Readers may acquire inspiration for future studies from the research articles in this Special Issue.

Conflicts of Interest: The authors declare no conflicts of interest.

Disclaimer/Publisher's Note: The statements, opinions and data contained in all publications are solely those of the individual author(s) and contributor(s) and not of MDPI and/or the editor(s). MDPI and/or the editor(s) disclaim responsibility for any injury to people or property resulting from any ideas, methods, instructions or products referred to in the content.

Citation: Shibata, Y. Continuous Research of Headache and Migraine. *Neurol. Int.* **2024**, *16*, 804. https://doi.org/10.3390/neurolint16040059

Received: 10 July 2024
Accepted: 15 July 2024
Published: 22 July 2024

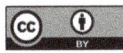

Copyright: © 2024 by the author. Licensee MDPI, Basel, Switzerland. This article is an open access article distributed under the terms and conditions of the Creative Commons Attribution (CC BY) license (https://creativecommons.org/licenses/by/4.0/).

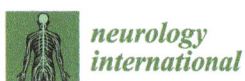

Review

Migraine: Advances in the Pathogenesis and Treatment

Horia Pleș [1], Ioan-Alexandru Florian [2,*], Teodora-Larisa Timis [3,*], Razvan-Adrian Covache-Busuioc [4], Luca-Andrei Glavan [4], David-Ioan Dumitrascu [4], Andrei Adrian Popa [4], Andrei Bordeianu [4] and Alexandru Vlad Ciurea [4]

1. Department of Neurosurgery, Centre for Cognitive Research in Neuropsychiatric Pathology (NeuroPsy-Cog), "Victor Babeș" University of Medicine and Pharmacy, 300041 Timișoara, Romania; ples.horia@umft.ro
2. Department of Neurosciences, "Iuliu Hatieganu" University of Medicine and Pharmacy, 400012 Cluj-Napoca, Romania
3. Department of Physiology, "Iuliu Hatieganu" University of Medicine and Pharmacy, 400012 Cluj-Napoca, Romania
4. Neurosurgery Department, "Carol Davila" University of Medicine and Pharmacy, 020021 București, Romania; razvan-adrian.covache-busuioc0720@stud.umfcd.ro (R.-A.C.-B.); luca-andrei.glavan0720@stud.umfcd.ro (L.-A.G.); david-ioan.dumitrascu0720@stud.umfcd.ro (D.-I.D.); andreiadrianpopa@stud.umfcd.ro (A.A.P.); andrei.bordeianu@stud.umfcd.ro (A.B.); prof.avciurea@gmail.com (A.V.C.)

* Correspondence: florian.ioan.alexandru@gmail.com (I.-A.F.); doratimis@gmail.com (T.-L.T.)

Abstract: This article presents a comprehensive review on migraine, a prevalent neurological disorder characterized by chronic headaches, by focusing on their pathogenesis and treatment advances. By examining molecular markers and leveraging imaging techniques, the research identifies key mechanisms and triggers in migraine pathology, thereby improving our understanding of its pathophysiology. Special emphasis is given to the role of calcitonin gene-related peptide (CGRP) in migraine development. CGRP not only contributes to symptoms but also represents a promising therapeutic target, with inhibitors showing effectiveness in migraine management. The article further explores traditional medical treatments, scrutinizing the mechanisms, benefits, and limitations of commonly prescribed medications. This provides a segue into an analysis of emerging therapeutic strategies and their potential to enhance migraine management. Finally, the paper delves into neuromodulation as an innovative treatment modality. Clinical studies indicating its effectiveness in migraine management are reviewed, and the advantages and limitations of this technique are discussed. In summary, the article aims to enhance the understanding of migraine pathogenesis and present novel therapeutic possibilities that could revolutionize patient care.

Keywords: migraine pathogenesis; molecular markers; calcitonin gene-related peptide (CGRP); migraine treatment; neuromodulation

1. Introduction

An overwhelming majority of the global population, approximately 95%, have suffered from a headache at some point in their lives, with an alarming annual prevalence that suggests nearly half of all adults have experienced a headache within a given year [1]. The ramifications of this health issue extend far beyond personal discomfort, with headaches accounting for one-tenth of consultations with general practitioners [2], and a significant portion, one-third, of referrals to neurologists [3]. Moreover, acute medical admissions related to headaches are alarmingly high, constituting one in every five cases.

The World Health Organization recognizes the debilitating nature of headaches, including them among the top ten global causes of disability. Interestingly, in women, the prevalence and impact of headaches are even more pronounced, ranking among the top five causes of disability [4]. It is pertinent to note that the debilitating impact of headaches is comparable to chronic conditions, such as arthritis and diabetes, and its severity exceeds that of conditions like asthma [5,6].

Taking the United Kingdom as an illustrative example, the socioeconomic implications of migraine, a specific type of headache, are vast. An estimated 25 million workdays are lost annually due to migraine, creating an indirect economic burden of nearly GBP 2 billion per year. This figure does not even include the direct healthcare costs associated with managing headaches, such as medication expenses, consultations with general practitioners, referrals to specialists, and visits to emergency care facilities [7].

Quantifying the influence of headaches, particularly migraine, on an individual's quality of life can be challenging. Yet, it is clear from reported data that the impact is substantial. A significant percentage, approximately 75% of patients, experience functional disability during a migraine attack. Additionally, half of the sufferers require the assistance of family members or friends during an attack, causing a significant disruption to their social lives [8]. The ripple effect of headaches extends beyond the individuals suffering from them, impacting society at large and requiring serious attention for more effective management strategies [9].

Migraine, a long-term headache disorder punctuated by episodic bouts, is characterized by repeated instances of severe headaches that present with unique associated symptoms. These include photophobia, a heightened sensitivity to light, and phonophobia, an increased sensitivity to sound [10]. The classification of episodic migraine—an intermittent but recurring form of this disorder—hinges on the frequency with which a patient experiences these debilitating headaches.

In the majority of cases, patients undergo fewer than 15 episodes of headaches per month, a condition identified as episodic migraine. Conversely, there is a subset of individuals who face a more frequent occurrence of headaches—on 15 or more days each month, spanning over three months. Importantly, at least eight of these days should either meet the diagnostic criteria for migraine without the accompanying aura or show responsiveness to treatment specifically designed for migraine. The International Headache Society recognizes this latter classification as chronic migraine [11].

Chronic migraine, although less common when compared to its episodic counterpart, remains a pervasive and incapacitating issue [12]. It poses a significant burden on those afflicted with the condition, dramatically impacting their daily lives and well-being [13,14]. This persistent form of migraine continues to be a widespread challenge, necessitating ongoing research and improved therapeutic strategies to ease the strain it puts on sufferers [15].

1.1. Brief Overview of Migraine as a Prevalent Neurological Condition

Over the past three decades, there has been a significant upsurge in the worldwide prevalence of migraine. As highlighted by the Global Burden of Disease (GBD) 2019 study, the estimated global occurrence of migraine escalated from 721.9 million (with a 95% uncertainty interval (UI) of 624.9–833.4) in 1990 to a staggering 1.1 billion (95% UI: 0.98–1.3) in 2019. The percentual shifts in global age-standardized prevalence rate and years lived with disability (YLDs) over these nearly three decades were recorded at 1.7 (95% UI: 0.7–2.8) and 1.5 (95% UI: −4.4 to 3.3), respectively [16].

In this time frame, the sharpest escalations in the age-standardized prevalence per 100,000 individuals were recorded in East Asia with a 7.9% increase (95% UI: 4.3–12%), and in Andean Latin America with an increase of 6.7% (95% UI: 2.1– 11.9%). Conversely, the most significant decreases were seen in high-income North America [−2.2% (95% UI: −5.3 to 1.1%)] and Southeast Asia [−2.2% (95% UI: −3 to −1.4%)]. Moreover, the age-standardized YLD rate due to migraine also saw an increase from 517.6 (95% UI: 82.0–1169.1) in 1990 to 525.5 (95% UI: 78.8–1194.0) in 2019.

The incidence of migraine consistently appeared higher in females than in males across all age groups. In 2019, the global age-standardized prevalence rate for females was 17,902.5 (95% UI: 15,588.3, 20,531.7) per 100,000 populations, in comparison to 10,337.6 (95% UI: 8948.0, 12,013.0) for males [16].

Notably, the most frequent incidence of migraine, both in terms of rate and absolute number of new cases, was seen in the age bracket of 10–14 years for both genders. Over the course of 2019, the number of YLDs due to migraine began to increase from birth, reaching a peak in the 30–34 age group, after which it slowly receded for both sexes [17].

Contrary to expectations, socioeconomic status did not appear to have a direct correlation with the burden of migraine. The study did not reveal any discernible link between the socio-demographic index (SDI) and the YLD rate associated with migraine. This lack of association suggests that migraine does not discriminate based on socioeconomic status, further underlining the pervasive nature of this debilitating condition [17].

The prevalence of migraine has been reported to fluctuate between 2.6% and 21.7%, with an estimated average prevalence close to 12%. However, these figures vary significantly across different nations and even between individual studies conducted within the same country [18–21].

Notably, there appears to be a strong familial connection among individuals suffering from migraine, suggesting that genetic factors significantly contribute to the risk of developing this condition [20,22–25]. Supporting this theory, twin studies have indicated that migraine represent a complex genetic disease that involves an intricate interplay between genetic and environmental factors. Remarkably, the heritability of migraine has been estimated to be as high as 65% [26–29].

However, in spite of the robust genetic implications suggested by these studies and several large-scale genome-wide association studies (GWAS) conducted over the years, the scientific community has yet to conclusively identify specific candidate genes responsible for migraine. A recent systematic re-evaluation of 27 proposed candidate genes found none to be statistically significant [30].

Interestingly, the prevalence of migraine among neurologists is significantly higher when compared to the general population, reaching prevalence rates as high as 48.6% in some studies. This elevated prevalence is most likely attributable to enhanced self-recognition of migraine symptoms among professionals who are extensively trained and experienced in diagnosing and treating the condition. This assertion is supported by a study revealing that just over half of individuals who were diagnosed with migraine actually recognized their headache as a migraine [31].

1.2. Prevalence of Migraine in Pediatric Patients

From a meta-analysis, in which data were sourced from 40 studies encompassing a sample of 15,626 pediatric and adolescent individuals diagnosed with migraines, an 11% prevalence rate was noted, displaying considerable heterogeneity. Among these, 27 studies delineated migraine prevalence based on gender. The aggregated prevalence rate for females stood at 4%, whereas for males it was 3%. Specific data concerning MwoA (migraine without aura) and MwA (migraine with aura) were gleaned from 13 studies, which covered 3481 and 1322 subjects diagnosed with MwoA and MwA, respectively. Prevalence for MwoA was identified at 8% and for MwA at 3%, with marked heterogeneity for both. Only six studies offered data on chronic migraines, revealing a prevalence that fluctuated between 0.2% and 12% [32].

From a separate dataset of 31 studies, information was extracted involving 13,105 pediatric and adolescent subjects diagnosed with TTH (tension-type headache). This cohort exhibited a prevalence of 17%, with notable heterogeneity. Out of these studies, 23 offered a gender-based breakdown of TTH prevalence, yielding a consolidated prevalence rate of 11% for females and 9% for males. Limited data on episodic and chronic TTH were derived from 7 studies, which presented a prevalence range of 4–29% and 0.2–12.9%, respectively [32].

Another set of data, obtained from 40 studies, encompassed 76,782 pediatric and adolescent participants diagnosed with primary headaches in general. The overall prevalence was determined at 62%, with significant heterogeneity observed. Gender-based prevalence data for primary headaches, extracted from 29 studies, showed an aggregated prevalence rate of 38% for females and 27% for males [32].

1.3. Medical Treatments of Migraine in Children

Recent advancements in the pharmaceutical sector have introduced a selective 5-HT1F agonist, lasmiditan, which serves as an efficacious acute treatment for adults, demonstrating no vasoconstrictor activity. This drug is currently under investigation for its applicability in pediatric populations. Additionally, several novel calcitonin gene-related peptide (CGRP) antibodies and antagonists, which have demonstrated efficacy in both the acute treatment and prevention of migraines in adults, are now being assessed in pediatric clinical trials. In adult medical practices, there is an increasing inclination towards peripheral nerve blocks and botulinum toxin; however, the need for robust evidence supporting their efficacy in children is paramount. Furthermore, the introduction of electroceuticals—therapeutic electric devices—has broadened the treatment horizon. These devices include the external trigeminal nerve stimulator (e-TNS), non-invasive vagal nerve stimulator (nVNS), single-pulse transcranial magnetic stimulator (sTMS), and remote electrical neuromodulation device (REN). Presently, substantial evidence supporting their effectiveness in pediatric populations remains elusive; furthermore, while significant progress has been observed, it predominantly benefits the adult demographic. There is an imperative need to expedite migraine research focusing on children [33].

2. Pathogenesis of Migraine: Role of Molecular Markers in Identifying Migraine Triggers and Mechanisms

2.1. Definition and Significance of Molecular Markers

Biomarkers, in the realm of medical and biological research, are defined as quantifiable indicators of biological conditions, representing either physical manifestations or results obtained from laboratory tests that correlate with biological processes. These markers have the potential to serve critical diagnostic or prognostic functions [34]. A more explicit definition of biomarkers was proposed during a conference hosted by the US Food and Drug Administration. In this context, biomarkers are characterized as quantifiable attributes that can be objectively measured and assessed, providing insights into standard biological, pathological, or pharmacological processes [35].

This clear and precise definition paves the way for a bifurcation of biomarkers into the following two unique types: diagnostic and therapeutic. Diagnostic biomarkers serve as flags for pathological conditions and bear a close association with the risk of developing a disease and its severity. They aid in identifying the presence of a disease and gauging its stage or intensity, thus playing a crucial role in guiding clinical decision-making [36].

On the other hand, therapeutic biomarkers hold a different but equally important role. They provide information on a treatment's response, effectively serving as indicators of the efficacy or success of a therapeutic intervention. These biomarkers help clinicians tailor treatments to individual patients, allowing for personalized medicine approaches. They offer a chance to predict whether a patient is likely to respond positively to a particular treatment, making them a powerful tool in the management and treatment of diseases. By providing an early indication of the effectiveness of a therapeutic regimen, these markers can guide healthcare professionals in adjusting treatments as necessary, minimizing the trial-and-error aspect of disease management and increasing the probability of successful outcomes [15].

Biomarkers represent objective physical traits that can be harnessed to illuminate and distinguish the biological nature and mechanisms of various diseases and syndromes. Essentially, they provide snapshots of the body's physiological state and can offer valuable insights into health and disease processes. Biomarkers have an extensive range of potential manifestations, which can include but are certainly not limited to, results obtained from the examination of blood, urine, muscle, nerve, skin, or cerebrospinal fluid [37].

Additionally, biomarkers may also be identified in the form of genes or gene products. These genetic markers offer a unique insight into an individual's inherent disease susceptibility or resistance and can often illuminate potential therapeutic pathways. Likewise, biomarkers can be identified through advanced imaging techniques such as X-rays, magnetic resonance imaging (MRI), or computed tomographic (CT) scans. These imaging biomarkers can provide a visual representation of disease progression, allowing clinicians to identify anatomical or functional changes in the body over time [34].

Another fascinating domain of biomarkers lies in the realm of electrophysiological measurements, such as those generated by electrocardiograms (ECGs), electroencephalograms (EEGs), or nerve conduction studies. These types of biomarkers record the electrical activity of the heart, brain, or nerves, respectively, offering a unique insight into the physiological function of these systems.

An important issue worth mentioning is those paraclinical investigations offer a new avenue for the management of migraine but are not proven to be of high sensibility and sensitivity for daily physician's practice. Even though neuroimaging and functional analyses of the brain activity might give a broader point of view regarding therapeutic possibilities, those should not be taken into consideration as absolute clinical criteria.

Ultimately, a biomarker could be virtually any characteristic that can be detected, quantified, and expressed in terms of physical qualities. These could include diverse measures, such as height, weight, depth, voltage, luminescence, resistance, viscosity, width, length, volume, or area. Each of these measures contributes to the vast array of biomarkers that hold promise for enhancing our understanding of diseases and guiding the development of effective therapeutic interventions. The utilization of such a wide array of biomarkers allows for a comprehensive, multi-faceted approach to understanding and treating diseases, ultimately leading to more effective and personalized healthcare solutions [38].

2.2. Identification of Potential Molecular Markers Associated with Migraine

The National Institutes of Health Biomarkers Definitions Working Group, in 1998, presented a definition for biomarkers. As per their definition, a biomarker refers to "a characteristic that can be objectively measured and evaluated as an indicator of normal biological processes, pathogenic processes, or pharmacological responses to a therapeutic intervention" [35]. Biomarkers may be classified based on their functional roles, such as diagnostic, therapeutic, risk, progression, and prognostic indicators.

The 'ideal' biomarker is characterized by the following features [39]:
- High sensitivity and specificity: this ensures that the biomarker can accurately identify individuals with a specific condition, and also correctly rule out those without the condition;
- High predictive value: the biomarker should be able to accurately forecast the course of the disease, providing valuable insights for disease management;
- Analytical stability: the biomarker should remain consistent over time and across different conditions, thereby ensuring reliable results;
- Easy, cost-effective, and minimally invasive analysis: the method of assessing the biomarker should be simple, economical, and cause minimal discomfort to the patient;
- Repeatability of method: the assessment method should yield consistent results when repeated, thereby ensuring the reliability of the biomarker.

In the context of migraine, however, there are no validated biomarkers due to the absence of substance or genetic variants that are exclusively associated with this condition or the lack of comprehensive studies on potential biomarkers.

2.2.1. Markers of Inflammation and Oxidative Stress

The markers of inflammation and oxidative stress have been associated with migraine in several studies. Proinflammatory cytokines, such as interleukin-1 (IL-1) and interleukin-6 (IL-6), have been implicated in this condition [40]. It has been found that the level of IL-1α is elevated in the blood of children suffering from migraine with aura (MA) [40]. Similarly, adults with MA have been found to exhibit higher plasma levels of IL-1β during headache-free periods and early stages of attacks as compared to those suffering from migraine without aura (MO) [40,41].

The concentration of IL-6 is reported to increase during the initial two hours of a migraine attack. Additionally, the levels of IL-10 and tumor necrosis factor alpha (TNF-α) are also found to be elevated during these attacks. It is believed that other inflammatory markers associated with vascular dysfunction, such as homocysteine (Hcy) and matrix metalloproteinase-9 (MMP-9), are also elevated in the blood of individuals with migraine [15].

Elevated serum Hcy concentration has been linked to migraine with aura (MA), and some studies have noted a relationship between increased Hcy levels and higher frequency and severity of migraine; however, these findings are not supported by all research. Hyperhomocysteinemia (elevated Hcy) is hypothesized to initiate migraine with aura attacks through changes in pain threshold [42,43].

2.2.2. Markers Associated with Pain Transmission and Emotions

Biochemical research has revealed several metabolic irregularities in the synthesis of neuromodulators and neurotransmitters associated with migraine, particularly migraine without aura (MO). Alterations in the metabolic pathway of tyrosine, for example, lead to abnormal production of neurotransmitters like noradrenaline (NE) and dopamine (DA). This process results in an increase in the levels of trace amines, such as tyramine, octopamine, and synephrine. Such changes compromise mitochondrial function and elevate glutamate concentrations within the central nervous system (CNS), as can be seen in Table 1 [43].

These imbalances in the neurotransmitter and neuromodulator levels within the dopaminergic and noradrenergic synapses of pain pathways could potentially activate the trigeminovascular system (TGVS), causing the release of the calcitonin gene-related peptide (CGRP). This chain of events is believed to directly trigger migraine attacks [44,45].

CGRP plays a key role in transmitting pain signals and promoting inflammation. Its release is stimulated by the activation of TGVS and severe migraine episodes. Infusion of CGRP has been observed to provoke migraine-like attacks in patients with migraine with aura (MA). It has been reported that during inter-attack periods, the saliva and plasma levels of CGRP in migraine patients are significantly higher compared to healthy individuals [43].

Research conducted on cultured trigeminal neurons suggests that migraine treatment strategies can inhibit CGRP transcription and curtail its release, while tumor necrosis factor alpha (TNF-α) may stimulate the transcription of this peptide [15]. Another study proposes that high levels of CGRP in saliva may correlate with a significantly improved response to rizatriptan treatment, suggesting that CGRP could serve as a valuable therapeutic marker [46].

Glutamate, which could potentially activate pathways involving both TGVS and cortical spreading depression (CSD), has been found in elevated concentrations in the plasma, platelets, and cerebrospinal fluid (CSF) of migraine sufferers, including those with chronic migraine. Research suggests that a reduction in plasma glutamate levels could be a marker of a positive response to prophylactic treatment in MO patients [43].

Serotonin (5-HT) release from platelets into the plasma may be implicated in the pathophysiology of the aura phase of migraine. Izzati-Zade observed a depletion of 5-HT stored in platelets during migraine attacks; moreover, a pattern has been observed in which the plasma level of 5-HT decreases between migraine attacks and the level of the corresponding metabolite, hydroxyindoleacetic acid (5-HIAA), increases. This pattern reverses during migraine attacks [47,48]. This correlation suggests that low 5-HT levels might enable the activation of the trigeminovascular nociceptive pathway triggered by CSD, thus supporting the hypothesis that migraines are a syndrome of low serotonergic disposition.

Additionally, a significantly higher concentration of hypocretin-1, a wakefulness-promoting neuropeptide, has been detected in the CSF of patients with chronic migraine, and this has been observed to correlate with painkiller usage [49,50]. Elevated hypocretin-1 levels may be indicative of the early stages of a migraine attack. Conversely, a study involving patients with cluster headaches reported reduced hypocretin-1 levels in the CSF, suggesting that low hypocretin-1 concentrations might reflect insufficient antinociceptive activity in the hypothalamus [51].

New therapeutic targets for migraine treatment, such as CGRP receptor antagonists, anti-CGRP antibodies, 5-HT1F agonists, glutamate antagonists, and dual hypocretin-1 receptor antagonists, are currently under investigation in phase II clinical trials [52,53]. These emerging therapies reflect the continuous exploration and evolution of our understanding of migraine pathophysiology.

Table 1. Molecules with altered CSF (cerebrospinal fluid) concentrations in patients with migraine.

Molecule	Migraine Type (Chronic Migraine [CM]/Episodic Migraine [EM])	Action in Relation to Migraine
Sodium [54,55]	EM	• During a migraine, there is an increase in cerebrospinal fluid (CSF) sodium concentration, while the blood plasma sodium concentration remains unchanged. Additionally, sodium excursions may follow a temporal pattern that worsens migraine in susceptible patients
Homocysteine [56]	EM	• High levels of homocysteine are potentially linked to migraine with aura and an increased risk of cardiovascular events in patients with migraine
3,4-Dihydroxyphenylacetic acid (DOPAC) [57]	EM	• Related with dopaminergic activity • Positive correlation between the concentration of DOPAC (3,4-dihydroxyphenylacetic acid) and the intensity of migraine, whether with or without aura
Phosphatidylcholine-specific phospholipase C [58]	EM	• The process involves the hydrolysis of phosphatidylcholine, resulting in the production of important second messengers, diacylglycerol, and phosphorylcholine
Transforming growth factor-β1 [59]	EM, CM	• An anti-inflammatory cytokine
Interleukin-1 receptor antagonist [59]	EM, CM	• Proinflammatory cytokine
Monocyte chemoattractant protein-1 [59]	EM, CM	• Proinflammatory cytokine
Corticotrophin-releasing factor [60]	CM, MOH	• May be involved in activation of hypocretin/orexin system.
Orexin-A (also referred to as hypocretin-1) [60]	CM, MOH	• Involved in the maintenance and regulation of various physiological functions, including arousal, sleep, appetite, drinking behavior, central control of autonomic activity, certain endocrine responses, and pain modulation
Glial cell line-derived neurotrophic factor [61]	CM	• It may play a role in pain relief by regulating the expression of sodium channel subunits, capsaicin VR1 receptors, and substance P release • Reduced levels found in patients with migraine
Somatostatin [61]	CM	• Regulatory anti-inflammatory and antinociceptive peptide
Glutamate [62]	CM	• The primary excitatory neurotransmitter in the central nervous system. It has been linked to various migraine-related processes, including cortical spreading depression, trigeminovascular activation, and central sensitization.

Table 1. Cont.

Molecule	Migraine Type (Chronic Migraine [CM]/Episodic Migraine [EM])	Action in Relation to Migraine
Tumor necrosis factor-α [63]	CM	• A proinflammatory cytokine that plays a significant role in brain inflammatory and immune processes, as well as in the initiation of pain
Taurine [64]	EM, CM	• Inhibitory effect on neuronal activity and vasodilating properties
Glycine [64]	EM, CM	• Inhibitory neurotransmitter
Glutamine [64]	EM, CM	• May be involved with initiation and propagation of spreading cortical depression
Neuropeptide Y [65]	Acute migraine	• Strong vasoconstrictor

3. Other Biomarkers Associated with Increased Risk for Migraine

3.1. Genetic Markers and Migraine

Many scientific investigations have striven to identify specific genetic mutations or polymorphisms that might contribute to an increased risk of developing migraine. However, as of now, none of these findings have been implemented in standard clinical practice. One rare subtype of migraine, known as familial hemiplegic migraine (FHM), which is characterized by aura and transient hemiplegia, has a well-understood genetic basis. There are three known genes where mutations have been linked with FHM—CACNA1A (FHM1), ATP1A2 (FHM2), and SCN1A (FHM3)—and this condition is inherited in an autosomal-dominant fashion [66].

The identified mutations connected to FHM lead to alterations in calcium and sodium channel functions, which are integral components of neuronal communication and excitability. Interestingly, these genetic variants have also been associated with other neurological disorders, including ataxia and childhood epilepsy [66]. Nevertheless, these mutations have not shown a strong correlation with common forms of migraine (with or without aura) or other types of headaches.

A recent study discerned a significant genetic correlation linking migraine risk to intracranial volume ($rG = -0.11$, $P = 1 \times 10^{-3}$). This correlation was not observed in relation to any subcortical region. Notwithstanding, the study pinpointed concurrent genomic overlap between migraines and all brain structures. Gene enrichment in these mutual genomic regions indicated potential associations with neuronal signaling and vascular regulation. Furthermore, the research suggested a potential causative link between reduced overall brain volume, as well as the volume of the hippocampus and ventral diencephalon, and heightened migraine risk. Additionally, a causative correlation was proposed between heightened migraine risk and an expanded amygdala volume. Through the utilization of comprehensive genome-wide association studies, the study illuminated shared genetic pathways influencing both migraine risk and various brain structures. This suggests that variances in brain morphology in individuals with elevated migraine susceptibility could be rooted in genetics. Delving deeper into these findings offers support to the neurovascular premise of migraine origin, highlighting prospective therapeutic avenues [67].

Another study elucidated the following genes associated with familial hemiplegic migraine [68]:

- FHM1: CACNA1A—This gene undergoes missense mutations resulting in a gain of function, alongside rare large exonic deletions or deletions at the 5′ non-coding end promoter. It codes for the Alpha-1 subunit of the neuronal Cav2.1 (P/Q type) voltage-gated calcium channels, crucial for modulating neuronal excitability at the presynaptic end of glutamatergic synapses;

- FHM2: ATP1A2—Characterized by missense mutations, rare small deletions, or truncating mutations and frameshifts. It encodes the catalytic alpha-2 subunit of glial and neuronal ATP-dependent transmembrane Na+/K+ pumps, pivotal for extracellular K+ clearance and establishing a Na+ gradient, which is indispensable for glutamate reuptake;
- FHM3: SCN1A—Experiences missense mutations (gain of function) and is responsible for the Alpha-1 subunit of neuronal Nav1.1 voltage-gated sodium channels. It plays a key role in propelling action potentials of cortical neurons, predominantly in GABAergic inhibitory interneurons;
- FMH4: PRRT2—Noted for missense mutations, this gene codes for the pre-synaptic proline-rich transmembrane protein. It interacts with the synaptosomal-associated protein 25 (SNAP25), implying a potential role in merging synaptic vesicles with the plasma membrane.

Two FHM1 knock-in (KI) transgenic mouse models have been established as per references [69,70]. The KI model for the R192Q mutation, linked with pure FHM1, does not exhibit clinical anomalies. In contrast, the KI for the S218L mutation, attributed to severe FHM1, presents cerebellar ataxia, transient hemiparesis, and epilepsy. As outlined in [71], these FHM1-KI mice demonstrate heightened CaV2.1 currents and neurotransmitter release, an imbalance in cortical neurotransmission, amplified excitatory transmission in the visual cortex, and a higher vulnerability to cortical spreading depression (CSD).

Various models of FHM2-KI transgenic mice have been developed. Heterozygous transgenic mice [72] display no clinical changes but have an elevated predisposition to CSD. Mice with a partial knock-out (KO) of ATP1A2 also demonstrate a heightened vulnerability to CSD [73]. Another model with a complete KO of ATP1A2 in astrocytes manifests episodic paralysis and spontaneous CSD waves coupled with diminished EEG activity. Aberrations in brain metabolism were observed with increased levels of serine and glycine. Interestingly, a diet devoid of serine and glycine curtailed paralysis episodes in these mutants [74].

For FHM3, multiple SCN1A mutations have been documented, with the majority being missense alterations leading to enhanced function [75]. A mouse model harboring the L1649Q variant exhibited an increased susceptibility to CSD, attributed to Na+ channel inactivation defects and augmented Na+ currents, causing hyperactivity in inhibitory interneurons.

With respect to FHM4, mutations in PRRT2 have been discovered in numerous instances as referenced in [76]. A significant portion of these cases were pure FHM, while others exhibited accompanying epilepsy, cognitive impairments, or dyskinesia. PRRT2-KO mice displayed paroxysmal abnormal movements early in life, progressing to unusual audiogenic motor behaviors in adulthood and a reduced seizure threshold. Notably, both human and mouse homozygous KO-PRRT2 neurons in culture exhibited hyperactive NaV1.2 and NaV1.6 channels, inferring PRRT2's inhibitory effect on voltage-gated sodium channels as described in [77].

Researchers have also employed genome-wide association studies (GWAS) to pinpoint genes linked to an elevated susceptibility for migraine (see Table 2). In one such investigation, genetic information from 5122 individuals afflicted with migraine and 18,108 control participants was scrutinized. This scrutiny led to the identification of several specific genetic variations known as single-nucleotide polymorphisms (SNPs), which displayed significant connections to migraine. Noteworthy among these were rs2651899 (positioned on chromosome 1p36.32, close to the PRDM16 gene), rs10166942 (situated on 2q37.1, near TRPM8), and rs11172113 (positioned on 12q13.3, near LRP1). It is important to highlight that although rs2651899 and rs10166942 could be differentiated between migraine and non-migraine headaches, these three SNPs did not exhibit exclusivity for migraine with or without aura, nor were they tied to specific migraine characteristics. Nonetheless, the biological significance of these connections is substantiated by the established functions of TRPM8 in neuropathic pain and LRP1 in glutamatergic synaptic transmission [78].

Another GWAS pinpointed the following two susceptibility loci for migraine without aura: MEF2D and TGFBR2 [79]. It is important to bear in mind that the results from GWAS carried out have not overlapped so far, and larger-scale studies are necessary to confirm and expand the findings of smaller investigations and to permit the use of meta-analytical methodologies.

A migraine GWAS study from 2021 [80] identified 79 independent loci significantly correlated with migraine. This study was ethnically diverse, encompassing participants of East Asian, African American, and Hispanic/Latino origin, and consisted of 28,852 cases versus 525,717 controls.

The latest migraine GWAS from 2022 by Hautakangas et al. comprised 102,084 cases against 771,257 controls. This study unearthed 123 unique loci associated with migraines, 86 of which were newly discovered post the 2016 GWAS. Further studies even expanded independent SNPs to 167. The 2022 GWAS [81] underscored both vascular and CNS tissues/cell types. Newly detected loci encoded migraine drug targets, such as CGRP (CALCA/CALCB) and serotonin 1F receptor (HTR1F). Significantly, CGRP is the objective for CGRP antibodies, and HTR1F is targeted by ditans. Moreover, an in-depth assessment of roughly 30,000 patients from the 2022 GWAS with a precise migraine diagnosis revealed unique risk variants for specific migraine types.

The research presented thus far suggests that, aside from FHM, we are only at the preliminary stage of identifying genes significantly associated with migraine risk [82]. This observation is further illustrated by the inconsistent findings from studies investigating specific associations in migraine patients with and without aura (summarized in Table 2). For instance, one study found a significant association between a polymorphism in the gene encoding the dopamine D2 receptor (see Table 2) and migraine without aura [83]. Meanwhile, another study supported the association of DBH and SLC6A3 genes with migraine with aura [62]. Contradictorily, other investigations did not corroborate these associations in migraine patients, whether with or without aura. This variability is not unusual in genetic studies investigating diseases with a multifactorial etiology. As such, further research is needed to unravel the complex genetic underpinnings of migraine [15].

Table 2. Genetic mutations/polymorphisms associated with increased risk for migraine and relation to migraine.

Gene Product	Migraine Type/Features	Action in Relation to Migraine
Dopamine type 2 (D2) receptor [23]	Migraine with and without aura [23,84]	• Vasoconstriction • Reduces trigeminal nerve activation • Inhibits release of vasoactive neuropeptide • Interrupts pain transmission centrally
Glutathione S-transferase [85]	Migraine without aura [85]	• Increases susceptibility to environmental xenobiotic-induced migraine attacks in GSTM1 genotype
Dopamine type 4 (D4) receptor [86]	Migraine without aura [86]	• A potential genetic association exists between dopamine D4 receptor gene and migraine without aura
Tumor necrosis factor-α [87]	Migraine without aura [88]	• Proinflammatory cytokine
Methyltetrahydrofolate reductase (MTHFR) C677T allele [89]	Migraine with aura [89]	• MTHFR C677T polymorphism may increase homocysteine levels associated with migraine with aura
Dopamine β-hydroxylase gene [90]	Migraine with aura [90]	• An intracellular enzyme catalyzing the conversion of dopamine to noradrenaline; imbalance may increase susceptibility to migraine
Angiotensin-converting enzyme allele [91]	Migraine with and without aura [92–94]	• Involved in vasoconstriction and vascular remodeling

Table 2. Cont.

Gene Product	Migraine Type/Features	Action in Relation to Migraine
Hypocretin receptor 1 [95]	Migraine without aura [95]	• Neuropeptide generated within the clusters of nerve cells in the hypothalamus that could potentially play a role in feelings of tiredness, frequent yawning, heightened drowsiness, and strong urges for food linked to migraine.
Syntaxin 1A [96]	Migraine without aura [96]	• Involved in the control of brain chemicals, such as serotonin and gamma-aminobutyric acid (GABA).
Cytochrome P450 (CYP) 1A2 [97]	Chronic migraine [97]	• CYP1A2*1F is connected to excessive use of triptan medications, and among those who misuse these drugs, it also impacts the drug response.

3.2. Recent Genetic Findings and Migraine

In a newly published family-based association study, significant markers connected to migraine were discovered, alongside genes believed to contribute to or modify the phenotypic expression of migraine within a substantial region of chromosome 6p12.2–p21.1. This region is recognized by the locus name MIGR3. Regrettably, due to the vastness of this area of interest, it is currently not feasible to pinpoint a singular gene; however, it is anticipated that future investigations employing more refined sequencing methodologies will eventually lead to the identification of a promising candidate gene implicated in migraine [98,99].

Despite the growing body of evidence suggesting that genetic factors play a pivotal role in the development of migraine, efforts to uncover the specific genes responsible for the common forms of migraine have only yielded modest success. As scientific collaboration expands on a global scale, the chances of identifying additional genetic variants linked to migraine are likely to increase. Furthermore, the unraveling of the genetic intricacies underlying polygenic diseases could potentially shed new light on the molecular pathways implicated in the pathophysiology of migraine. By extending our understanding of the genetic aspects of migraine, we may pave the way for the development of more effective diagnostic tools and therapeutic interventions.

3.3. Inflammatory Indicators and Migraine

Interleukins, specifically IL-1 and IL-6, have been linked with the occurrence of migraine. These cytokines, characterized by their proinflammatory nature, are believed to play a role in vascular dysfunction. Studies indicate that children experiencing migraine have raised plasma levels of IL-1α compared to those who do not suffer from migraine, and these concentrations are markedly higher in individuals with migraine accompanied by aura compared to those without aura [40]. Furthermore, adults experiencing aura migraine have significantly elevated plasma levels of IL-1β during periods free from headaches and during the early onset of migraine attacks, in comparison to individuals with migraine that do not present with aura [41]. IL-6 levels also exhibit a surge in the initial two hours of a migraine attack when measured from blood samples taken from the jugular vein [50].

Other cytokines, including IL-10 and tumor necrosis factor alpha (TNF-α), have shown associations with migraine. During migraine attacks, there are elevated serum levels of IL-10 and TNF-α [100]; moreover, between attacks, TNF-α levels in plasma are higher in children who suffer from migraine compared to those who do not. The connection between TNF-α and migraine is particularly noteworthy, given the repeated association of elevated levels of this cytokine with endothelial dysfunction [63]. While some studies propose that patients with migraine may have compromised endothelial function, others contradict these findings [15].

Further inflammatory markers, which are considered to be linked to vascular dysfunction, are found to be elevated in the blood of migraine patients. Research has demonstrated that average plasma levels of C-reactive protein and homocysteine are higher in children who suffer from migraine compared to those who are not plagued by headaches [54]. Evidence also suggests that premenopausal women with migraine, especially those with aura, show signs of increased endothelial activation—a component of endothelial dysfunction—evidenced by elevated levels of von Willebrand factor, C-reactive protein, nitrate/nitrite, and tissue-type plasminogen activator antigen [55]. Markers linked to vascular repair and remodeling processes have also shown an association with migraine.

Investigations in both human subjects and animal models have proposed that matrix metalloproteinase-9 (MMP-9) might protect against the development and destabilization of plaques [61]. Moreover, patients experiencing migraine have been found to have significantly higher plasma levels of MMP-9 compared to healthy individuals and those with tension-type headaches. The average plasma MMP-9 levels were highest in subjects who had their blood samples taken between two and four days post their latest attack, implying that the elevated MMP-9 might be an indication of structural damage and subsequent remodeling associated with migraine attacks [64].

While the findings summarized here point to a relationship between various inflammatory mediators and migraine, additional research aimed at understanding the biological implications of these inflammatory mediators is necessary to confirm the validity of these potential indicators.

3.4. Contribution of Imaging Techniques in Understanding Migraine Pathology

3.4.1. Overview of Imaging Methods Used in Migraine Research

The advent of neuroimaging technologies has brought significant advancements in our understanding of migraine mechanisms and has enabled us to pinpoint secondary structural and functional impacts resulting from migraine. Imaging conducted during a migraine episode has helped the scientific community progress from a strictly vascular understanding of migraine pathophysiology, to a neurovascular theory, and currently towards a central nervous system (CNS) model.

Through the lens of neuroimaging, we have gained substantial ground towards unearthing the elusive "migraine generator"—the structure that triggers the initiation of a migraine episode. The investigative power of neuroimaging has shed light on the role of central sensitization in the pathophysiology of individual migraine attacks and in the progression of the disease. It has also enhanced our understanding of medication overuse headaches, along with the mechanisms by which abortive and prophylactic medications for migraine work [58].

One pivotal discovery has been the identification of cortical spreading depression (CSD) during migraine, with or perhaps without the accompaniment of an aura. This phenomenon is a wave of hyperactivity followed by a wave of inhibition in neuronal activities, which spreads across the cortex of the brain. It has been increasingly recognized as an important part of migraine pathophysiology [65].

Moreover, it has become evident through neuroimaging that individuals prone to migraine undergo structural and functional brain alterations in the periods between migraine attacks. These alterations appear to be correlated with both the duration of the disease and its severity, suggesting a possible link between more severe disease manifestation and persistent abnormalities between migraines. In essence, the affliction may not be limited to the episodes of the migraine attack but may present as a continuous, cyclic process with long-term impacts on brain structure and function. Neuroimaging has revolutionized the exploration and understanding of migraine, enabling us to visualize the structural and functional impacts of this condition on the brain, refine our understanding of its pathophysiology, and develop more effective therapeutic strategies. However, despite these strides, the complex nature of migraine warrants further research to fully understand the intricate interplay between genetic, environmental, and neurobiological factors in the manifestation and progression of the disease [101].

3.4.2. Findings and Insights Gained through Imaging Studies

Given the episodic and largely unpredictable nature of individual migraine attacks, conducting imaging during a spontaneous migraine has posed substantial challenges. To circumvent this issue, some researchers have induced migraine attacks in subjects by exposing them to known triggers, such as photic stimulation, physical exertion, or nitroglycerin [102]. A handful of investigators have successfully captured the onset of a migraine headache, while others have performed imaging immediately after the headache's initiation. Nevertheless, the total number of studies that have managed to image a migraine attack in progress remains relatively small.

4. Central Sensitization

The phenomenon of central sensitization in individuals prone to migraine leads to heightened pain perception during a migraine, a condition known as cutaneous allodynia, and may contribute to the progression from episodic to chronic migraine [102]. Approximately 65% of migraine sufferers develop cutaneous allodynia during individual headache episodes [103–105]. Patients with allodynia experience the skin becoming painfully sensitive to stimuli that are normally harmless, such as a light touch. Developing ways to block or reverse central sensitization could potentially alleviate migraine pain and lower the likelihood of episodic migraine evolving into chronic migraine.

One of the challenges in neuroimaging of central sensitization is differentiating between changes that arise from the increased pain sensation of cutaneous allodynia and those from structures that may specifically mediate the onset and maintenance of central sensitization. Recent advances in functional magnetic resonance imaging (fMRI) studies offer some progress in this regard. Utilizing the heat/capsaicin model of sensitization, fMRI studies have identified activation in the midbrain reticular formation region that appears specific to central sensitization [106,107]. Investigators propose that this activation occurs in the nucleus cuneiformis and the rostral superior colliculi/periaqueductal gray area.

Further fMRI studies investigated the influence of gabapentin, a medication commonly used to treat nerve pain, on brain activations following painful mechanical stimulation of normal skin compared to skin with capsaicin-induced secondary hyperalgesia [92]. Under both conditions, gabapentin reduced activations in the operculoinsular cortex. Interestingly, it was only in the presence of central sensitization that gabapentin was able to reduce activations in the brainstem and suppress stimulus-induced deactivations, suggesting that gabapentin might be more effective at reducing painful transmission when central sensitization is present. These insights set the foundation for additional investigations aimed at pinpointing the site where gabapentin acts to affect central sensitization. Unraveling this could provide valuable information for the development of future therapies aimed at inhibiting central sensitization, thereby offering a potential new avenue for migraine treatment [101].

Insights into Migraine Pathology: From Current Pathophysiological Understanding to Peripheral Interactions and Plasma Protein Extravasation

A number of laboratory studies conducted during the 1990s postulated that the pain associated with migraine might arise from a sterile, neurogenically mediated inflammation of the dura mater, the thick membrane that surrounds the brain. Evidence of neurogenic plasma extravasation, the process whereby plasma proteins pass out of small blood vessels into surrounding tissues, has been observed during the electrical stimulation of the trigeminal ganglion in rat models. Interestingly, this process of extravasation can be halted by substances such as ergot alkaloids, indomethacin, acetylsalicylic acid, and the serotonin 5HT1B/1D agonist, sumatriptan [84].

Adding to this, preclinical research has suggested that a phenomenon known as cortical spreading depression, a wave of hyperactivity followed by a wave of inhibition in the brain, could act as a potent trigger for the activation of trigeminal neurons [85]. However, this notion has been a subject of controversy and ongoing debate in the scientific community.

Notably, post-stimulation of the trigeminal ganglion, researchers have observed structural changes in the dura mater, including mast cell degranulation, a process by which mast cells release granules rich in histamine and other molecules, and modifications in postcapillary venules, including platelet aggregation [86].

While it is widely accepted that such changes—particularly the initiation of a sterile inflammatory response—would be likely to cause pain, it remains uncertain whether these alterations alone are sufficient or whether they necessitate the presence of other stimulators or promoters. One of the limitations of neurogenic dural plasma extravasation as a theory is its inability to predict whether novel therapeutic targets would be effective in either the acute or preventative treatment of migraine. Indeed, the blockade of neurogenic plasma protein extravasation (PPE) has not been proven to be a reliable indicator of antimigraine efficacy in humans. This observation is substantiated by the unsuccessful outcomes of clinical trials of several potential treatments such as substance P, neurokinin 1 receptor antagonists, specific PPE blockers, CP122,288 and 4991w93, an endothelin antagonist, a neurosteroid, and an inhibitor of the inducible form of nitric oxide synthase (iNOS) named GW274150 [87].

5. Investigations into Neuropeptides

Through the application of electrical stimulation to the trigeminal ganglion, observable increases in extracerebral blood flow and the local release of calcitonin gene-related peptide (CGRP) and substance P (SP) have been noted in both human and cat subjects. In felines, such stimulation not only enhances the cerebral blood flow but also prompts the release of vasoactive intestinal polypeptide (VIP), a potent vasodilator peptide, via the greater superficial petrosal branch of the facial nerve. Intriguingly, the VIP ergic innervation of cerebral vessels is mainly anterior as opposed to posterior, which may make these regions more susceptible to spreading depression, possibly accounting for the common posterior onset of aura symptoms. A more specific pain-inducing area, the superior sagittal sinus, when stimulated, raises the cerebral blood flow and jugular vein CGRP levels. In human studies, elevated CGRP levels have been observed during the headache phase of severe migraine, though not in less intense attacks, as well as in cluster headaches and chronic paroxysmal hemicranias, corroborating the hypothesis that the trigeminovascular system might serve a protective function in such conditions. Migraine triggered by nitric oxide (NO) donors, which mimic typical migraine, also lead to CGRP increases that can be blocked by sumatriptan, as is the case in spontaneous migraine. Significantly, certain compounds that have been proven ineffective for migraine treatment, such as the conformationally restricted analogs of sumatriptan, CP122,288, and zolmitriptan, 4991w93, were also unable to inhibit CGRP release following superior sagittal sinus stimulation in cats. The development and successful trials of specific non-peptide CGRP receptor antagonists underscore the significance of this as a novel principle in the treatment of acute migraine. Nonetheless, considering the variability, it is unlikely to serve as a reliable migraine biomarker. Also, the lack of effect of CGRP receptor antagonists on plasma protein extravasation (PPE) explains, in part, why this model has not successfully translated into human therapeutic strategies [88].

Migraine triggers in patients include cAMP-mediated mechanisms via cilostazol, even when the CGRP receptor is blocked with erenumab. Additionally, cranial artery dilation from cilostazol remains unaffected by CGRP receptor blockage. These insights imply that migraine attacks induced by cAMP do not need CGRP receptor activation, hinting at potential novel avenues for mechanism-based migraine drug development [89].

In the realm of preclinical research, there is evidence suggesting that PACAP-specific active transport systems cross the blood–brain barrier (BBB) [90]. Yet, after crossing the BBB, PACAP isoforms either degrade quickly or re-enter the bloodstream, pointing to its primary peripheral effect. In vitro data [91] highlighted PACAP38's ability to relax vascular smooth muscle cells post-abluminal application, but not after luminal application in cerebral arteries. In contrast, in vivo tests showed no significant change in regional cerebral blood flow due to PACAP38 intravenous infusion [93].

Throbbing headaches during migraines probably stem from pain signals from both intra- and extracranial (when vasodilated) vessels, especially arteries. No studies have focused on selective VIP blockage for migraine treatment yet. However, recent findings hint that prolonged vasodilation from VIP might induce migraine-like episodes, suggesting that VIP blockage could be a promising migraine treatment [94].

The receptors (AM1, AM2, or CGRP) that might mediate migraine-like reactions due to adrenomedullin remain unidentified [95]. AM22-52, the only known adrenomedullin antagonist, appears limited in its ability to antagonize adrenomedullin effects in rat cells, though it has shown potential in inhibiting CGRP effects [96]. No specific treatments to counteract adrenomedullin or its receptors exist currently. However, an in vitro research [97] indicated that the CGRP-receptor targeting antibody erenumab and the CGRP-receptor antagonist telcagepant opposed not only CGRP but also adrenomedullin signaling at the CGRP receptor.

Research on arresting the NO-cGMP cascade for drug development shows potential. A mouse study [56] illustrated that the sGC stimulator VL-102 induced both acute and prolonged hyperalgesia. This effect was blocked by the sGC inhibitor (ODQ) and by several antimigraine drugs (sumatriptan, topiramate, and propranolol).

Lastly, migraine patient studies have identified mutations in the TRESK potassium channel. TRESK works by inhibiting TREK1 and TREK2, amplifying the TG's excitability. As mentioned in [59,60], decreasing TG excitability using the TREK1/TREK2 agonist ML67-33 countered an NO donor-triggered migraine-like phenotype in mice similarly to the CGRP receptor antagonist olcegepant. Furthermore, it entirely reversed TG-induced facial allodynia in rats due to NO donors.

Our understanding of alternative targets leading to intracranial artery vasodilation is expanding. However, we have yet to develop successful therapies to tackle CGRP-independent mechanisms. For instance, an antibody designed to inhibit PACAP (a peptide part of the VIP, secretin, and glucagon superfamily) was developed as an alternative treatment but did not show efficacy in trials. Additionally, the results from attempts to block NO-induced reactions have been mixed. Using glibenclamide did not alleviate headaches caused by PACAP38 and levcromakalim. Still, TRPV1 agonists like capsaicin and civamide demonstrated some effectiveness due to their capacity to desensitize nerve endings hosting these channels. There is a pressing need for more research to craft alternative targeted migraine therapies, such as those focusing on VIP, amylin, adrenomedullin, PDE3, PDE5, calcium channels, and ASICs. In theory, targeting the most downstream elements like KATP channels, being the cascade's "final link", might yield better results; however, this could also bring about severe and unwanted side effects. The high induction rate of levcromakalim possibly being a result of this remains to be confirmed [57].

Changes in the connection between the hypothalamus and brainstem with the spinal trigeminal nuclei and the dorsal rostral pons have been observed during the premonitory phase of a migraine, lasting up to 48 h before pain begins [108]. The exact process that makes the hypothalamus 'overactive' in migraine situations, leading to the sensitization of trigeminal nociceptors, remains undefined. Moreover, the hypothalamus houses chemosensitive neurons that can recognize metabolic alterations in the brain and the body. External stimuli causing disruptions in balance and the brain's inherent biorhythm could potentially push the brain toward a migraine episode through hypothalamic activation [109].

NSAIDs are a reliable choice for managing acute migraine flare-ups, but care must be taken due to potential side effects like stomach issues and kidney problems. Beta-blockers serve as effective preventative measures against migraines, but they come with their own drawbacks, such as causing dizziness and fatigue. Moreover, they are not recommended for patients with specific health conditions like asthma, heart failure, and certain cardiac rhythm disorders. While calcium channel blockers have been considered for migraine prevention, the current evidence does not strongly support their use for this purpose. Antiseizure medications, like topiramate and divalproex sodium, and certain antidepressants, namely, venlafaxine and amitriptyline, have been found effective in preventing migraine attacks, but users must be wary of associated side effects. In deciding on a treatment course, it is crucial to weigh the potential benefits against the risks. Open dialogue between the patient and the physician will ensure the most suitable therapeutic choice is made [110].

6. Headache Physiology: Central Connections and the Trigeminocervical Complex

6.1. Migraine Neuronal Activation and Therapeutic Implications

Utilizing Fos immunohistochemistry, researchers have been able to discern the activation of cells by detecting Fos protein expression within the trigeminocervical complex. Following the irritation of meningeal with blood, there was a significant upregulation of Fos expression within the trigeminal nucleus caudalis. Additionally, upon stimulation of the superior sagittal sinus, Fos-like immunoreactivity was observed not only in the trigeminal nucleus caudalis but also in the dorsal horn at the C1 and C2 levels in both feline and simian subjects [58]. These findings are consistent with results obtained from 2-deoxyglucose analyses in congruent experiments [65]. Similarly, the activation of the greater occipital nerve, an offshoot of the C2, amplifies the metabolic activity in the aforementioned regions. It has been documented in animal-based studies that it is feasible to directly obtain readings from trigeminal neurons receiving input from both the supratentorial trigeminal and the greater occipital nerve. A mere 5 min stimulation of the greater occipital nerve resulted in a pronounced escalation in response to supratentorial dural stimuli, with the effects lasting for more than 60 minutes [101]. Conversely, the stimulation of the dura mater of the middle meningeal artery utilizing mustard oil as a C fiber irritant augmented the responses to occipital muscle stimulation [102]. Additional data derived from the Fos technique posit that such interactions likely necessitate the activation of the NMDA subtype of glutamate receptors [103]. Taken together, these findings suggest that the cervical and ophthalmic inputs intersect at the level of the second-order neuron [104]. It is worth nothing that bilateral Fos expression was observed when a lateralized structure, specifically the middle meningeal artery, was stimulated in both feline and simian models [105]. This particular group of neurons from the superficial laminae of the trigeminal nucleus caudalis and C1/2 dorsal horns is functionally recognized as the "trigeminocervical" complex. Such insights indicate that the transmission of nociceptive information from the trigeminovascular system predominantly occurs via the most caudal cells, which provides an anatomical elucidation for the referral of migraine-associated pain to the posterior cranial region. It is imperative to highlight that pharmacological experimentation has unveiled that migraine-abating drugs, such as ergot derivatives, acetylsalicylic acid, sumatriptan, eletriptan, naratriptan, rizatriptan, zolmitriptan, and novel CGRP receptor antagonists, have the potential to modulate these second-order neurons, thereby decreasing their activity [106]. This proposes another plausible avenue for therapeutic interventions in migraine. The modus operandi of triptans is believed to engage the 5-HT1B, 5-HT1D, and 5-HT1F receptor subtypes, which correlates with the positioning of these receptors on peptidergic nociceptors.

Subsequent exploration into neuropeptides has underscored the potential of CGRP receptor antagonists for migraine treatment. Elevated levels of CGRP and SP subsequent to trigeminal ganglion stimulation, observed in both humans and felines, might serve as a protective mechanism in severe migraine, cluster headaches, and chronic paroxysmal hemicranias. Additionally, an upswing in CGRP levels was documented during a NO donor-triggered migraine episode, but this surge was mitigated by sumatriptan, further corroborating the implication of the trigeminovascular system in these conditions. Nevertheless, specific compounds, such as CP122,288 and 4991w93, which were ineffective against migraine, failed to inhibit CGRP release post-superior sagittal sinus stimulation in feline subjects. In spite of these observations, the advent and ensuing triumphant clinical trial outcomes of particular CGRP receptor antagonists for acute migraine have emphasized the significance of this therapeutic strategy [64,107].

In studies involving the trigeminocervical complex, Fos immunohistochemistry has been utilized to identify activated cells by mapping the Fos protein expression. This method revealed an increased Fos expression in the trigeminal nucleus caudalis after meningeal irritation with blood and in the trigeminal nucleus caudalis and the C1 and C2 levels in the dorsal horn of cats and monkeys after stimulation of the superior sagittal sinus [111]. Moreover, the stimulation of the greater occipital nerve, a branch of C2, resulted in increased metabolic activity in these regions [112]. This suggests that inputs from the cervical and ophthalmic regions converge at the level of the second-order neuron. Pharmacological research indicates that drugs like ergot derivatives, acetylsalicylic acid, sumatriptan, eletriptan, naratriptan, rizatriptan, zolmitriptan, and CGRP receptor antagonists may help reduce cell activity at these second-order neurons and therefore could be a potential therapeutic approach for migraine [88].

Studies into serotonin–5 HT1F receptor agonists and their relation to migraine have shown that some triptans, including naratriptan, are also potent 5 HT1F receptor agonists. This suggests that 5 HT1F activation could potentially inhibit trigeminal nucleus Fos activation and neuronal firing in response to dural stimulation without affecting cranial vascular effects. These findings further support the idea that vascular mechanisms are not necessarily required for acute migraine treatments [113].

Glutamatergic transmission in the trigeminocervical complex has also been explored as a potential target for antimigraine drugs. The family of glutamate receptors (GluRs) is particularly interesting, with studies showing that NMDA receptor channel blockers can reduce nociceptive trigeminovascular transmission in vivo. Furthermore, the AMPA/kainate receptor antagonists CNQX and 2,3-Dioxo-6-nitro-1,2,3,4-tetrahydrobenzoquinoxaline-7-sulfonamide decreased Fos protein expression after the activation of structures involved in nociceptive pathways [114]. Notably, the iGluR5 kainate receptors may play a role in trigeminovascular physiology, suggesting a potential target for future treatments. In clinical trials, the iGluR5 kainate receptor antagonist LY466195 demonstrated efficacy in acute migraine treatment, reinforcing the pursuit of glutamate targets for treatment, albeit with caution regarding potential side effects [115].

6.2. Discussion of Key Pathological Processes Involved in Migraine

6.2.1. Neurophysiology of Migraine as a Backdrop to Imaging

The utilization of neurophysiological techniques in migraine patients has yielded significant knowledge about the condition. These techniques prioritize time resolution over spatial resolution and, until the advent of MRI, and to some extent even now, provided a higher chance for repeated trials. Research across the visual, somatosensory, auditory, and nociceptive domains has consistently shown activation patterns that differ markedly from non-migraine. These findings have led to the theory that thalamocortical dysrhythmia plays a significant role in migraine pathophysiology [116,117] (see Figure 1).

An intriguing observation from these studies is the abnormal habituation in migraine patients between attacks, as exemplified by the increased intensity of auditory evoked potentials in these periods [118]. Interestingly, this abnormality seems to normalize just before a migraine attack [119]. It is worth noting that this metric appears to be serotonin-dependent and can be modulated by triptans, which are serotonin 5-HT1B/1D receptor agonists [120]. The amplification of the passive "oddball" auditory event-related potential and an interictal habituation deficit measured by the nociceptive blink reflex, further suggest that the brain of a migraineur does not habituate in the same way as a non-migraineur's brain does [121].

These observations have given rise to the idea that the brain of a person with migraine reacts more intensely, rather than simply being hyperexcitable [121].

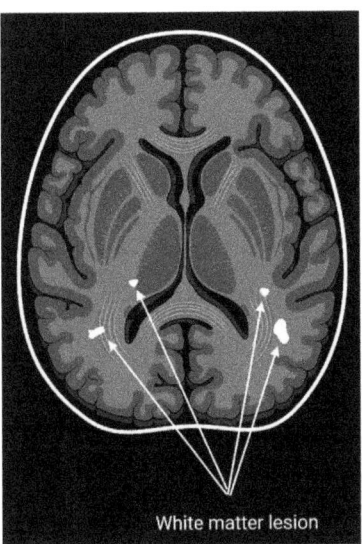

Figure 1. The two main types of lesions found in migraine include: white matter hyperintensities and silent brain infarcts.

6.2.2. Inter-Attack Imaging Studies

1. Structural Studies

Numerous research endeavors have revealed structural disparities between the brains of those who suffer from migraine and those who do not. Structural investigations, often cross-sectional, should be analyzed with consideration to the functional interactions of pain-processing areas and the trigeminal system. Voxel-based morphometry has showcased decreased grey matter in areas involved in pain processing, such as the anterior cingulate cortex, amygdala, insula, operculum, and the frontal, temporal, and precentral gyri. Interestingly, grey matter reduction in the anterior cingulate cortex has been found to be correlated with the frequency of migraine episodes [122]. On the other hand, a greater grey matter volume was seen in the bilateral caudate nuclei in high-frequency migraine sufferers compared to those with low-frequency migraine [123]. Additionally, there was an observed thickening in the somatosensory cortex, particularly in the portion responsible for mapping sensations from the head and face. This thickening was more pronounced compared to individuals who did not exhibit these changes and served as controls [124]. Research involving diffusion tensor imaging has revealed decreased fractional anisotropy in the thalamocortical pathway of individuals with migraine. Specifically, this reduction was observed in the ventral trigeminothalamic tract for those experiencing aura, and in the ventrolateral periaqueductal gray (PAG) for those without aura [124]. Other studies found only minor diffusivity changes in grey matter, while changes in white matter and brain volume were similar in both groups. Nevertheless, a more extensive investigation discovered that individuals with migraine accompanied by aura exhibited a shorter T1 relaxation time in the thalamus compared to those without aura and individuals without migraine who were in good health. In a separate study, a reduction in brain volume was detected across multiple regions when comparing migraine sufferers to control subjects. Significantly, it remains uncertain whether these alterations stem from recurrent migraine episodes or are intricately connected to the underlying mechanisms of migraine. It is worth noting that certain changes tend to revert to a more typical state during a migraine, implying a potential connection between the most recent attack and these structural modifications [125]. Taken together, these findings suggest that the structural alterations seen in migraine patients, particularly in the anterior cingulate cortex and the trigeminal somatosensory system, reflect the brain's ability to develop migraine attacks and may underlie the progression of the disorder.

2. Functional Studies

Functional studies serve to supplement structural brain imaging, focusing on the resting migrainous brain and its response to external stimuli.

(A) Metabolism and Receptor Pharmacology

Functional differences between two groups at rest can be evaluated using 18F-FDG PET to assess regional brain metabolism. Kim et al. [126] found that migraine was associated with reduced metabolism in central pain processing areas, suggesting a dysfunction of central pain processing in the interictal state. No area showed hypermetabolism.

(B) Stimulated Blood Flow Changes

Photophobia, a common non-head pain symptom in migraine, can result in light being perceived as overly bright or painful. Individuals suffering from migraine, even when not experiencing an attack, have been shown to tolerate less luminance than healthy individuals [127]. A study using H215O-PET revealed that exposure to different light intensities activated the visual cortex in migraine but not in controls. Moreover, applying trigeminal pain activated the same areas in control subjects, suggesting a facilitation of the retino-geniculate-cortical pathway of visual processing and/or a dysfunction of visual association areas causing photophobia. Other studies found differences in response to heat stimuli and painful heat stimulation in migraine compared to controls. Demarquay et al. [128] evaluated olfactory processing in migraine and found unique cortical responses associated with olfactory hypersensitivity. These findings suggest that the brains of migraine respond differently to external stimuli compared to healthy controls, possibly due to pre-existing functional abnormalities that worsen during a migraine attack, leading to a "dys-excitable" state [129].

(C) Studies focused on resting-state brain activity

Resting-state studies offer a unique perspective on brain function, especially in the context of disorders like migraine. These investigations focus on how the brain operates when it is not performing any particular task, thereby providing insights into the intrinsic communication patterns within the brain. They represent a significant departure from other neuroimaging techniques as follows: while structural brain imaging helps identify disparities in grey and white matter, and stimulus-driven functional magnetic resonance imaging (fMRI) pinpoints distinct dysfunctional areas, resting-state studies evaluate the interaction, or "cross-talk", among different brain regions [121].

One such study by Mainero et al. found that individuals suffering from migraine exhibit heightened connectivity between the periaqueductal gray (PAG) and multiple areas significant to nociceptive and somatosensory processing. These findings were further linked with the frequency of migraine episodes, signifying the pathophysiological relevance of this enhanced connectivity in the modulation of pain during migraine [130].

Another vital aspect of migraine is the presence of cutaneous allodynia, considered a reflection of central sensitization during migraine attacks. When comparing resting-state connectivity between migraine with and without cutaneous allodynia, distinctive patterns were identified. Specifically, connectivity differences were noted between the PAG/nucleus cuneiformis and various discriminative pain processing centers, such as the brainstem, thalamus, insula, cerebellum, and higher-order pain-modulating areas located in frontal and temporal regions [131]. This evidence suggests that individual symptoms during a migraine attack might be determined by abnormal communication between pain-modulating areas during interictal periods.

While all participants in the study had migraine with normal routine investigation results, the presence of ictal allodynia seems to delineate different subtypes of migraine. This implies that migraine itself could also be pathophysiologically diverse. In terms of headache phase studies, seed-based resting-state fMRI has exhibited increased connectivity between primary visual and auditory cortices and the right dorsal anterior insula, and between the dorsal pons and the bilateral anterior insulae. Interestingly, these findings did not correlate with migraine frequency, suggesting that these changes were inherent characteristics of migraine pathophysiology rather than episodic manifestations [121].

Expanding the scope, resting functional connectivity of certain brain regions, including the right middle temporal, posterior insula, middle cingulate, left ventromedial prefrontal, and bilateral amygdala regions, was found to effectively distinguish between the brains of migraine and non-migraine [132]. Despite being grounded in clinical observation, these techniques have the potential to yield insights into migraine biology, contribute to the development of NextGen treatments, and offer biomarkers of change, particularly for preventive studies.

Resting-state studies are not limited to the seed-based approach, which focuses on the connectivity of specific "seed" areas, such as the PAG or nucleus cuneiformis. Task-free resting-state studies employing independent component analysis without a priori hypothesis have also been conducted. One such study by Tessidore et al. [133] examined the default mode network in patients with migraine without aura. They found decreased connectivity in the prefrontal and temporal regions of the default mode network among these patients. The authors speculated that this could indicate a dysfunction of the default mode network, potentially tied to maladaptive responses to stress or environmental triggers, which are often characteristic of migraine.

In conclusion, being a migraineur suggests the presence of nuanced differences in brain structure and function, even outside of active migraine attacks. Notably, most areas showing such differences belong to the non-specific pain processing areas or the trigeminal system. A significant challenge moving forward is understanding how these differences predispose individuals to migraine, and identifying which structures drive the transition from the interictal phase, through the premonitory phase, to the headache phase, and eventually, the postdrome period that returns to the interictal phase.

(D) Studies focusing on mitochondrial energy metabolism

Considering the recognition of migraine as a component of mitochondrial cytopathies, exploring how this biological aspect influences the onset and development of migraine provides a promising research avenue. Although initial studies on mitochondrial DNA did not find any typical MELAS or MERRF mutations, a successfully conducted randomized controlled trial of riboflavin (vitamin B2) as a preventive treatment for migraine supports the hypothesis that metabolic dysfunction could increase susceptibility in some patients [134].

Utilizing 31P-NMR spectroscopy, Welch et al. [135] identified changes in the phosphate metabolism in patients with migraine with aura during an attack. Later studies using the same technique found similar metabolic shifts in patients with migraine without aura and even in children [136]. Furthermore, by employing 3T MRI and 31P-NMR spectroscopy, researchers were able to identify alterations in energy metabolism in the occipital cortex of patients with migraine without aura [137]. Given the observed variations in energy changes among patients, these findings could potentially explain some, but not all, of the biological mechanisms contributing to the manifestation of migraine.

3. Premonitory Phase Studies

From a clinical perspective, the premonitory phase—the transitional period between the asymptomatic interictal phase and the onset of a headache attack—is crucial for understanding what triggers migraine. An essential fMRI study in this regard examined the activation and deactivation patterns induced by the trigemino-nociceptive stimulation of the nasal mucosa as the day of the headache approached [138]. In comparison to control subjects, interictal migraine showed reduced activation of the spinal trigeminal nuclei. Interestingly, this deactivation demonstrated the following cyclic behavior throughout a migraine interval: normalization prior to the next attack and a significant reduction of deactivation during the attack. This cyclical behavior may reflect the brain's increased susceptibility to initiate the next attack, with the identification of its pacemaker critical to our understanding of the initiation of a migraine attack.

Clinically, the earliest indicators of an impending migraine attack are known as premonitory symptoms, which manifest before the onset of head pain and signal to the patient that a headache is imminent. These symptoms, likely tied to the hypothalamus [139], include concentration problems, fatigue, irritability, and depression. A recent study by Maniyar et al. [140] induced migraine attacks in eight patients who could predict the onset of a headache by a pronounced premonitory phase. During this phase, which occurs before the onset of head pain, H215O-PET showed activation of the hypothalamus, midbrain ventral tegmental area, and the PAG. This functional representation of premonitory symptoms hints at the potential role of the hypothalamus in triggering migraine. Additional data from a single patient tracked with BOLD-fMRI over a 30-day period showed increased hypothalamic responses as the attack approached, and the effects were coupled with the dorsolateral pons [141]. Additionally, the hypothalamus could play a crucial role in non-headache symptoms during the pain phase since its activation was observed in spontaneous migraine attacks using H215O-PET [142]. Interestingly, activations reported in trigeminal-autonomic cephalalgias are more posterior than those reported in migraine [121].

4. The Aura Phase

Typically, a visual aura in the context of a migraine presents itself before the onset of the headache phase, although there are instances where it coincides with the headache or even occurs without any headache at all. The manifestation of this aura often begins as a scintillating or blind spot situated in the center of the individual's field of vision [121]. Personal experiences reported by Lashley [143] indicated that this visual disturbance or scotoma progressively expanded over a period of approximately one hour, moving in a C-shaped trajectory towards one side's temporal visual field. Based on his observations, the estimated speed of this phenomenon over the visual cortex was calculated to be approximately 3 mm per minute.

A few years later, the concept of a potential underlying mechanism emerged from the work of Leão, who stimulated the cortices of rabbits electrically. He observed a depression in the electroencephalogram (EEG) readings that spread out from the stimulation site at a similar speed of 3 mm per minute. Leão postulated that this cortical phenomenon could possibly serve as the foundation for the migraine aura [144]. This theory sustained for several decades that the occurrence of a typical visual aura could be associated with this phenomenon, termed "cortical spreading depression" (CSD) [145].

The validation of the CSD occurrence in humans was conjectural until a groundbreaking study by Olesen et al. [146]. They injected Xenon-133 into the carotid artery during a human migraine aura and found an observable progressive alteration of regional cerebral blood flow (rCBF). Fast forward two decades later, patients who could self-trigger their visual aura or who were capable of reaching a medical facility during the early stages of a visual aura were included in a functional magnetic resonance imaging (fMRI) study using checkerboard stimulation. The change in blood oxygenation level-dependent (BOLD) signal in the visual cortex in response to checkerboard stimulation during the progression of a visual aura showed characteristics similar to those of the CSD observed in animal models. This included a signal spread at a velocity of roughly 3.5 mm per minute, aligning with the earlier clinical predictions and the CSD observed in rabbit cortices [147]. These findings suggest that the visual aura experienced in migraine might indeed be the result of a CSD-like event. Additionally, the study by Hadjikhani et al. [148] pinpointed the origin of this unique response to checkerboard stimulation to be located in the visual association cortex V3A.

5. The Headache Stage

Renowned as the most prominent symptom of a migraine attack, the headache stage is often the defining phase for many patients. To diagnose a migraine, however, additional symptoms need to be present. These can range from nausea, photophobia (light sensitivity), phonophobia (sound sensitivity), to sensitivity to movement [149]. The imaging patterns observed during a migraine are typically a composite of these symptoms, with some possibly reflecting individual symptoms like head pain, photophobia, or allodynia (an increased response to pain), and others hinting at underlying mechanisms that trigger the migraine.

(a) The Experience of Head Pain: The complexity of primary headache disorders extends beyond head pain that is typically triggered by harmful stimuli on the skin. However, the sensation of pain is a shared experience in harmful head pain and spontaneous migraine attacks. Therefore, the markers identified in functional brain imaging of experimental head pain should also be observable in migraine headaches. Thus, any additional regions highlighted in primary headache disorders may provide specific insights into migraine, potentially revealing symptoms beyond head pain or even mechanisms that drive migraine attacks. Functional brain imaging of harmful pain in the head is a significant focus as it could improve our understanding of functional brain imaging of migraine. May et al. [150] used $H_2^{15}O$-PET to measure rCBF in seven healthy subjects after injecting a small amount of capsaicin into the forehead. They noticed an increase in rCBF in several brain areas during the pain state, including the bilateral insula, the anterior cingulate cortex, the cavernous sinus, and the cerebellum. Notably, there was no activation of the brainstem.

(b) Migraine Attacks: Over the past two decades, a seminal study employing positron emission tomography sought to evaluate regional cerebral blood flow utilizing 15C-labeled O2 inhalation in a cohort of nine individuals experiencing spontaneous right-lateralized migraine episodes. Relative to the non-painful interlude, the migraine episodes were concomitant with augmented rCBF in regions, such as the cingulate cortex, auditory association cortex, and the parieto-occipital juncture proximate to the visual association cortex. Furthermore, the migraine-afflicted state manifested with escalated rCBF in the midbrain, the dorsal rostral pons adjacent to the periaqueductal gray, and the raphe nuclei [128]. Contrasting the generalized pain signature derived from the capsaicin experiment, this investigation attributed diverse migraine-related symptoms to distinct cerebral domains as follows: the experience of cephalic pain was associated with the cingulate cortex, photophobia was linked to the visual association cortex, and phonophobia was ascribed to the auditory association cortex. The cessation of these symptoms was synchronous with the waning of the aforementioned signals. Yet, the elevated rCBF in the brainstem endured during the nascent non-painful phase, implying that this anatomical region might not merely be symptomatic but could also typify a dysfunction pivotal for initiating or perpetuating a migraine episode. Clinical research, coupled with fundamental studies, further bolsters the centrality of the brainstem in the pathogenesis of migraine. An illustrative point being the emergence of migraine episodes in individuals previously devoid of migraine who underwent deep brain stimulation targeting the PAG for unrelated pain conditions. Moreover, the progressive accumulation of iron in the PAG over the disease's tenure intimates the indispensable role of the PAG in migraine genesis. Corroborating this notion, a plethora of animal-centric studies have delineated how brainstem nuclei, specifically the PAG and raphe nuclei, profoundly modulate trigeminovascular pathways in laboratory-induced migraine paradigms [91,129].

Functional brain imaging employing advanced techniques of enhanced spatial and temporal resolutions have corroborated the pivotal role of the brain stem in the pathophysiology of migraine. In a comparative study, Bahra et al. [130] distinguished migraine from cluster headaches, underscoring the specificity of brain stem activation to migraine. Examining the lateralization of this activation during unilateral migraine episodes, Afridi et al. [131] ascertained that the activation was ipsilateral to the side of the headache. This suggests the possibility that unilateral migraine might be attributed to unilateral dysfunction of the brain stem. In a preceding discourse, Maniyar et al. [117] detected activation in the dorsal rostral pons, the PAG, and the hypothalamus during the preliminary premonitory phase of migraine, buttressing the hypothesis of a central "migraine mediator" located in these regions. Melding the clinical manifestations of migraine—typified by altered sensory, nociceptive, photic, acoustic, and olfactory perceptions—with functional imaging insights, it becomes evident that either the brain stem, hypothalamic structures, or a combination of both are instrumental in migraine pathophysiology. Such structures potentially pinpoint the anatomical epicenters of cerebral dysfunction engendering the multifaceted dynamics of migraine episodes.

(c) Photophobia: Denuelle et al. [119] conducted research on eight individuals suffering from migraine, evaluating them during headache episodes, post-sumatriptan alleviation, and interictal periods. Utilizing continuous light stimulation, they discerned that low luminance provocation elevated rCBF as indicated by H215O-PET scans. During the headache phase, hyperperfusion was detected in the cuneus, and post-relief, both the cuneus and lingual gyrus demonstrated this phenomenon; conversely, such changes were absent interictally. This might insinuate an augmented excitability of the visual cortex amidst migraine occurrences. Notably, even post-headache alleviation, the persistence of this hyperperfusion, unrelated to the headache's presence, hints at the structural foundation of photophobia potentially residing in primary and ancillary visual cortices. Moreover, zones responsive to minimal luminance during migraine were equivalently reactive interictally to escalated luminous intensities, further substantiating the cyclic nature underpinning migraine and their concomitant symptoms.

In studies targeting the premonitory phase, focusing on non-painful symptoms, pivotal insights have emerged, emphasizing the separation of such phenomena from pain while highlighting their integral role in migraine biology. When contrasting individuals with provoked premonitory symptoms, those exhibiting photophobia (or perhaps more aptly termed photic hypersensitivity due to the absence of pain) demonstrated activation within the extrastriate visual cortex, specifically Brodman area 18 [117]. Interictal connectivity within the visual system, manifested in the lingual gyrus, was also identified using resting-state methodologies. Furthermore, in experiments distinguishing migraine with and without nausea, those experiencing nausea showcased activation in the rostral dorsal medulla encompassing regions like the nucleus tractus solitarius, the dorsal motor nucleus of the vagus nerve, and the nucleus ambiguous; moreover, activation in the PAG was also evident. These research endeavors have enriched our comprehension of cerebral regions implicated in migraine, unequivocally indicating mechanisms transcending mere pain dependency [91].

Different visual migrainous phenomena are associated with dysfunctions in different areas of the visual association cortex. For instance, the cuneus and lingual gyrus are involved in photophobia, while V3A might be the origin of a typical visual aura. When comparing the imaging results during the migraine premonitory phase, such as hypothalamic and brain stem activation, with those of cortical activation during a typical migraine aura, it appears likely that the aura and migraine are distinct phenomena [121].

6. Blood–Brain Barrier (BBB): The integrity of the BBB in migraine

In postdrome, patients often describe fatigue, difficulty with concentration, and a need for sleep. Some patients also report a feeling of elation and well-being and a return of appetite. The symptoms are not always perceived as bothersome and are commonly overlooked by patients and doctors. Often, the patient is just relieved that the headache phase is over.

More work is needed to understand the nature and cause of the postdromal phase. It would be especially helpful to understand the brain's role in postdromal phase symptoms, whether the brain goes back to normal after a migraine attack, and if not, why not. Also, more understanding of how the brain recovers and how quickly it recovers would be very helpful. Whether this phase represents a therapeutic opportunity is unknown but should be explored [121].

6.3. Calcitonin Gene-Related Peptide (CGRP) in Migraine

6.3.1. Role of CGRP in Migraine Development and Progression

1. Introduction to CGRP and its significance in migraine

Calcitonin gene-related peptide (CGRP) is an incredibly potent neuropeptide comprised of 37 amino acids. It serves as a vasodilator and is produced within neurons located in both the peripheral and central nervous systems. This neuro-peptide binds to a complex heterodimer receptor, which is primarily composed of a class B G-protein coupled receptor, commonly referred to as CLR (calcitonin receptor-like receptor) [151].

Within the central nervous system, empirical research has identified elevated levels of CGRP in the blood and saliva of patients who experience certain headache disorders. Such disorders include migraine and cluster headaches, as well as neuralgias like trigeminal neuralgia, chronic paroxysmal hemicranias, and even rhinosinusitis. It is noteworthy that the levels of CGRP remain heightened during a migraine episode and continue to be elevated in-between these attacks for patients suffering from chronic migraine. Additionally, studies have revealed that exogenous infusions of CGRP can initiate a migraine episode [152].

CGRP's role extends to the pathogenesis of migraine, which is an intricate neurovascular disorder. This is typically characterized by a throbbing or pounding headache, which affects one side of the head. It is often accompanied by other symptoms, such as photophobia (light sensitivity), phonophobia (sound sensitivity), nausea, vomiting, and even disability. Additionally, the duration of a typical migraine episode can last between 4 and 72 h [153]. Researchers have found that CGRP triggers the release of vasoactive neuropeptides in trigeminal neurons, leading to vasodilation of the cerebral vasculature, thereby contributing to the emergence of a migraine.

The Food and Drug Administration (FDA) has sanctioned several medications specifically targeting CGRP or its receptor for the management and prevention of migraine. Prominent among these are monoclonal antibodies including erenumab, eptinezumab, galcanezumab, and fremanezumab, which zero in on the CGRP receptor. In addition, CGRP receptor antagonists, like rimegepant and ubrogepant, have been incorporated into therapeutic regimens. Two other receptor antagonists, atogepant and vazegepant, remain under clinical evaluation and anticipate FDA endorsement. Prophylactic interventions for both episodic and chronic migraine commonly incorporate erenumab, eptinezumab, galcanezumab, and fremanezumab. For addressing acute migraine manifestations, with or without the presence of an aura, rimegepant and ubrogepant are the preferred choices. Presently, the efficacy of galcanezumab and fremanezumab in precluding cluster headaches is a subject of active research [135].

Interestingly, CGRP has been shown to have cardio-protective properties in pathological conditions. For instance, research conducted on rodent models of various cardiovascular diseases has revealed this beneficial action of CGRP. Human studies also support this notion by showing that CGRP can reduce afterload and increase inotropy, which are potentially cardioprotective effects, particularly in cases of heart failure. Despite these findings, no drugs have yet been developed to harness this cardio-protective effect of CGRP on the cardiovascular system [154].

Recent research has also begun to uncover CGRP's involvement in numerous other physiological and pathological phenomena. These include peripheral nerve regeneration, Alzheimer's disease, regulation of vascular tone in mesenteric arteries, and even pregnancy. Despite these promising findings, no medications have been developed to date to leverage these potential beneficial effects of CGRP [155].

Preclinical studies have demonstrated that calcitonin gene-related peptide (CGRP) exhibits activity in both the central and peripheral nervous systems (CNS and PNS), making it a crucial element in the pathophysiology of migraine. In the periphery, CGRP acts on a number of targets, such as mast cells, blood vessels, glial cells, and trigeminal afferents located in the meninges, along with neural cell bodies and satellite glia found in the trigeminal ganglia. Within the meninges, CGRP is thought to contribute to neurogenic inflammation by stimulating mast cells to release neuron-sensitizing agents. This cascade effect can lead to enhanced vasodilation in the dura. Consequently, the modulation of neural activity within the meninges may instigate a feedback loop, ultimately leading to peripheral sensitization of nociceptors [156]. The notion of CGRP playing a peripheral role in migraine is strongly supported by the effectiveness of systemically administered CGRP-targeting monoclonal antibodies, which exhibit poor permeability to the blood–brain barrier (BBB) [157]. It is clear that peripheral sensitization is critical for CGRP's actions and likely establishes the foundation for CGRP actions in the CNS.

Within the central nervous system (CNS), the distribution of CGRP and its receptor spans various pathways postulated to play pivotal roles in migraine pathophysiology. Situated externally to the blood–brain barrier (BBB), the trigeminal ganglion extends its projections to the trigeminal nucleus caudalis (TNC). From here, second-order neurons transmit signals to the posterior thalamic area (PTA), an umbrella term denoting all nuclei within this specific thalamic region. Serving ostensibly as a hub for sensory integration, the PTA exhibits functional aberrations during migraine occurrences. Neurons in the thalamus receive inputs from both the TNC and retinal ganglion cells. Crucial rodent studies have accentuated the import of the PTA in photophobia's onset, proposing its role as a nexus for light and pain integration [139].

Situated in select nuclei of the PTA, CGRP and its receptors are postulated to be integral to this pathway—a hypothesis fortified by research showing that CGRP infusion into the PTA augments neuronal activity. Additionally, ascending pathways carrying somatosensory and nociceptive stimuli converge upon the CGRP-expressing neurons located in the subparafascicular and intralaminar nuclei. In human subjects, during migraine attacks, activation is discerned in the posterior thalamus, which also manifests altered connectivity patterns with various brain areas. Taken together, this suggests that the neuromodulatory actions of CGRP, observed in distinct neural networks, might be instrumental in rendering the PTA hyperresponsive to sensory input [140].

Further elucidating this sensory hyperreactivity, pathways potentially involve the parabrachial nucleus (PBN), colloquially termed the "general alarm" system. Functioning as an intermediary for pain and assorted sensory signals en route to the forebrain, the PBN receives direct extensions from the trigeminal nucleus, influencing the emotional facet of pain. Given the abundance of CGRP in the PBN and its extensive projections to brain regions implicated in migraine pathophysiology, modified signaling within this conduit might underlie the heightened sensory perception characteristic of migraine. CGRP's dual—peripheral and central—actions likely synergize to precipitate a migraine. Considering the disorder's multifaceted nature, it is improbable that a singular action of CGRP singularly instigates migraine [141].

2. Mechanisms by which CGRP contributes to migraine symptoms

The role of CGRP in migraine symptomatology is primarily deciphered through preclinical investigations. Recognized as a paramount instigator of migraine, CGRP can elicit an array of migraine-reminiscent symptoms in animals that parallel the effects observed when humans are infused with CGRP, encompassing pain-related symptoms. In rodents, mechanical hypersensitivity, an often-reported migraine symptom, can be instigated following CGRP administration. For instance, CGRP's dural administration in mice provoked periorbital touch hypersensitivity, whereas its intrathecal introduction led to heightened pain sensitivity in rat hindpaws and amplified mechanical allodynia in mice upon pinch [140].

For an extended period, the challenge of gauging spontaneous pain in animals persisted due to the absence of an apt assessment method. However, in 2010, Mogil and his team pioneered a method, illustrating that specific pain forms could be evaluated via facial grimace scales without necessitating an evoked response [142]. Building on this foundation, our research demonstrated that injecting CGRP peripherally in mice culminates in spontaneous, migraine-analogous pain, which sumatriptan could substantially mitigate. We employed an uninterrupted, objective appraisal of eye closure to assess the grimace induced by CGRP. Our findings also elucidated that CGRP-induced pain was not influenced by light levels, positing that pain and light aversion, another symptom induced by CGRP, operate independently [143].

Photophobia, characterized by an augmented sensitivity or discomfort in light conditions usually deemed non-painful, stands as a diagnostic hallmark of migraine. Those afflicted with migraine often perceive even subdued light as unsettling, gravitating away from luminous environments [144]. This human experience has been adeptly mirrored in a mouse paradigm where exposure to light becomes aversive post-CGRP administration, both centrally and peripherally, in conventional mice. This aversive reaction to light can be palliated by triptans, insinuating that the murine aversion to light resonates with human migraine. Intriguingly, in a specialized mouse model sensitized to CGRP—where human RAMP1 (an essential component of the CGRP receptor) is overexpressed within the nervous system—a mere 55 lux light intensity suffices to trigger light aversion post central CGRP administration. Notably, this aversive reaction to light is not an offshoot of anxiety, as evidenced by the unaffected performance of these mice in a light-agnostic anxiety assessment (the open field test) [145,146]. Furthermore, post-CGRP injection, these mice exhibit diminished mobility, but this inertia is predominantly observed in dimly lit sections of their enclosure. Such a preference for darker locales and a proclivity to rest mirrors human behavioral tendencies during migraine episodes.

6.3.2. CGRP as a Therapeutic Target

1. Overview of CGRP-targeted treatments in migraine management—Evaluation of the effectiveness of CGRP inhibitors

Over recent years, a plethora of molecules aiming to obstruct CGRP signaling pathways have been developed, with the objective of mitigating migraine symptoms. The first molecules that showed promise were CGRP receptor antagonists, known as "gepants." These substances demonstrate a high affinity for the canonical CGRP receptor, blocking the CGRP from binding and obstructing the subsequent signal transduction. Importantly, gepants do not incite direct vasoconstriction, making them potentially safer than triptans for a migraine population that statistically exhibits a higher prevalence of cardiovascular diseases [158].

Numerous clinical trials have established that both intravenous and orally administered gepants can effectively alleviate acute migraine symptoms (Table 3); however, the efficacy of gepants in preventing migraine is currently a matter of debate. Some clinical trials had to be halted due to adverse effects, while others are still in progress [159]. The development of some gepants was ceased for various reasons. For example, olcegepant demonstrated low oral bioavailability, and both telcagepant and MK-3207 were discontinued due to liver toxicity associated with frequent use [159].

In spite of these initial safety concerns, the apparent efficacy of gepants has encouraged continued efforts to devise safe molecules that block CGRP. Currently, three gepants—rimegepant, ubrogepant, and atogepant—are still under clinical development. In phase 2b clinical trials, the efficacy of rimegepant for acute migraine treatment was assessed using various endpoints, such as freedom from pain, migraine, photophobia, phonophobia, and nausea remission [76]. Medium doses of rimegepant (75, 150, and 300 mg) were found to be significantly more effective than the placebo, and unlike the previously terminated gepants, rimegepant did not exhibit any adverse effects on liver function. Interestingly, a higher dose of rimegepant (600 mg) did not yield significant benefits over the placebo, leading the researchers to hypothesize that this could be attributed to inherent variability among patients randomized to this dose group [160].

Post this investigation, a series of three phase 3 double-blind, randomized, placebo-controlled trials (NCT03235479, NCT03237845, NCT03461757) alongside a safety investigation (NCT03266588) were commenced, with outcomes yet to be unveiled [150]. In parallel, ubrogepant showcased a favorable dose-effect correlation for acute migraine treatment in a phase 2b double-blind, randomized, placebo-controlled trial [151], exhibiting negligible side effects. However, these findings are somewhat overshadowed by the heightened placebo group response and the study's restricted patient count. Two subsequent phase 3 double-blind, randomized, placebo-controlled trials (NCT02867709, NCT02828020) wrapped up in December 2017 and February 2018, respectively. The initial findings echo the results of the earlier phase 2b study. Atogepant, possessing a molecular structure distinct from its gepant counterparts, is currently under examination for migraine prevention. Initial data from a phase 2b/3 trial (NCT02848326) indicate that adults administered atogepant underwent a more pronounced decline in their monthly migraine days average compared to those receiving a placebo. There were no reported grave side effects tied to the treatment. As of the time this review was drafted, ubrogepant emerged as the inaugural gepant to secure FDA sanctioning for acute migraine intervention, encompassing cases with or devoid of an aura [140].

Table 3. Clinical trials investigating drugs that target CGRP (calcitonin gene-related peptide): both completed and currently underway.

Drug Name, Type of Molecule	Indication (Acute or Prophylactic)	Development Stage
Atogepant, CGRP antagonist	Prophylactic	FDA-approved
BI 44370 TA, CGRP antagonist	Acute	Abandoned
Eptinezumab, CGRP monoclonal antibody	Prophylactic	FDA-approved EMA-approved
Erenumab, CGRP receptor monoclonal antibody	Prophylactic	FDA-approved
Fremanezumab, CGRP monoclonal antibody	Prophylactic	FDA-approved
Galcanezumab, CGRP monoclonal antibody	Prophylactic	FDA-approved
MK-3207, CGRP antagonist	Acute	Abandoned for liver toxicity
Olcegepant, CGRP antagonist	Acute	Abandoned for lack of oral availability
Rimegepant, CGRP antagonist	Acute	FDA-approved
Telcagepant, CGRP antagonist	Acute and prophylactic	Abandoned for liver toxicity
Ubrogepant, CGRP antagonist	Acute	FDA-approved

Monoclonal antibodies aimed at CGRP (such as fremanezumab, galcanezumab, and eptinezumab) and its receptor (like erenumab) form a separate molecular category adept at obstructing CGRP signaling pathways. Three among these antibodies (fremanezumab, galcanezumab, and erenumab) recently achieved FDA endorsement for preventive migraine therapy, while a verdict on a fourth candidate, eptinezumab, is anticipated in 2020. Remarkably, about half of the patients administered these antibodies witnessed a 50% downturn in their migraine days. Notably, no discernible efficacy disparity was observed across antibodies, irrespective of whether they latch onto the receptor or isolate CGRP. These antibodies also maintain their therapeutic effectiveness for an extended period beyond a month post-application, thus qualifying as prophylactic agents administered monthly or even on a quarterly schedule to patients. This mode of application stands in stark contrast to the daily oral dosing demanded by gepants [140].

Drawing from extensive clinical trials and nearly a year's presence in the market, CGRP and its receptor antibodies seem to have a good safety profile and are generally well-tolerated. Yet, the ramifications of the prolonged CGRP blockade remain to be understood. A glimmer of optimism emerges from Amgen/Novartis's findings, which indicate that their antibody remained safe up to the three-year mark in an ongoing five-year open-label study [152]. Moreover, an examination focusing on patients diagnosed with angina did not highlight any detrimental effects of the antibody [153]. Still, this study is not without its constraints. It predominantly featured male participants in a disorder that chiefly affects females, roped in patients with stable angina pectoris instead of those with microvascular disease (who would better mirror the vulnerable population), and gauged drug implications rather prematurely before the receptor antibody could adequately attach to the receptor (see Figure 2) [154].

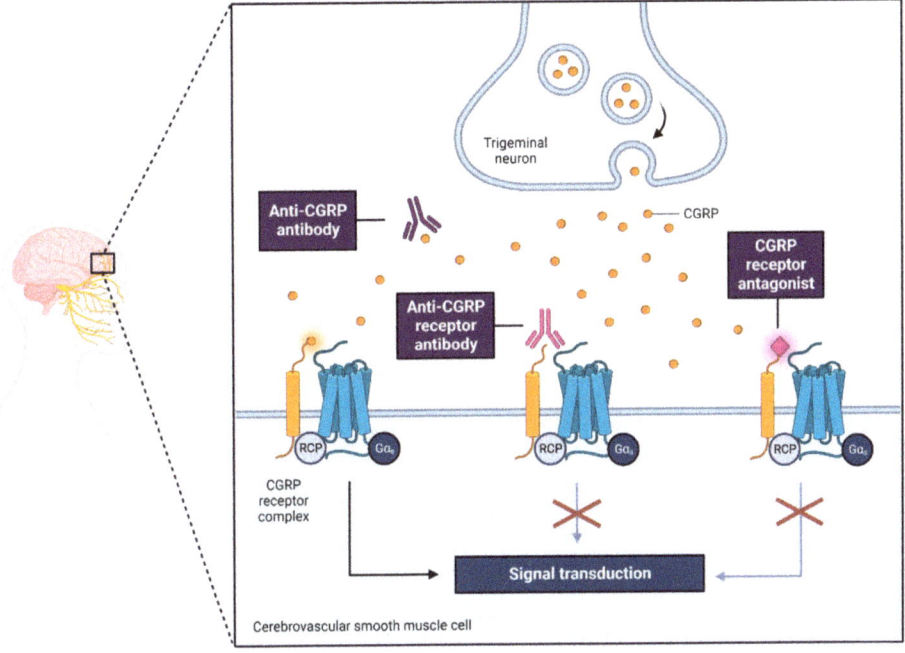

Figure 2. Calcitonin gene-related peptide-targeting drugs for migraine.

Cardiovascular risks loom large, especially considering that migraine patients are identified as high-risk candidates for stroke and cardiovascular complications. The following pressing question arises: might a CGRP blockade amplify the intensity of a stroke episode? A recent case study highlighted a patient who encountered an ischemic incident post the administration of a CGRP antagonist medication [155]. Still, it is pivotal to understand that conclusions can not be hastily drawn from a solitary patient's experience. Rigorous, long-duration studies centered on cardiovascular wellness are imperative. A prudent starting point would be animal-based research endeavors, delving into the impacts of CGRP blockade on ischemic conditions (see Figure 2).

6.4. Medical Treatment of Migraine

6.4.1. Overview of Conventional Medical Treatments for Migraine

1. Medications commonly prescribed for migraine relief—Discussion of their mechanisms of action and limitations (Figure 3)

    Therapeutic Interventions for Migraine Cessation

    (a) Anti-Inflammatory Agents: NSAIDs and Acetaminophen

    Non-steroidal anti-inflammatory drugs (NSAIDs) serve as the primary selection for mitigating the intensity and duration of migraines and are supported by an extensive body of evidence. Various NSAIDs, such as ibuprofen, naproxen sodium, acetylsalicylic acid (ASA), diclofenac potassium, aspirin, tolfenamic acid, piroxicam, ketoprofen, and ketorolac, have all exhibited their efficacy in treating migraine through evidence gleaned from randomized controlled trials and systematic reviews. Acetaminophen, as well as a combination formula of acetaminophen, aspirin, and caffeine, has also displayed significant efficacy in the acute treatment of migraine [161].

Mechanism of Action

NSAIDs primarily act by hindering the synthesis of prostaglandins. They act to reversibly block cyclooxygenase (COX) enzymes 1 and 2. The NSAIDs that inhibit prostaglandin E2 synthesis are particularly effective in mitigating acute migraine attacks. Aspirin, for instance, serves as an irreversible inhibitor of both COX 1 and 2 enzymes.

The complete mode of action of acetaminophen is not fully understood yet; however, it is believed to exert its effects on central processes, like enhancing the serotonergic descending inhibitory pathways. Acetaminophen may also interact with opioidergic systems, eicosanoid systems, and the nitric oxide-containing pathways [162].

(b) Triptans

The U.S. Food and Drug Administration (FDA) has given the green light to a total of seven triptans specifically designed for the immediate relief of migraine episodes. This lineup includes sumatriptan, eletriptan, naratriptan, zolmitriptan, rizatriptan, frovatriptan, and almotriptan. In terms of pricing, triptans tend to be on the higher side compared to NSAIDs. As a result, they are generally selected as a treatment strategy when alternatives like NSAIDs or acetaminophen do not produce the desired outcomes, or when the intensity of the migraine demands their application [158].

Mechanism of Action

Triptans function as serotonin-receptor agonists. They possess high affinity for the 5-HT1B and 5-HT1D receptors, and they have variable affinity for the 5-HT1F receptors. The supposed mode of action involves binding to postsynaptic 5-HT1B receptors located on the smooth muscle cells of blood vessels and to presynaptic 5-HT1D receptors situated on trigeminal nerve terminals and dorsal horn neurons [163].

(c) Antiemetics

Antiemetics are frequently chosen for migraine treatment when symptoms include nausea or vomiting. These medications can be administered either alongside NSAIDs or triptans, or used as monotherapy. Metoclopramide and prochlorperazine are two commonly employed antiemetics. Metoclopramide has the most significant body of evidence supporting its efficacy in treating migraine and is less likely to cause extrapyramidal side effects compared to prochlorperazine. Other antiemetics used for migraine management include domperidone, promethazine, and chlorpromazine [161].

Mechanism of Action

Metoclopramide is a benzamide that antagonizes the D2 receptor at lower doses and the 5HT-3 receptor at higher doses, providing both antiemetic and migraine relief effects. Both prochlorperazine and chlorpromazine function as dopamine antagonists, interacting with the D2 receptor, which helps in mitigating the symptoms of migraine and controlling nausea and vomiting.

(d) Ergotamines

With the advent of triptans, the usage of ergotamines has declined as triptans have shown superior efficacy. Dihydroergotamine has shown some efficacy in treating migraine, while the effectiveness of ergotamine remains unclear. A systematic review revealed that dihydroergotamine was not as effective as triptans; however, when combined with an antiemetic, dihydroergotamine was found to be as effective as ketorolac, opiates, or valproate [164]. Dihydroergotamine might be a useful alternative when patients do not respond to other medications, including triptans.

Mechanism of Action

Ergotamines, similar to triptans, are potent agonists of 5-HT 1b/1d receptors. Their mechanism of action is thought to involve the constriction of the presumed pain-causing intracranial extracerebral blood vessels at the 5-HT1B receptors and inhibition of trigeminal neurotransmission at both peripheral and central 5-HT1D receptors; moreover, they interact with other serotonin, adrenergic, and dopamine receptors. They induce the constriction of peripheral and cranial blood vessels [165].

Interventions Aimed at Migraine Prevention

(a) Beta-Blockers

Beta-blockers, such as propranolol, timolol, bisoprolol, metoprolol, atenolol, and nadolol, have been explored for their prophylactic role in preventing migraine attacks and have shown positive results in clinical studies. However, beta-blockers exhibiting intrinsic sympathomimetic activity, like acebutolol, alprenolol, oxprenolol, and pindolol, do not appear to demonstrate efficacy for migraine prevention [166].

Mechanism of Action

The exact mechanisms underlying the preventive effect of beta-blockers on migraine are not completely understood. One prevailing theory suggests that their migraine prevention abilities may be linked to their beta-1 mediated effects, which inhibit the release of noradrenaline and activity of tyrosine hydroxylase, thereby contributing to their prophylactic action. Other potential mechanisms may involve the serotonergic blockade, inhibiting thalamic activity, and blocking the effect of nitrous oxide.

(b) Antiepileptic Drugs

Several antiepileptic drugs (AEDs) have been investigated for their efficacy in migraine prevention, with topiramate and valproate demonstrating the most substantial evidence of effectiveness [166].

Mechanism of Action

The precise mode of action of antiepileptic drugs in preventing migraine remains elusive. For topiramate, it is known to block several channels, such as voltage-dependent sodium and calcium channels. In addition, it has been shown to reduce glutamate-mediated excitatory neurotransmission, enhance the inhibition mediated by GABA-A, inhibit carbonic anhydrase activity, and decrease CGRP secretion from trigeminal neurons, all of which could potentially contribute to its preventive effects on migraine. Similarly, for valproate, a multifaceted approach is likely involved in preventing migraine. These mechanisms might encompass enhancing GABAergic inhibition, blocking excitatory ion channels, and downregulating the expression of CGRP in brain tissue. These multifactorial actions collectively could underpin the migraine preventive effects of these antiepileptic drugs.

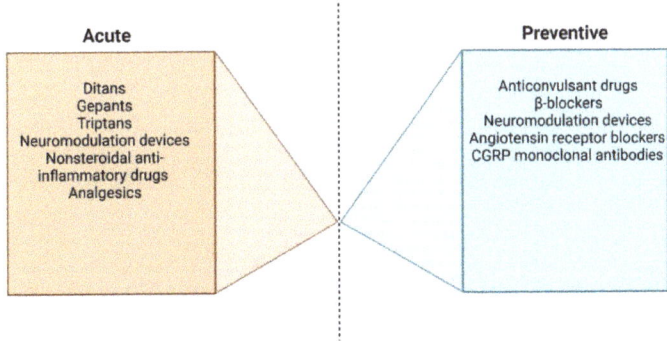

Figure 3. Migraine management.

6.4.2. Emerging Therapeutic Approaches in Migraine Management

1. Introduction to novel medications and treatment strategies and Potential benefits and challenges associated with these approaches

Goals of present research

The goals of present research in migraine treatment are manifold and multifaceted, particularly in the context of elucidating and exploring the role of peptides or their respective receptors that emerge during a migraine episode. Simultaneously, there is an unflagging pursuit of methods to obstruct the activation of the trigeminovascular system and the receptors of the neurotransmitters, which are intricately linked to the cascade of events leading to a migraine. These avenues of exploration are deemed paramount for the inception of innovative, effective, and targeted pharmacological interventions. These treatments are intended to serve both as acute therapeutic options and preventive strategies against migraine.

In light of the challenges and limitations associated with the use of triptans, a class of drugs conventionally employed in the treatment of migraine, there is a concerted effort within research and development programs to discover and develop new acute treatments. The aim here is to ensure these novel treatments are as effective as, if not more so, than triptans, whilst also being better tolerated by patients; furthermore, these treatments should ideally possess a distinctive, migraine-specific neural mechanism of action. An ideal feature of these new treatments would be the ability to avoid manipulating the vascular tone, thereby reducing potential side effects associated with vascular modulation [167].

In pursuit of these objectives, two primary biochemical pathways have been subjected to rigorous scrutiny—the calcitonin gene-related peptide (CGRP) pathway and the serotonin pathway. This intensive research has yielded two promising new classes of drugs, known as the gepants and the ditans, respectively. Both of these drug families are targeted interventions designed to alleviate the symptoms of migraine. In addition to their potential as acute treatments, the studies focusing on the CGRP pathway have also unearthed potential preventative strategies. This has culminated in the development of anti-CGRP monoclonal antibodies, which are being recognized as potential prophylactic treatments for migraine.

These promising new treatments are currently in an advanced stage of development, undergoing rigorous clinical trials. Some of these therapies are anticipated to be launched into the market in the near future, ushering in a new era of migraine management. This continued research endeavors to deliver more personalized and effective therapeutic options, minimizing the distress and impairment that migraine bring into the lives of those afflicted by them [167].

6.5. Competitive Environment

6.5.1. The Role of Calcitonin Gene-Related Peptide in Migraine

Regarded as one of the most potent vasodilators known, the calcitonin gene-related peptide (CGRP) exists in the following two forms within the human body: the alpha-CGRP, a 37-amino acid peptide that is predominantly expressed in primary sensory neurons of the dorsal root ganglia, trigeminal ganglia, and vagal ganglia; and the beta-CGRP, which is found primarily within intrinsic enteric neurons. The ubiquity of CGRP is seen in its widespread distribution across the cerebral and cerebellar cortex, thalamus, hypothalamus, inhibitory nociceptive nuclei of the brainstem, trigemino-cervical complex, and the trigeminovascular system [168].

Within the trigeminal ganglia, CGRP is found in cells that generate thinly myelinated A-delta fibers as well as unmyelinated C-fibers. Receptors for CGRP are present within the cortical and subcortical structures mentioned earlier. On trigeminal fibers, these receptors operate as autoreceptors, thereby governing CGRP release. Elevated levels of CGRP are detected during migraine attacks, although some research suggests conflicting evidence [167].

Notably, an intravenous infusion of CGRP was found to induce migraine attacks in about 60% of the patients studied. Interestingly, patients diagnosed with familial hemiplegic migraine, a rare type of migraine accompanied by aura, showed no sensitivity to CGRP. This could potentially be attributed to alterations in the levels of CGRP within their trigeminal system [169].

Experimental activation of trigeminal ganglion cells has been found to cause the release of CGRP. This release is inhibited in a dose-dependent manner by 5-HT1B/D agonists, underscoring the importance of the trigeminal system as a potential target for CGRP receptor antagonists and triptans. CGRP, in addition to its vascular effects, has emerged as a key regulator of neuronal function, significantly influencing neurotransmitter systems like the glutamatergic system [170].

Drawing from these findings, drugs that modulate CGRP activity have shown promise in the future treatment of migraine. These include CGRP receptor antagonists, which compete with the body's naturally occurring CGRP at receptor binding sites and have been shown to be effective in the treatment of acute migraine attacks. Other approaches to modulate CGRP activity, such as the development of monoclonal antibodies against CGRP and the CGRP receptor, have been introduced recently [167].

6.5.2. CGRP Receptor Antagonists (The Gepants)

CGRP receptor antagonists, referred to as gepants, are small compounds that vie with the body's endogenous CGRP for receptor binding sites. The ability of these CGRP receptor antagonists to cross the blood–brain barrier remains uncertain. Despite their promise, the development journey of new emerging CGRP antagonists has been beset by challenges. Initial antagonists, such as olcegepant (BIBN4096BS), telcagepant (MK-0974), and MK-3207, demonstrated efficacy as acute treatments for migraine. However, they were burdened by unfavorable safety profiles.

In an initial proof-of-concept study in acute migraine treatment, the intravenously administered olcegepant at a dosage of 2.5 mg significantly outperformed placebo at a 2-h response rate, marking a potential breakthrough in acute migraine treatment [171]. Following this, telcagepant, an orally administered CGRP receptor antagonist, underwent a phase II proof-of-concept study that showcased the efficacy of a 300–600 mg dose. However, when telcagepant was tried as a daily preventive migraine treatment, it led to liver enzyme derangement, leading to the discontinuation of trials [172]. MK-3207, the third oral CGRP receptor antagonist developed and tested in migraine, showed superiority to placebo above the dose of 10 mg in 2-h pain freedom, but was discontinued due to liver toxicity issues.

A promising CGRP receptor antagonist, BI 44370 TA, was utilized in a phase II study to evaluate its safety, tolerability, and efficacy in the treatment of an acute migraine attack in episodic migraine sufferers [173]; however, studies on this agent have been discontinued as well.

6.5.3. Ubrogepant (MK-1602)

Ubrogepant (MK-1602) is a novel oral CGRP receptor antagonist that is chemically distinct from both telcagepant and MK-3207. The safety and efficacy of ubrogepant at varying doses was evaluated in a Phase IIb, multicenter, randomized, double-blind, placebo-controlled trial. Results showed a positive trend across all doses of ubrogepant for the 2-h pain freedom endpoint. Importantly, there were no observed post-treatment elevations of ALT > 3 ULN hand and no other abnormal laboratory values of clinical relevance, as found with the earlier CGRP antagonists. The success of this study led to the initiation of phase 3 clinical trials. Positive preliminary efficacy and safety results of two phase III multicenter randomized, double-blind, placebo-controlled clinical trials comparing ubrogepant 50 mg and 100 mg versus placebo (Achieve 1) and ubrogepant 25 mg and 50 mg versus placebo (Achieve 2) were recently presented at the American Headache Society (AHS) conference [174]. Despite these promising findings, further data on consistency of effect and safety in patients for whom triptans are contraindicated are needed to solidify its role as a viable alternative to triptans.

6.5.4. Rimegepant (BMS-927711): Overview and Clinical Trials

Rimegepant is a pioneering and unique calcitonin gene-related peptide (CGRP) receptor antagonist that bears a distinct chemical structure from telcagepant. In the sphere of migraine treatment, rimegepant's effectiveness and safety have been evaluated in a rigorous phase II clinical trial. This trial was double-blind, randomized, placebo-controlled, and dose-ranging, involving a total of 885 participants.

The participants of the study were allocated randomly to receive one of six doses of BMS-927711 (10 mg, 25 mg, 75 mg, 150 mg, 300 mg, or 600 mg), sumatriptan (100 mg), or a placebo for the treatment of moderate to severe migraine attacks. The study was designed with the primary endpoint of achieving pain freedom two hours after the dose. Secondary endpoints were more comprehensive, including an endpoint consisting of the absence of headache pain, as well as a lack of symptoms, such as photophobia, phonophobia, and nausea, at two hours post-dose.

Along with these endpoints, the trial studied several other secondary efficacy and safety measures. Interestingly, a higher proportion of participants who received rimegepant 150 mg achieved the primary endpoint of being pain-free at two hours, amounting to 32.9%, which was significantly higher than the percentage observed for other doses of rimegepant ($p < 0.001$). For instance, the respective proportions were 31.4% for the 75 mg dose, 29.7% for the 300 mg dose, and 15.3% for the placebo group. Sumatriptan 100 mg proved superior to all doses of rimegepant, with a success rate of 35%.

With regards to the secondary efficacy endpoint of total migraine freedom, the dose of rimegepant 75 mg was the most effective, with a success rate of 28.2%. This dose was statistically superior to the placebo. However, sumatriptan 100 mg outperformed each dose of rimegepant at this secondary endpoint. The trial also reported that the proportion of patients who were headache-free for up to 24 h after dosing was higher for several doses of rimegepant and for sumatriptan compared to the placebo group.

In terms of safety, most adverse events (AEs) were mild to moderate, and none of the patients had to discontinue due to AEs. Two patients experienced increased hepatic enzymes reported as an adverse event, one in the rimegepant group and the other in the placebo group.

The results of this trial suggest that rimegepant's effectiveness is similar to sumatriptan 100 mg in treating migraine attacks, but with potentially fewer triptan-related side effects, such as paresthesia and chest discomfort. A phase III trial comparing the efficacy of rimegepant 75 mg with a placebo has recently been concluded. Moreover, an ongoing prospective multicenter open-label long-term safety study is expected to complete recruitment by late 2019. These two studies will contribute to understanding the consistency and safety of rimegepant in migraine therapy [160].

6.5.5. Atogepant (AGN-241689): The Future of Migraine Prevention

Atogepant, a small molecule with a distinct structure similar to that of ubrogepant, is the only CGRP receptor antagonist currently under investigation for migraine prevention. Its higher potency and longer half-life compared to ubrogepant make it suitable for preventive treatment.

The safety, efficacy, and tolerability of atogepant were evaluated in a phase II/III multicenter, randomized, double-blind, placebo-controlled, parallel-group study (NCT02848326). In this trial, adult patients were randomized to receive placebo, 10 mg QD, 30 mg QD, 30 mg BID, 60 mg QD, and 60 mg BID, respectively, and were treated for 12 weeks for the prevention of episodic migraine.

The primary efficacy endpoint was the change from baseline in mean monthly migraine/probable migraine headache days across the 12-week treatment period. All active treatment groups showed a statistically significant reduction from baseline in the primary efficacy parameter. In terms of safety, atogepant was well tolerated, with the most common adverse events being nausea, fatigue, constipation, nasopharyngitis, and urinary tract infection. The liver safety profile for atogepant was similar to placebo, with no indications of hepatotoxicity with daily administration over 12 weeks. The development program of this treatment is set to advance to the next stage [167].

6.5.6. Anti-CGRP and Anti-CGRP Receptor Monoclonal Antibodies

The CGRP pathway has also been targeted through the development of antibodies against CGRP and the CGRP receptor. This marks the first use of engineered antibodies in the field of migraine, and their development was initially met with some skepticism.

These monoclonal antibodies (mAbs), including galcanezumab (LY2951742), a fully humanized mAb anti-CGRP, fremanezumab (TEV-48125), a fully humanized mAb anti-CGRP, and eptinezumab, a genetically engineered humanized anti-CGRP antibody, target the ligand to prevent the binding of CGRP to its receptor. Erenumab (AMG 334) is a fully humanized mAb that targets the CGRP receptor.

These compounds have a favorable pharmacological profile that includes a long half-life, the absence of a vasoconstrictive effect or other significant hemodynamic changes [80]. Because of their high molecular weight, they do not cross the blood–brain barrier, suggesting a reduced likelihood of central nervous system-related side effects, which are commonly observed with current pharmacological prophylaxis treatments used in migraine.

Further enhancing their potential for long-term patient compliance, these mAbs can be administered either subcutaneously (sc) or intravenously (IV) at different rates ranging from once every three months to twice a month, depending on the compound.

In a series of methodologically similar randomized, double-blind, placebo-controlled Phase II and III clinical trials, the efficacy and safety of these novel treatments in the prevention of episodic and chronic migraine (CM) were explored [167].

6.5.7. Erenumab (AMG334)

Erenumab, marketed as Aimovig, is a novel migraine prophylactic belonging to the monoclonal antibody class of drugs. It operates by specifically targeting and blocking the calcitonin gene-related peptide (CGRP) receptor, a crucial element in the neurochemical pathway believed to play a role in migraine pathogenesis. The initial efficacy of erenumab was established through a phase II trial where participants suffering from episodic migraine received monthly doses of 70 mg over three months. The study outcomes exhibited a promising reduction in the number of monthly migraine days by 3.4 days compared to placebo [167].

This was further substantiated in the STRIVE study, a multicenter, phase III trial, which compared two doses of erenumab (70 mg and 140 mg) with a placebo over six months. The primary objective was to assess the change in the mean number of migraine days per month, while secondary objectives were to evaluate reductions in the severity of migraine and their impacts on physical function and daily activities. Both doses showed statistically significant reductions in the number of migraine days and severity compared to placebo. Notably, patients' disability scores, measuring the impact of migraine on daily activities, were also significantly improved [175].

A similar study, the ARISE trial, evaluated only the 70 mg dose of erenumab and confirmed its superior efficacy compared to placebo; however, unlike the STRIVE study, it did not reveal a significant improvement in the migraine disability scores. In both trials, erenumab demonstrated an excellent safety and tolerability profile with common side effects being minor, such as upper respiratory tract infection, injection site pain, and nasopharyngitis.

The long-term safety and efficacy of erenumab were further evaluated in a 5-year open-label extension of the phase II clinical trial. Here, participants with a history of inadequate response to up to two previous preventive treatments received erenumab 70 mg. This study demonstrated a reduction of 5 migraine days on average from an initial baseline of 8.8 migraine days per month. In addition, significant improvements were observed in disability and quality of life scores, indicating the long-term benefit of erenumab treatment [176].

Erenumab's performance was also assessed in chronic migraine patients in a randomized, double-blind, placebo-controlled phase II clinical trial. The participants received subcutaneous injections of either placebo, erenumab 70 mg, or erenumab 140 mg every

4 weeks for 12 weeks. Erenumab significantly reduced the number of monthly migraine days and monthly acute migraine treatments compared to placebo, thereby validating its preventive role in chronic migraine management [177]. As a result of these studies, erenumab was granted FDA approval in May 2018 for the prevention of migraine in adults.

6.5.8. Galcanezumab (LY2951742)

Like erenumab, galcanezumab is a humanized monoclonal antibody but differs in its mechanism. It inhibits the activity of CGRP by binding to the ligand itself rather than the receptor. The phase II proof-of-concept trials conducted in episodic migraine patients showed a mean reduction of 4.2 monthly migraine days with galcanezumab (150 mg) compared to a reduction of 3.0 days in the placebo group. The most commonly reported adverse events were erythema, upper respiratory tract infections, and abdominal pain [178].

A subsequent phase IIb clinical trial assessed the superiority of galcanezumab at varying doses (5, 50, 120, 300 mg) administered subcutaneously monthly for three months compared to placebo. The primary outcome was the mean change in migraine days from week 9 to 12 post-randomization. The 120 mg dosage significantly reduced migraine headache days compared with placebo [179].

Two phase III trials, EVOLVE-1 and EVOLVE-2, confirmed the efficacy of galcanezumab in reducing migraine days and improving the quality of life. Participants received monthly subcutaneous injections of galcanezumab at doses of 120 and 240 mg versus placebo for 6 months. Both studies met the primary and secondary efficacy endpoints at 6 months for both doses. The REGAIN study (NCT02614261), a 3-month double-blind study with a 9-month open-label extension for preventing migraine in chronic migraine patients, echoed the previous findings. The study met the primary endpoint at 3 months, showing that galcanezumab was significantly more effective in reducing monthly migraine days than placebo. Notably, it also showed a higher incidence of injection site reactions, erythema, and sinusitis in the galcanezumab groups [180]. These results highlight the promising role of galcanezumab in managing migraine, with long-term safety and efficacy data eagerly awaited.

6.5.9. Examination of Fremanezumab (TEV48125)

Fremanezumab, a fully humanized monoclonal antibody that targets the calcitonin gene-related peptide (CGRP), has been investigated for its potential use in the prevention of migraine. Its development was initially spurred by promising results from phase I studies, echoing the progress of other monoclonal antibodies against CGRP. To evaluate its efficacy and safety, a phase IIb study was carried out. The experimental protocol included a multicenter, randomized, double-blind, placebo-controlled design where participants were assigned to receive either 225 mg or 675 mg of subcutaneous (sc) TEV-48125 or a placebo. This was to be administered every 28 days for three months.

The primary objective of the study was to observe the mean decrease from the baseline in the number of migraine days during the third treatment cycle (weeks 9–12). In addition to this, safety parameters were also evaluated. In post-hoc analyses, investigators assessed the percentage of participants who achieved at least a 50% and 75% decrease in the number of migraine days relative to baseline. Both dosage levels of TEV48125 were found to meet the primary efficacy outcome, and no issues regarding safety or tolerability were identified. The most common adverse events associated with the treatment were mild pain or erythema at the injection site.

Following this, a phase III trial was conducted to further investigate the preventative effects of TEV-48125 (fremanezumab) in episodic migraine. This study was a randomized, double-blind, placebo-controlled, parallel-group trial that tested monthly sc fremanezumab injections of 225 mg or 675 mg following a quarterly dose regimen, against a placebo. The primary outcome was the mean change in the number of monthly migraine days per month over a 12-week period. Secondary efficacy endpoints included the proportion of patients achieving at least a 50% reduction in the mean number of monthly migraine days from baseline to week 12, along with changes in migraine-related disability scores [181].

Both the monthly and quarterly regimens of fremanezumab met the primary efficacy endpoint, showing superiority over the placebo in reducing mean migraine days. No significant difference was found between the two fremanezumab regimens. Adverse events were most commonly injection site reactions, but the proportion of participants who discontinued due to these events was small (2%). This study also shed light on the possibility of using a single dose therapy given quarterly for migraine prevention, which is significant as the results were similar to those from monthly injections. This may open up new potential for multi-injection regimens in migraine prevention [182].

TEV-48125 (fremanezumab) was also tested for chronic migraine (CM) in a multicenter, randomized, double-blind, placebo-controlled, phase IIb study. Here, TEV-48125 was administered at different doses from those used in the episodic migraine trials as follows: 675 mg in the first treatment cycle and 225 mg in the second and third treatment cycles, or 900 mg monthly for three months, against a placebo. The efficacy endpoints for this trial varied from those of the episodic migraine studies. The primary outcome was the change from baseline in the number of headache-hours during the third treatment cycle (weeks 9–12), while the secondary endpoint was the change in the number of moderate or severe headache days. Both doses showed a significant reduction in the number of headache-hours compared to placebo and a significantly greater reduction in mean number of headache days [183].

After the promising results of the phase II study, a randomized, double-blind, placebo-controlled, parallel-group trial was conducted to further confirm the efficacy of fremanezumab for CM prevention. Participants with CM were randomized to receive fremanezumab either quarterly (a single dose of 675 mg at baseline and placebo at weeks 4 and 8) or monthly (675 mg at baseline and 225 mg at weeks 4 and 8) or a placebo. The primary endpoint was the mean change from baseline in the average number of headache days, as defined by the International Headache Society (IHS). Both doses met the primary endpoint and showed a significantly greater percentage of participants obtaining at least a 50% reduction in headache days compared to placebo.

Fremanezumab was found to be associated with a higher incidence of injection-site reactions than placebo, but the severity of these reactions did not significantly differ among the trial arms. Following these studies, fremanezumab (Ajovy) received FDA approval on 14 September 2018, making it the second anti-CGRP monoclonal antibody approved for preventing migraine in adults. Notably, it became the first drug of its kind to offer both quarterly and monthly dosing options [184].

6.5.10. Eptinezumab (ALD403)

Eptinezumab (ALD403) is an innovative product of genetic engineering, specifically, a humanized antibody that is designed to target both isoforms of human CGRP. CGRP, a molecule implicated in the pathophysiology of migraine, serves as a significant focal point for novel migraine therapeutics, including eptinezumab (see Figure 4) [65].

This novel therapeutic agent has been put through a phase II proof-of-concept study to evaluate its potential in managing episodic migraine. This study was designed with the primary objective of ascertaining the safety of eptinezumab following the intravenous administration of a single 1000 mg dose. As secondary objectives, the researchers investigated efficacy outcomes and gauged the extent of disability induced by migraine at the 12-week mark following infusion. They were particularly interested in discerning changes in the frequency of migraine days from the baseline to weeks 5–8.

Participants in the trial experienced an average of 8.4–8.8 migraine days per month at baseline, and adverse events were reported by 57% of eptinezumab recipients, compared to 52% in the placebo group. The adverse events included conditions like upper respiratory tract infection, urinary tract infection, fatigue, back pain, nausea, vomiting, and arthralgia, most of which were of mild to moderate severity. Importantly, none of the serious adverse events reported were linked to the study drug.

When it came to efficacy, eptinezumab outperformed the placebo by achieving a statistically significant reduction in the mean number of migraine days from the baseline to weeks 5–8. The results also underscored a significant finding—a large proportion of participants receiving eptinezumab achieved a 50% reduction in migraine days at weeks 5–8. Interestingly, this trial observed a high placebo response rate, which might have been influenced by the intravenous administration of the drug, a departure from the delivery methods used in previous trials with anti-CGRP monoclonal antibodies.

Motivated by these promising findings, a phase III study was designed. Titled PROMISE 1, this randomized, double-blind, placebo-controlled trial sought to evaluate the efficacy and safety of various doses of eptinezumab in participants suffering from episodic migraine. The primary endpoint of this study was to identify changes in the mean frequency of migraine days over weeks 1–12, relative to a 28-day baseline period. In this study, participants were randomized to receive one of three doses of eptinezumab (300 mg, 100 mg, or 30 mg) or a placebo. The medication was administered via intravenous infusion every 12 weeks.

In the PROMISE 1 study, all doses of eptinezumab met the primary efficacy endpoint, demonstrating a significantly greater reduction in migraine days compared to the placebo group. Further, a significantly greater proportion of participants administered with eptinezumab experienced a 50% reduction in migraine days, providing more evidence for the drug's efficacy. The study did not find any significant safety issues, further supporting the suitability of eptinezumab as a therapeutic option.

Several studies with anti-CGRP monoclonal antibodies, including eptinezumab, have highlighted a remarkably rapid response to the active drug, usually noticeable within the first month following administration. Eptinezumab, in particular, demonstrated the ability to reduce migraine from the very first day post-administration and maintained similar improvement levels at 4- and 12-weeks post-infusion.

The evaluation of eptinezumab's efficacy, safety, and tolerability continued with phase II and phase III trials in patients with chronic migraine (CM). In a randomized, double-blind, placebo-controlled phase II study, different doses of eptinezumab were administered to test their effects against a placebo. Unique to this study, the primary endpoint was the percentage of patients achieving a 75% reduction in migraine days per month from baseline to week 12. Eptinezumab doses of 300 mg and 100 mg significantly outperformed the placebo group in achieving this endpoint.

These results paved the way for a phase III trial, known as PROMISE 2, to further investigate the safety and efficacy of eptinezumab for the prevention of chronic migraine. In this study, patients received either eptinezumab (300 mg or 100 mg) or a placebo, administered via infusion every 12 weeks. This study found that both doses of eptinezumab outperformed the placebo in reducing the mean number of monthly migraine days during the 12-week, double-blind treatment period. Notably, as early as day one post-infusion, a significant percentage of patients receiving eptinezumab demonstrated a reduction in migraine prevalence that was sustained through day 28.

Taken together, these studies affirm the potential of eptinezumab as a promising, efficacious, and well-tolerated therapeutic option for the management of episodic and chronic migraine. The drug's safety profile aligns well with that observed in previous studies, further bolstering its candidacy as an effective addition to the array of available migraine therapeutics [185].

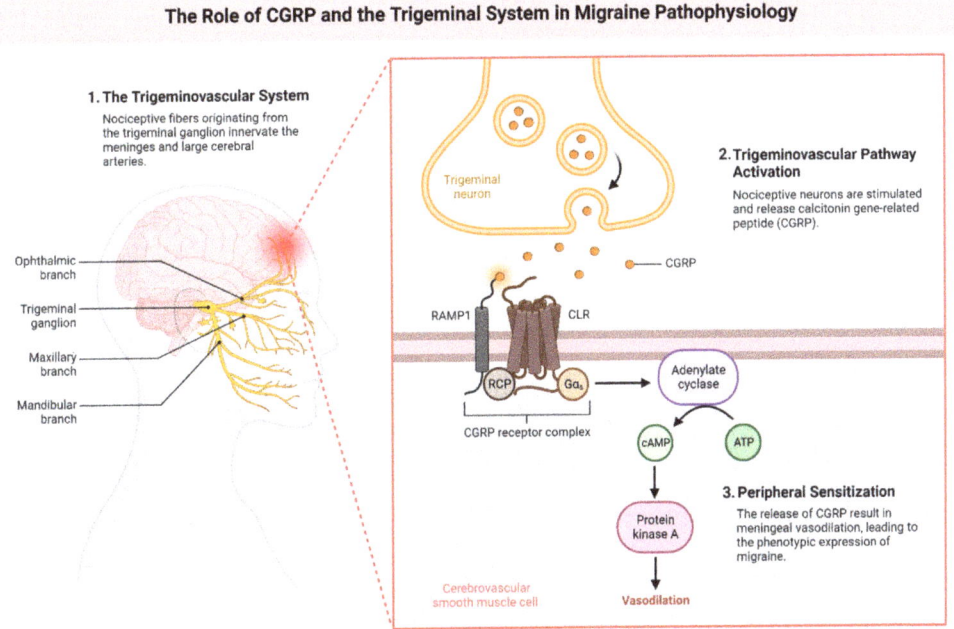

Figure 4. The role of CGRP and the trigeminal system in migraine pathophysiology.

6.6. Neuromodulation in Migraine

6.6.1. Definition and Concept of Neuromodulation in Migraine Therapy

1. Explanation of neuromodulation as a treatment modality

Neuromodulation is an innovative biomedical technique that manipulates or modulates the activities of the central or peripheral nervous system through the use of various stimuli such as electrical, magnetic, or chemical agents [186]. The technique hinges on the targeted delivery of these stimuli to specific neural sites within the body, with the express aim of altering nerve activity. Fundamentally, neuromodulation is non-destructive, reversible, and adaptable, highlighting its potential as a safe and effective approach for therapeutic interventions.

Recently, there has been an increased recognition of neuromodulation as a potentially superior treatment for migraine, compared to traditional medication therapies. The efficacy and safety of this technology are driving a paradigm shift in how both clinicians and patients approach the management of migraine. Instead of relying solely on pharmacological interventions, there is a growing interest in non-invasive neuromodulation therapies.

Among these therapies, non-invasive vagus nerve stimulation (nVNS) and single-pulse transcranial magnetic stimulation have gained notable attention due to their demonstrated effectiveness and safety profiles. These methods represent significant advancements in neuromodulation and are changing the landscape of migraine management [187].

In the modern healthcare context, neuromodulation technology holds substantial promise, particularly for vulnerable patient populations. For instance, expectant mothers, who need to avoid certain medications due to potential harm to the fetus, and patients who struggle with tolerating medications or find them ineffective, may greatly benefit from non-invasive neuromodulation therapies. The potential benefits extend not just to the realm of improved health outcomes, but also to the sphere of healthcare economics.

In specific circumstances, non-pharmacological neuromodulation techniques may prove to be a cost-effective alternative to traditional treatment modalities [188]. By reducing dependency on medications, these techniques can help circumvent the long-term costs associated with drug therapy, such as costs related to side effects and long-term use. Furthermore, as these therapies improve in effectiveness and efficiency, they may help reduce the indirect costs of migraine, such as lost productivity and reduced quality of life.

In conclusion, neuromodulation represents a pioneering field in neuroscience that has the potential to revolutionize the treatment of migraine and other neurological disorders. Through the targeted use of electrical, magnetic, or chemical stimuli, this technique can modulate nerve activity in a way that is non-destructive, reversible, and adaptable. As research in this area continues to unfold, the healthcare industry will likely see an increasing shift toward these non-invasive, cost-effective, and patient-friendly treatment options.

2. Overview of different types of neuromodulation techniques

Neuromodulation operates through the application of electrical or magnetic pulses to interact with or stimulate the central or peripheral pain pathways. This technique essentially targets the pain mechanisms in the human body with the aim of reducing the intensity of experienced pain. The application of electrical or magnetic stimuli can alter central neurotransmitters when they engage with pain circuits [189]. These modifications, in the context of treating acute migraine attacks, may potentially halt the processes that lead to the onset of an attack. For preventative purposes, these neuromodulatory changes aim to lessen the central sensitization that culminates in chronic headaches.

Traditional neuromodulation techniques engage the neurological system either centrally or peripherally through the skin, employing a changing magnetic field or an electric current to manipulate the mechanisms associated with headache-related pain. Both modes of delivery demonstrate rapid effectiveness, making them suitable for addressing acute symptoms; moreover, sustained application of these modalities might confer long-term preventative benefits [190]. Figure 5 offers a visualization of various neuromodulation techniques alongside their respective targets or sites of action.

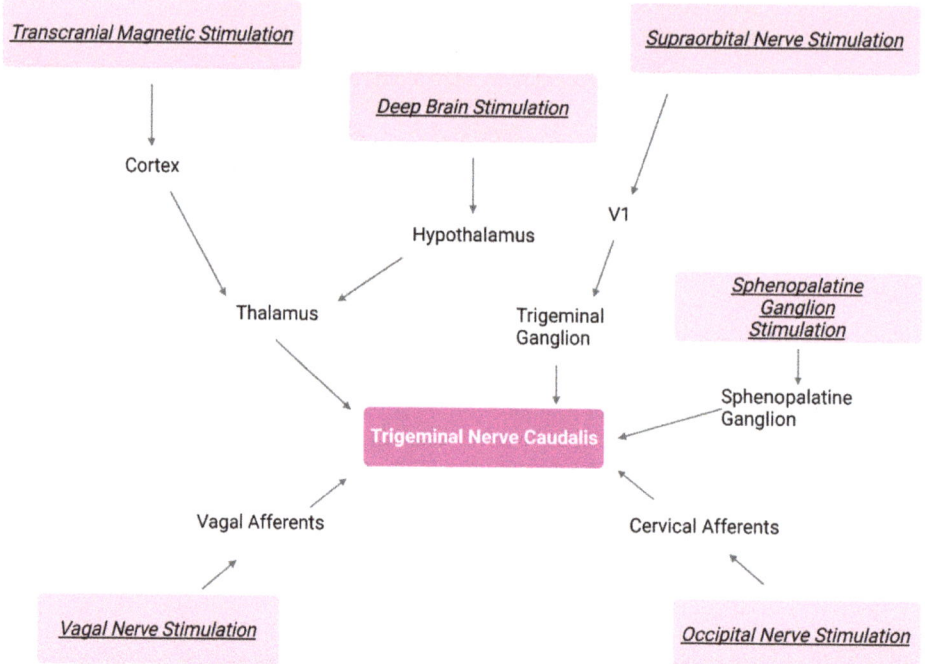

Figure 5. Several neuromodulation techniques and their respective site of action or targets.

Neuromodulation is implemented via a device that modifies brain cell activity utilizing electrical or magnetic stimulations. These devices exhibit diversity in their modes of operation. Some are designed to halt attacks, while others are utilized for preventative purposes. The commonality among them lies in the principle of altering the activity within nerve pathways. These devices, alternatively referred to as stimulators, can be categorized based on their operational parameters. Neuromodulation devices may employ magnetic, electrical, or temperature-changing stimuli. They may be invasive or non-invasive, and their design may range from portable, easy-to-use devices to those that necessitate surgical placement [187].

In the realm of neuromodulation, different techniques and devices offer a range of options to tailor treatments according to the patient's specific needs. As our understanding of the mechanisms behind migraine deepens, the applications of neuromodulation will continue to evolve, potentially offering more effective and personalized treatments for patients suffering from migraine and other neurological conditions.

3. Neuromodulation Modalities

With the emergence of neuromodulation and the recognition of its potential for preventative treatment in chronic pain conditions, such as migraine and cluster headaches, there has been significant development in the field of non-invasive neuromodulation techniques. These advancements offer alternative treatments that pose minimal risk to the patient while maximizing the potential for pain management and relief. Not only have several of these techniques successfully passed through clinical trial phases, but they have also found their way into the marketplace where they are actively being utilized for patient treatment.

Simultaneously, numerous other neuromodulation techniques are currently in various stages of clinical trials, showing the ongoing growth and exploration in this sector of medicine. These techniques, aimed at managing acute migraine attacks and chronic pain, are progressing towards market utilization, continually broadening the treatment options available for these conditions [191].

Figure 6 offers a visual representation of the different non-invasive neuromodulation techniques employed in the management of acute migraine episodes. This visual aid helps provide a better understanding of the variety and extent of non-invasive techniques available, each with its distinct advantages and specific use-cases, contributing to the expansive repertoire of neuromodulation methods.

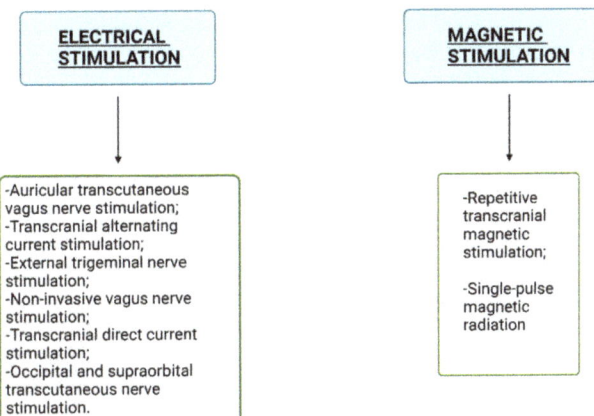

Figure 6. Different non-invasive neuromodulations in the management of acute attacks of migraine.

The evolution and diversity in neuromodulation techniques symbolize the adaptability and progressive nature of contemporary medicine. Through continuous research and development, these techniques are becoming increasingly refined, potentially providing better, more targeted treatment for patients suffering from acute migraine and other chronic pain conditions. It signifies a remarkable shift in our approach to pain management, with techniques that prioritize patient safety and comfort while not compromising on effectiveness [187].

6.6.2. Effectiveness of Neuromodulation in Managing Migraine: Review of Clinical Studies on the Use of Neuromodulation for Migraine—Assessment of the Benefits and Limitations of Neuromodulation

1. Vagus Nerve Stimulation

The gammaCore Sapphire™, crafted by electroCore, Inc. (Basking Ridge, NJ, USA), is a handheld non-invasive vagus nerve stimulator (nVNS) designed for transcutaneous application to the vagus nerve on either side of the neck. The FDA first granted clearance to this device in April 2017, initially for the treatment of acute pain associated with episodic cluster headaches in adults. Now, it has expanded FDA approval, covering both the acute and preventive treatment of migraine-related pain for individuals aged 12 or older.

Four major nVNS trials have been conducted concerning migraine, consisting of two studies for episodic migraine (EM), one tailored for chronic migraine (CM), and another one incorporating CM. The EVENT study, which was the first nVNS trial for CM, primarily sought to assess safety and tolerability in a pilot feasibility format. This randomized double-blind sham-controlled research focused on CM prevention. Though the efficacy endpoints (a change in monthly headache days after 2 months; -1.4 vs. -0.2, $p = 0.59$) did not show statistical significance, there were hints of potential benefits with prolonged use. After an 8-month treatment period, 15 subjects witnessed a mean change of -7.9 (95% CI -11.9 to -3.8, $p < 0.01$) [186].

Another noteworthy trial was the PREMIUM II study, a randomized sham-controlled double-blind study that included both CM and EM subjects. Unfortunately, it was cut short due to the COVID-19 pandemic. With a total of 300 participants enrolled and a modified intention-to-treat (mITT) subgroup of 113 subjects analyzed, the PREMIUM II study discovered a non-significant reduction in monthly migraine days (verum vs. sham: -3.1 vs. -2.3 headache days, $p = 0.233$) in the mITT cohort. However, 44.9% of verum-treated individuals experienced at least a 50% decrease in migraine days, in contrast to 26.8% in the sham group ($p = 0.048$) [187].

Clinical trials have demonstrated that the gammaCore Sapphire™ is safe and generally well-tolerated, with no significant treatment-linked adverse events. Some common side effects reported in the CM trials were facial pain, gastrointestinal symptoms, and upper respiratory tract infections. While the preliminary data indicate that nVNS may hold promise for treating CM, further exploration and evidence are needed to solidify these findings.

2. Remote Electronic Neuromodulation

Nerivio® (Theranica Bio-Electronics Ltd., Montclair, NJ, USA) is a remote electronic neuromodulation (REN) device that has been FDA-approved for the acute treatment of migraine (both EM and CM) in patients aged 12 years and older. The device comprises an armband that emits electronic stimuli controlled by a smartphone app. It is recommended that patients begin use within 60 min of the onset of a migraine or aura. The stimulation lasts for 45 min and can be adjusted for intensity by the individual user via the app, which also features a migraine diary for logging headaches and usage sessions.

Following two randomized double-blind sham-controlled trials that led to the initial FDA clearance of Nerivio for use in EM in 2019, two subsequent open-label observational studies (TCH-005, TCH-006) contributed to the FDA clearance for CM in 2020. In the TCH-005 study, 42 subjects were enrolled, with 210 evaluable treatments carried out by 38 participants. The TCH-006 study evaluated a total of 493 evaluable treatments from 91 participants out of the 126 enrolled [192].

The device-related adverse events were generally related to topical peripheral sensations such as warmth, itching, arm pain, redness, and numbness.

3. Electrical Stimulation of the Trigeminal Nerve

The CEFALY DUAL device, a next-generation evolution of the original electrical trigeminal nerve stimulation (eTNS) unit designed by CEFALY-Technology (Seraing, Belgium), received the stamp of approval from the FDA for the acute as well as preventive management of migraine in adults. As of late 2020, this device is available over-the-counter. CEFALY DUAL offers two customizable settings—an ACUTE program, which utilizes a 100 Hz frequency over a 60 min session for instant relief, and a PREVENTIVE program, which operates at a lower frequency of 60 Hz for 20 min daily to thwart the onset of migraine [193,194].

The therapeutic potential of the CEFALY device for both acute and preventive treatment of migraine is supported by two randomized controlled trials, with one trial specifically mentioning CM [8]. The ACME study, a randomized double-blind sham-controlled trial involving patients with migraine (likely including but not specifying CM), revealed that using CEFALY during the onset of a headache provided more significant pain reduction compared to the sham group (-3.46 ± 2.32 vs. -1.78 ± 1.89; $p < 0.001$). The study likely comprised mostly patients with episodic migraine (EM), as those who had used Botox in the previous four months were excluded [193,194].

Three open-label observation studies, two involving CEFALY and one using supraorbital transcutaneous electrical nerve stimulation (TENS), have specifically targeted CM. In these studies, the CEFALY device was found to decrease monthly migraine days and acute medication consumption. The adverse events were minimal and reversible, with the most common being paresthesia (2.03%), changes in arousal (mostly fatigue, sometimes insomnia, 0.82%), headache (0.52%), and skin allergy to the electrode (0.09%) [13]. These findings suggest that eTNS could be beneficial for CM treatment [192].

4. Single-Pulse Transcranial Magnetic Stimulation

eNeura Inc.'s sTMS mini™, hailing from Baltimore, MD, USA, is an innovative device that administers single-pulse stimulation to the rear of the head. This stimulation method is believed to modify the excitability of the cerebral cortex by halting cortical spreading depolarization waves and curbing thalamocortical signaling [190]. Initially conceived for episodic migraine patients exhibiting aura, the device has secured FDA clearance for both the acute and prophylactic treatment of migraine in individuals aged 12 years and up. The preventive regimen necessitates a twice-daily treatment involving 4 pulses (a pair of consecutive pulses, a pause of 15 min, followed by another 2 pulses). For acute treatment, the procedure entails three successive pulses when a migraine begins, with an option to administer more pulses at quarter-hour intervals if required [191].

The FDA endorsement of this device came on the heels of a randomized, double-blind, sham-controlled trial. Following this, an open-label observational investigation, dubbed the ESPOUSE study, was conducted. This study saw participation from 13 (amounting to 10%) chronic migraine sufferers who used the device daily for both preventive measures (the aforementioned 4 pulses administered twice daily) and acute relief (3 pulses with the possibility of repetition every 15 min for two subsequent sessions). Although the specific effects of daily sTMS application on chronic migraine were not delineated in detail, the research indicated that sTMS effectively slashed monthly headache days, reduced the need for acute medication, and brought down the Headache Impact Test-6 (HIT-6) score. The treatment regimen involving sTMS was generally well-received by participants. The predominant side effects cataloged were sensations of lightheadedness, tingling, and the occurrence of tinnitus [191].

5. Combined Occipital and Trigeminal Nerve Stimulation

The Relivion® is a user-operated stimulation device that secured FDA clearance in the early months of 2021. It is adept at delivering electrical surges to six branches spanning both the occipital and trigeminal nerves. The device comes equipped with pre-set settings, allowing for six treatment cycles (providing uninterrupted stimulation for a 48-h window) as and when needed, primarily for delivering swift relief from migraine episodes. The green light for its market entry was largely due to findings from a widespread study dubbed the RIME study. This investigation involved 131 episodic migraine sufferers who underwent stimulation for a one-hour period [187].

A look back at previous studies revealed that the concurrent stimulation of both occipital and trigeminal nerves, executed via an implanted mechanism, yielded positive results both in the immediate aftermath and over extended periods. Specifically, 75% (or 4 out of 16) of the subjects with stubborn CM observed short-term benefits, while half of the participants (8 out of 16) reported sustained relief [192]. These initial findings hint at the potential of Relivion® as a viable therapeutic avenue for CM. However, a more comprehensive dataset is required to substantiate these preliminary yet promising outcomes.

7. Investigational Devices

7.1. Transcranial Direct Current Stimulation (tDCS)

Transcranial direct current stimulation (tDCS) employs a gentle current, typically ranging from 1 to 2 milliamperes, delivered through sponge electrodes arranged in a variety of montages. This technology has been investigated as a potential treatment for headache disorders. Despite the exact mechanism of action remaining unclear, it is believed that tDCS may influence network-level neural information processing without directly affecting neural spiking or membrane potential. This process could potentially modify brain connectivity, thereby enhancing placebo effects while reducing nocebo effects. However, it is important to note that many of the tDCS trials for migraine were pilot studies of low to moderate quality. These trials have employed varying stimulation duration, current ampere, polarity, montage, and the number of sessions, thus, a universally optimized stimulation protocol has not yet been established [192].

In recent years, spanning half a decade, four rigorously designed, sham-controlled trials have honed in on transcranial direct current stimulation (tDCS) as a possible treatment route for chronic migraine (CM). These studies, distinct in design, likely adhered to a single-blind methodology. Complementing these, two studies adopting an open-label approach were undertaken. Noteworthy findings were presented by Andrade and team, pinpointing that anodal stimulation, targeted either at the left primary motor area (M1) or the dorsolateral prefrontal cortex (DLPFC), as opposed to sham procedures, significantly diminished HIT-6 scores and alleviated pain intensity [193]. In a contrasting study spearheaded by Dalla Volta and colleagues, it was discovered that cathodal stimulation, specifically targeting the coolest forehead point, surpassed sham stimulation in terms of reducing monthly headache occurrences, the frequency of attacks, and their duration. Adding to this narrative, two niche open-label research initiatives underscored a notable reduction in headache episodes observed 30 days post anodal stimulation [194]. In stark contrast, findings documented by Cerrahoglu Sirin and team indicated no discernible difference in the monthly headache frequencies a month subsequent to either anodal or sham stimulation [195]. Further amplifying the narrative of inconclusive results, a comprehensive investigation by Grazzi et al. failed to delineate any significant differences when comparing anodal tDCS, cathodal tDCS, and sham stimulation at the 6 and 12-month mark. This was specifically observed in CM patients who were in the throes of abrupt medication withdrawal due to overuse [196].

Conclusively, the true efficacy of tDCS in offering a preventive strategy against CM, especially when gauged several months post-intervention, remains shrouded in ambiguity. For future tDCS trials to shed more clarity and establish therapeutic consistency, there is an imperative need to adopt a standardized protocol, meticulously outlining the polarity, montage, number of sessions, repetition intervals, and the definitive endpoints.

7.2. Repetitive Transcranial Magnetic Stimulation (rTMS)

Repetitive transcranial magnetic stimulation (rTMS) devices deliver a sequence of rapid pulses. These pulses are engineered to generate a minute, focused cortical electric current targeting specific brain areas like the M1 and DLPFC. Intriguingly, these areas are pivotal in modulating motor-thalamus-brainstem as well as prefrontal-thalamic-cingulate signaling pathways. As a general rule of thumb, high-frequency stimulations, ranging from 5 to 20 Hz, are believed to amplify cortical excitability, interact with diverse neurotransmitter and opioidergic networks, and mold neuronal plasticity [197,198]. The therapeutic potential of rTMS has been officially recognized by the FDA for the management of severe depression and obsessive-compulsive disorders. Even with a solid safety track record, the efficacy of rTMS in tackling pain disorders, post-traumatic headaches, and primary headache syndromes is currently under the microscope. Recent comprehensive reviews propose that high frequency rTMS, specifically targeting the motor cortex, might emerge as a promising migraine management strategy. However, the need of the hour is robust, high-quality randomized controlled trials (RCTs) with unified protocols to substantiate this therapeutic proposition [199,200].

In the recent half-decade, both open-label and randomized controlled trials have delved deep into the potential of rTMS for CM management [187]. Though certain open-label initiatives incorporated CM, they steered clear of presenting efficacy data and, hence, will not be the focus here [201]. An exploratory study helmed by Rapinesi et al. broadcasted a marked dip in migraine episodes, dependency on rescue medications, pain intensity, and scores measuring depression. This was observed after the combination of deep TMS, targeting the left DLPFC with a specific protocol, and conventional treatments [202]. A comparative study by Shehata et al., juxtaposing rTMS with onabotulinumtoxin A, revealed that rTMS, designed with a specific frequency and targeting the left M1, echoed the therapeutic efficacy of onabotulinumtoxin-A in managing CM; however, the rTMS effects waned noticeably after a span of eight weeks [203]. A research endeavor by Kalita et al., contrasting left M1 rTMS over a three-month period in CM and chronic tension-type headache patients, underscored a significant reduction in headache episodes post rTMS treatment within the group; however, when pitting the two groups against each other, the results were not statistically significant [204]. Granato et al., in their research with CM patients also grappling with medication overuse headache (MOH), could not identify any clear advantages of rTMS over its sham counterpart, especially when metrics like monthly headache days, symptomatic drug dependency, and Migraine Disability Assessment (MIDAS) scores were evaluated after a 120-day span [205]. An intriguing facet of this study was the sham stimulator's capacity to mimic the vibratory sensation of actual stimulation. Whether this mimicry carries any real therapeutic value remains an enigma.

7.3. Occipital Nerve Stimulation (ONS)

Occipital nerve stimulation (ONS) is a form of treatment that involves the use of an implantable device with electrodes positioned near the occipital nerves and a pulse generator in the chest. This type of treatment has been researched for many years for conditions like occipital neuralgia and refractory chronic migraine (CM). While the precise mechanism is not fully understood, it is believed that ONS may counterbalance trigeminally mediated central sensitization or restore the lost conditional pain modulation in these patients. A number of multi-center randomized sham-controlled trials, published over five years ago, showed improvements in areas such as headache frequency, intensity, and disability [192].

Within the last five years, open-label studies have been published on the use of ONS for chronic migraine [195–197]. However, the specific parameters of the stimulation and the study endpoints were quite varied between studies. Miller et al. analyzed a group of 53 intractable CM patients and discovered an 8.51-day reduction in monthly moderate-to-severe headache days after bilateral ONS electrodes implantation [195]. Similarly, Garcia-Ortega et al. studied 37 refractory CM patients and reported significant pain reduction [196]. However, it is worth noting that up to 20% of patients reported adverse events such as infection, lead migration, and stimulation-related symptoms one year after treatment [197].

Despite the potential side effects, ONS seems to be a promising device for chronic migraine; however, no ONS device has been cleared by the FDA for use in treating migraine yet.

7.4. Spinal Cord Stimulation (SCS)

Spinal cord stimulation (SCS) is another method that has been utilized to manage intractable headache. It involves placing SCS electrodes into the high-cervical epidural space (C2/3) with a pulse generator implanted subcutaneously. This technique has shown promising results, with patients experiencing a significant reduction in mean pain intensity and a decrease in the median number of migraine days. Nevertheless, issues such as infections and lead dislocations have been reported. Despite these concerns, the effectiveness of SCS for chronic migraine is still under investigation [198].

Another interesting approach being explored is the exposure to green light. This might help modulate nociception and anxiety. While non-green light stimuli seemed to exacerbate pain intensity during a migraine attack, exposure to green light was seen to reduce pain intensity in around 20% of the patients. In a small crossover study, daily green light exposure resulted in a significant reduction in the number of headaches in CM patients. Due to its potential effectiveness and safety, this approach warrants further investigation [192].

8. Clinical Perspective

There are presently almost half a dozen devices cleared by the U.S. Food and Drug Administration (FDA) specifically for treating migraine. Interestingly, the clearance for several of these devices has also been extended to cover adolescent patients aged 12 or older. However, it is crucial to note that not all of these FDA-cleared devices have been thoroughly investigated for use in chronic migraine (CM). The only randomized sham-controlled trial conducted for CM was undertaken utilizing the gammaCore device, and unfortunately, it failed to meet its primary efficacy endpoint.

Various open-label observational studies have employed devices, such as CEFALY or Nerivio, to assess pain reduction in patients with CM. However, these studies lack blinding and are subject to potential selection and reporting biases. Furthermore, certain studies have included both episodic migraine (EM) and CM patients, yet failed to provide a detailed breakdown of the number of CM cases or any response data specifically related to CM.

In addition, the absence of established trial guidelines that address the unique aspects and challenges associated with neuromodulation device trials for migraine has led to substantial variation in study endpoints, types of control, and the populations analyzed (intention-to-treat vs. per-protocol). As a result, it can be difficult to compare the outcomes of different studies. In an effort to address these issues, the International Headache Society has published recommendations for evaluating neuromodulation devices in both the acute and preventive treatment of migraine [199].

As the application of these devices becomes more common, we anticipate the emergence of larger, higher-quality studies that adhere to established clinical trial guidelines. These studies are essential to fully establish the benefits of these devices in the treatment of CM. Furthermore, the conduct of high-quality trials should also ideally encourage insurance companies to broaden their coverage to include more neuromodulation devices.

9. Discussion

Migraine remains an intriguing neurological disorder with complex mechanisms and pathophysiology that are still being researched extensively. Migraines are believed to be hereditary conditions characterized by increased responsiveness of cortical and subcortical networks; however, the triggers and factors contributing to its onset and progression remain unknown.

Migraine's multidimensionality can be seen through the following various phases: premonitory phase, headache pain, postdromal phase, and sometimes aura phase. Each of these involves interactions among hypothalamus nuclei, cortical regions, and trigeminovascular pathways, resulting in characteristic symptoms experienced during an attack.

Despite these challenges, migraine research has made significant advances, providing light on potential therapeutic targets and validating CGRP as an effective target for both acute and preventative treatments—giving hope of the better management of migraine episodes as well as improved quality of life for affected individuals.

However, much work remains to be performed in understanding its intricate processes and developing effective treatment and prevention measures. More awareness, additional funding for research, collaboration among scientists, healthcare providers, and patients, as well as increased collaboration, will all play an integral role in increasing understanding and alleviating migraine's burden.

As we discover more about migraine, it is crucial that we provide empathy, support, and personalized care to those living with this neurological challenge. By harnessing the collective knowledge and dedication of scientific communities worldwide, we can make significant advances in migraine research that ultimately benefit millions living with this neurological disorder [200].

Author Contributions: Conceptualization, H.P. and A.V.C.; methodology, T.-L.T.; soft-ware, I.-A.F.; validation, R.-A.C.-B., L.-A.G. and H.P.; formal analysis, D.-I.D.; investigation, A.A.P.; resources, A.B.; data curation, L.-A.G.; writing—original draft preparation, R.-A.C.-B. and A.V.C.; writing—review and editing, R.-A.C.-B., L.-A.G and A.V.C.; visualization, A.B.; supervision, D.-I.D.; project administration, A.V.C.; funding acquisition, A.V.C. All authors have read and agreed to the published version of the manuscript.

Funding: This research received no external funding.

Institutional Review Board Statement: Not applicable.

Informed Consent Statement: No requirement for ethical approval.

Data Availability Statement: All Data is available on PubMed.

Conflicts of Interest: The authors declare no conflict of interest.

References

1. Stovner, L.; Hagen, K.; Jensen, R.; Katsarava, Z.; Lipton, R.; Scher, A.; Steiner, T.; Zwart, J.-A. The Global Burden of Headache: A Documentation of Headache Prevalence and Disability Worldwide. *Cephalalgia* **2007**, *27*, 193–210. [CrossRef] [PubMed]
2. Bateman, D. The future of neurology services in the UK. *Pract. Neurol.* **2011**, *11*, 134–135. [CrossRef] [PubMed]
3. Sender, J.; Bradford, S.; Watson, D.; Lipscombe, S.; Rees, T.; Manley, R.; Dowson, A. Setting up a Specialist Headache Clinic in Primary Care: General Practitioners with a Special Interest (GPwSI) in Headache. *Headache Care* **2004**, *1*, 165–171. [CrossRef]
4. WHO. *The World Health Report 2001: Mental Health: New Understanding, New Hope*; WHO: Geneva, Switzerland, 2001.
5. Solomon, G.D.; Price, K.L. Burden of Migraine: A Review of its Socioeconomic Impact. *Pharmacoeconomics* **1997**, *11*, 1–10. [CrossRef]
6. Terwindt, G.M.; Ferrari, M.D.; Tijhuis, M.; Groenen, S.M.A.; Picavet, H.S.J.; Launer, L.J. The impact of migraine on quality of life in the general population: The GEM study. *Neurology* **2000**, *55*, 624–629. [CrossRef] [PubMed]
7. Steiner, T.; Scher, A.; Stewart, W.; Kolodner, K.; Liberman, J.; Lipton, R. The Prevalence and Disability Burden of Adult Migraine in England and their Relationships to Age, Gender and Ethnicity. *Cephalalgia* **2003**, *23*, 519–527. [CrossRef]
8. Clarke, C.E.; MacMillan, L.; Sondhi, S.; Wells, N.E. Economic and social impact of migraine. *QJM Mon. J. Assoc. Physicians* **1996**, *89*, 77–84. [CrossRef]
9. Ahmed, F. Headache disorders: Differentiating and managing the common subtypes. *Br. J. Pain* **2012**, *6*, 124–132. [CrossRef]
10. Haut, S.R.; Bigal, E.M.; Lipton, R.B. Chronic disorders with episodic manifestations: Focus on epilepsy and migraine. *Lancet Neurol.* **2006**, *5*, 148–157. [CrossRef]
11. Olesen, J. Preface to the Second Edition. *Cephalalgia* **2004**, *24*, 9–10. [CrossRef]
12. Stewart, W.F.; Wood, G.C.; Manack, A.; Varon, S.F.; Buse, D.C.; Lipton, R.B. Employment and Work Impact of Chronic Migraine and Episodic Migraine. *J. Occup. Environ. Med.* **2010**, *52*, 8–14. [CrossRef] [PubMed]
13. Natoli, J.; Manack, A.; Dean, B.; Butler, Q.; Turkel, C.; Stovner, L.; Lipton, R. Global prevalence of chronic migraine: A systematic review. *Cephalalgia* **2009**, *30*, 599–609. [CrossRef]
14. Blumenfeld, A.; Varon, S.; Wilcox, T.; Buse, D.; Kawata, A.; Manack, A.; Goadsby, P.; Lipton, R. Disability, HRQoL and resource use among chronic and episodic migraineurs: Results from the International Burden of Migraine Study (IBMS). *Cephalalgia* **2010**, *31*, 301–315. [CrossRef] [PubMed]

15. Durham, P.; Papapetropoulos, S. Biomarkers Associated with Migraine and Their Potential Role in Migraine Management. *Headache J. Head Face Pain* **2013**, *53*, 1262–1277. [CrossRef] [PubMed]
16. Safiri, S.; Pourfathi, H.; Eagan, A.; Mansournia, M.A.; Khodayari, M.T.; Sullman, M.J.M.; Kaufman, J.; Collins, G.; Dai, H.; Bragazzi, N.L.; et al. Global, regional, and national burden of migraine in 204 countries and territories, 1990 to 2019. *Pain* **2021**, *163*, e293–e309. [CrossRef] [PubMed]
17. Amiri, P.; Kazeminasab, S.; Nejadghaderi, S.A.; Mohammadinasab, R.; Pourfathi, H.; Araj-Khodaei, M.; Sullman, M.J.M.; Kolahi, A.-A.; Safiri, S. Migraine: A Review on Its History, Global Epidemiology, Risk Factors, and Comorbidities. *Front. Neurol.* **2022**, *12*, 800605. [CrossRef]
18. Burch, R.C.; Loder, S.; Loder, E.; Smitherman, T.A. The Prevalence and Burden of Migraine and Severe Headache in the United States: Updated Statistics from Government Health Surveillance Studies. *Headache J. Head Face Pain* **2015**, *55*, 21–34. [CrossRef]
19. Lipton, R.B.; Stewart, W.F.; Diamond, S.; Diamond, M.L.; Reed, M. Prevalence and Burden of Migraine in the United States: Data from the American Migraine Study II. *Headache J. Head Face Pain* **2001**, *41*, 646–657. [CrossRef]
20. Merikangas, K.R. Contributions of Epidemiology to Our Understanding of Migraine. *Headache J. Head Face Pain* **2013**, *53*, 230–246. [CrossRef]
21. Wang, S.-J. Epidemiology of migraine and other types of headache in Asia. *Curr. Neurol. Neurosci. Rep.* **2003**, *3*, 104–108. [CrossRef]
22. Dzoljic, E.; Vlajinac, H.; Sipetic, S.; Marinkovic, J.; Grbatinic, I.; Kostic, V. A survey of female students with migraine: What is the influence of family history and lifestyle. *Int. J. Neurosci.* **2013**, *124*, 82–87. [CrossRef] [PubMed]
23. Hernandez-Latorre, M.; Roig, M. Natural History of Migraine in Childhood. *Cephalalgia* **2000**, *20*, 573–579. [CrossRef] [PubMed]
24. Russell, M.B.; Olesen, J. Increased familial risk and evidence of genetic factor in migraine. *BMJ* **1995**, *311*, 541–544. [CrossRef] [PubMed]
25. Stewart, W.F.; Staffa, J.; Lipton, R.B.; Ottman, R. Familial risk of migraine: A population-based study. *Ann. Neurol.* **1997**, *41*, 166–172. [CrossRef] [PubMed]
26. Gervil, M.; Ulrich, V.; Kaprio, J.; Olesen, J.; Russell, M.B. The relative role of genetic and environmental factors in migraine without aura. *Neurology* **1999**, *53*, 995. [CrossRef]
27. Honkasalo, M.-L.; Kaprio, J.; Winter, T.; Heikkila, K.; Sillanpaa, M.; Koskenvuo, M. Migraine and Concomitant Symptoms Among 8167 Adult Twin Pairs. *Headache J. Head Face Pain* **1995**, *35*, 70–78. [CrossRef]
28. Mulder, E.J.; van Baal, C.; Gaist, D.; Kallela, M.; Kaprio, J.; Svensson, D.A.; Nyholt, D.R.; Martin, N.G.; MacGregor, A.J.; Cherkas, L.F.; et al. Genetic and Environmental Influences on Migraine: A Twin Study Across Six Countries. *Twin Res.* **2003**, *6*, 422–431. [CrossRef]
29. Svensson, D.A.; Larsson, B.; Waldenlind, E.; Pedersen, N.L.; Msc, D.A.S. Shared Rearing Environment in Migraine: Results from Twins Reared Apart and Twins Reared Together. *Headache J. Head Face Pain* **2003**, *43*, 235–244. [CrossRef]
30. De Vries, B.; Anttila, V.; Freilinger, T.; Wessman, M.; Kaunisto, A.M.; Kallela, M.; Artto, V.; Vijfhuizen, L.S.; Göbel, H.; Dichgans, M.; et al. Systematic re-evaluation of genes from candidate gene association studies in migraine using a large genome-wide association data set. *Cephalalgia* **2015**, *36*, 604–614. [CrossRef]
31. Yeh, W.Z.; Blizzard, L.; Taylor, B.V. What is the actual prevalence of migraine? *Brain Behav.* **2018**, *8*, e00950. [CrossRef]
32. Onofri, A.; Pensato, U.; Rosignoli, C.; Wells-Gatnik, W.; Stanyer, E.; Ornello, R.; Chen, H.Z.; De Santis, F.; Torrente, A.; Mikulenka, P.; et al. Primary headache epidemiology in children and adolescents: A systematic review and meta-analysis. *J. Headache Pain* **2023**, *24*, 8. [CrossRef] [PubMed]
33. Loh, N.R.; Whitehouse, W.P.; Howells, R. What is new in migraine management in children and young people. *Arch. Dis. Child.* **2022**, *107*, 1067–1072. [CrossRef] [PubMed]
34. Loder, E.; Rizzoli, P. Biomarkers in Migraine: Their Promise, Problems, and Practical Applications. *Headache J. Head Face Pain* **2006**, *46*, 1046–1058. [CrossRef] [PubMed]
35. Biomarkers Definitions Working Group; Atkinson, A.J., Jr.; Colburn, W.A.; DeGruttola, V.G.; DeMets, D.L.; Downing, G.J.; Hoth, D.F.; Oates, J.A.; Peck, C.C.; Spilker, B.A.; et al. Biomarkers and surrogate endpoints: Preferred definitions and conceptual framework. *Clin. Pharmacol. Ther.* **2001**, *69*, 89–95. [CrossRef]
36. Phillips, K.A.; Van Bebber, S.; Issa, A.M. Diagnostics and biomarker development: Priming the pipeline. *Nat. Rev. Drug Discov.* **2006**, *5*, 463–469. [CrossRef]
37. Lesko, L.; Atkinson, A. Use of Biomarkers and Surrogate Endpoints in Drug Development and Regulatory Decision Making: Criteria, Validation, Strategies. *Annu. Rev. Pharmacol. Toxicol.* **2001**, *41*, 347–366. [CrossRef]
38. Packer, C.S. Biochemical markers and physiological parameters as indices for identifying patients at risk of developing pre-eclampsia. *J. Hypertens.* **2005**, *23*, 45–46. [CrossRef]
39. Mayeux, R. Biomarkers: Potential uses and limitations. *NeuroRx* **2004**, *1*, 182–188. [CrossRef]
40. Boćkowski, L.; Sobaniec, W.; Żelazowska-Rutkowska, B. Proinflammatory Plasma Cytokines in Children with Migraine. *Pediatr. Neurol.* **2009**, *41*, 17–21. [CrossRef]
41. Kaciński, M.; Gergont, A.; Kubik, A.; Steczkowska-Klucznik, M. Proinflammatory cytokines in children with migraine with or without aura. *Przegląd Lek.* **2005**, *62*, 1276–1280.
42. Kara, I.; Sazci, A.; Ergul, E.; Kaya, G.; Kilic, G. Association of the C677T and A1298C polymorphisms in the 5,10 methylenetetrahydrofolate reductase gene in patients with migraine risk. *Mol. Brain Res.* **2003**, *111*, 84–90. [CrossRef] [PubMed]

43. Kowalska, M.; Prendecki, M.; Kozubski, W.; Lianeri, M.; Dorszewska, J. Molecular factors in migraine. *Oncotarget* **2016**, *7*, 50708–50718. [CrossRef] [PubMed]
44. D'Andrea, G.; D'Arrigo, A.; Carbonare, M.D.; Leon, A. Pathogenesis of Migraine: Role of Neuromodulators. *Headache J. Head Face Pain* **2012**, *52*, 1155–1163. [CrossRef] [PubMed]
45. D'andrea, G.; D'amico, D.; Bussone, G.; Bolner, A.; Aguggia, M.; Saracco, M.G.; Galloni, E.; De Riva, V.; Colavito, D.; Leon, A.; et al. The role of tyrosine metabolism in the pathogenesis of chronic migraine. *Cephalalgia* **2013**, *33*, 932–937. [CrossRef] [PubMed]
46. Cady, R.K.; Vause, C.V.; Ho, T.W.; Bigal, M.E.; Durham, P.L. Elevated Saliva Calcitonin Gene-Related Peptide Levels During Acute Migraine Predict Therapeutic Response to Rizatriptan. *Headache J. Head Face Pain* **2009**, *49*, 1258–1266. [CrossRef]
47. Sicuteri, F.; Testi, A.; Anselmi, B. Biochemical Investigations in Headache: Increase in the Hydroxyindoleacetic Acid Excretion During Migraine Attacks. *Int. Arch. Allergy Immunol.* **1961**, *19*, 55–58. [CrossRef]
48. Ferrari, M.D.; Odink, J.; Tapparelli, C.; Van Kempen, G.; Pennings, E.J.; Bruyn, G.W. Serotonin metabolism in migraine. *Neurology* **1989**, *39*, 1239. [CrossRef]
49. Tsujino, N.; Sakurai, T. Orexin/Hypocretin: A Neuropeptide at the Interface of Sleep, Energy Homeostasis, and Reward System. *Pharmacol. Rev.* **2009**, *61*, 162–176. [CrossRef]
50. Sarchielli, P.; Rainero, I.; Coppola, F.; Rossi, C.; Mancini, M.; Pinessi, L.; Calabresi, P. Involvement of Corticotrophin-Releasing Factor and Orexin-A in Chronic Migraine and Medication-Overuse Headache: Findings from Cerebrospinal Fluid. *Cephalalgia* **2008**, *28*, 714–722. [CrossRef]
51. Barloese, M.; Jennum, P.; Lund, N.; Knudsen, S.; Gammeltoft, S.; Jensen, R. Reduced CSF hypocretin-1 levels are associated with cluster headache. *Cephalalgia* **2014**, *35*, 869–876. [CrossRef]
52. Tso, A.R.; Goadsby, P.J. New Targets for Migraine Therapy. *Curr. Treat. Options Neurol.* **2014**, *16*, 318. [CrossRef]
53. Diener, H.-C.; Charles, A.; Goadsby, P.J.; Holle, D. New therapeutic approaches for the prevention and treatment of migraine. *Lancet Neurol.* **2015**, *14*, 1010–1022. [CrossRef] [PubMed]
54. Nelson, K.B.; Richardson, A.K.; He, J.; Lateef, T.M.; Khoromi, S.; Merikangas, K.R. Headache and Biomarkers Predictive of Vascular Disease in a Representative Sample of US Children. *Arch. Pediatr. Adolesc. Med.* **2010**, *164*, 358–362. [CrossRef] [PubMed]
55. Tietjen, G.E.; Herial, N.A.; White, L.; Utley, C.; Kosmyna, J.M.; Khuder, S.A. Migraine and Biomarkers of Endothelial Activation in Young Women. *Stroke* **2009**, *40*, 2977–2982. [CrossRef] [PubMed]
56. Ben Aissa, M.; Tipton, A.F.; Bertels, Z.; Gandhi, R.; Moye, L.S.; Novack, M.; Bennett, B.M.; Wang, Y.; Litosh, V.; Lee, S.H.; et al. Soluble guanylyl cyclase is a critical regulator of migraine-associated pain. *Cephalalgia* **2017**, *38*, 1471–1484. [CrossRef]
57. Al-Hassany, L.; Boucherie, D.M.; Creeney, H.; van Drie, R.W.A.; Farham, F.; Favaretto, S.; Gollion, C.; Grangeon, L.; Lyons, H.; Marschollek, K.; et al. Future targets for migraine treatment beyond CGRP. *J. Headache Pain* **2023**, *24*, 76. [CrossRef]
58. Matharu, M.S.; Bartsch, T.; Ward, N.; Frackowiak, R.S.J.; Weiner, R.; Goadsby, P.J. Central neuromodulation in chronic migraine patients with suboccipital stimulators: A PET study. *Brain* **2004**, *127*, 220–230. [CrossRef]
59. Royal, P.; Andres-Bilbe, A.; Prado, P.Á.; Verkest, C.; Wdziekonski, B.; Schaub, S.; Baron, A.; Lesage, F.; Gasull, X.; Levitz, J.; et al. Migraine-Associated TRESK Mutations Increase Neuronal Excitability through Alternative Translation Initiation and Inhibition of TREK. *Neuron* **2019**, *101*, 232–245.e6. [CrossRef]
60. Prado, P.; Landra-Willm, A.; Verkest, C.; Ribera, A.; Chassot, A.-A.; Baron, A.; Sandoz, G. TREK channel activation suppresses migraine pain phenotype. *iScience* **2021**, *24*, 102961. [CrossRef]
61. Lim, C.S.; Shalhoub, J.; Gohel, M.S.; Shepherd, A.C.; Davies, A.H. Matrix Metalloproteinases in Vascular Disease-A Potential Therapeutic Target. *Curr. Vasc. Pharmacol.* **2010**, *8*, 75–85. [CrossRef]
62. Todt, U.; Netzer, C.; Toliat, M.; Heinze, A.; Goebel, I.; Nürnberg, P.; Göbel, H.; Freudenberg, J.; Kubisch, C. New genetic evidence for involvement of the dopamine system in migraine with aura. *Hum. Genet.* **2009**, *125*, 265–279. [CrossRef]
63. Naya, M.; Tsukamoto, T.; Morita, K.; Katoh, C.; Furumoto, T.; Fujii, S.; Tamaki, N.; Tsutsui, H. Plasma Interleukin-6 and Tumor Necrosis Factor-.ALPHA. Can Predict Coronary Endothelial Dysfunction in Hypertensive Patients. *Hypertens. Res.* **2007**, *30*, 541–548. [CrossRef] [PubMed]
64. Imamura, K.; Takeshima, T.; Fusayasu, E.; Nakashima, K. Increased Plasma Matrix Metalloproteinase-9 Levels in Migraineurs. *Headache J. Head Face Pain* **2007**, *48*, 135–139. [CrossRef] [PubMed]
65. Olesen, J.; Friberg, L.; Iversen, H.K.; Lassen, N.A.; Andersen, A.R.; Karle, A.; Olsen, T.S. Timing and topography of cerebral blood flow, aura, and headache during migraine attacks. *Ann. Neurol.* **1990**, *28*, 791–798. [CrossRef] [PubMed]
66. Thomsen, L.L.; Kirchmann, M.; Bjornsson, A.; Stefansson, H.; Jensen, R.M.; Fasquel, A.C.; Petursson, H.; Stefansson, M.; Frigge, M.L.; Kong, A.; et al. The genetic spectrum of a population-based sample of familial hemiplegic migraine. *Brain* **2006**, *130*, 346–356. [CrossRef] [PubMed]
67. Mitchell, B.L.; Diaz-Torres, S.; Bivol, S.; Cuellar-Partida, G.; Gormley, P.; Anttila, V.; Winsvold, B.S.; Palta, P.; Esko, T.; Pers, T.H.; et al. Elucidating the relationship between migraine risk and brain structure using genetic data. *Brain* **2022**, *145*, 3214–3224. [CrossRef]
68. Grangeon, L.; Lange, K.S.; Waliszewska-Prosół, M.; Onan, D.; Marschollek, K.; Wiels, W.; Mikulenka, P.; Farham, F.; Gollion, C.; Ducros, A.; et al. Genetics of migraine: Where are we now. *J. Headache Pain* **2023**, *24*, 12. [CrossRef]
69. van den Maagdenberg, A.M.; Pietrobon, D.; Pizzorusso, T.; Kaja, S.; Broos, L.A.; Cesetti, T.; van de Ven, R.C.; Tottene, A.; van der Kaa, J.; Plomp, J.J.; et al. A Cacna1a Knockin Migraine Mouse Model with Increased Susceptibility to Cortical Spreading Depression. *Neuron* **2004**, *41*, 701–710. [CrossRef]

70. Maagdenberg, A.M.J.M.v.D.; Pizzorusso, T.; Kaja, S.; Terpolilli, N.; Shapovalova, M.; Hoebeek, F.E.; Barrett, C.F.; Gherardini, L.; van de Ven, R.C.G.; Todorov, B.; et al. High cortical spreading depression susceptibility and migraine-associated symptoms in $Ca_V2.1$ S218L mice. *Ann. Neurol.* **2010**, *67*, 85–98. [CrossRef]
71. Meneghetti, N.; Cerri, C.; Vannini, E.; Tantillo, E.; Tottene, A.; Pietrobon, D.; Caleo, M.; Mazzoni, A. Synaptic alterations in visual cortex reshape contrast-dependent gamma oscillations and inhibition-excitation ratio in a genetic mouse model of migraine. *J. Headache Pain* **2022**, *23*, 125. [CrossRef]
72. Leo, L.; Gherardini, L.; Barone, V.; De Fusco, M.; Pietrobon, D.; Pizzorusso, T.; Casari, G. Increased Susceptibility to Cortical Spreading Depression in the Mouse Model of Familial Hemiplegic Migraine Type 2. *PLoS Genet.* **2011**, *7*, e1002129. [CrossRef] [PubMed]
73. Unekawa, M.; Ikeda, K.; Tomita, Y.; Kawakami, K.; Suzuki, N. Enhanced susceptibility to cortical spreading depression in two types of Na^+,K^+-ATPase α2 subunit-deficient mice as a model of familial hemiplegic migraine 2. *Cephalalgia* **2017**, *38*, 1515–1524. [CrossRef] [PubMed]
74. Smith, S.E.; Chen, X.; Brier, L.M.; Bumstead, J.R.; Rensing, N.R.; Ringel, A.E.; Shin, H.; Oldenborg, A.; Crowley, J.R.; Bice, A.R.; et al. Astrocyte deletion of α2-Na/K ATPase triggers episodic motor paralysis in mice via a metabolic pathway. *Nat. Commun.* **2020**, *11*, 6164. [CrossRef] [PubMed]
75. Bertelli, S.; Barbieri, R.; Pusch, M.; Gavazzo, P. Gain of function of sporadic/familial hemiplegic migraine-causing SCN1A mutations: Use of an optimized cDNA. *Cephalalgia* **2018**, *39*, 477–488. [CrossRef]
76. Suzuki-Muromoto, S.; Kosaki, R.; Kosaki, K.; Kubota, M. Familial hemiplegic migraine with a PRRT2 mutation: Phenotypic variations and carbamazepine efficacy. *Brain Dev.* **2020**, *42*, 293–297. [CrossRef]
77. Michetti, C.; Castroflorio, E.; Marchionni, I.; Forte, N.; Sterlini, B.; Binda, F.; Fruscione, F.; Baldelli, P.; Valtorta, F.; Zara, F.; et al. The PRRT2 knockout mouse recapitulates the neurological diseases associated with PRRT2 mutations. *Neurobiol. Dis.* **2016**, *99*, 66–83. [CrossRef]
78. Chasman, D.I.; Schürks, M.; Anttila, V.; De Vries, B.; Schminke, U.; Launer, L.J.; Terwindt, G.M.; van den Maagdenberg, A.M.J.M.; Fendrich, K.; Völzke, H.; et al. Genome-wide association study reveals three susceptibility loci for common migraine in the general population. *Nat. Genet.* **2011**, *43*, 695–698. [CrossRef]
79. Freilinger, T.; International Headache Genetics Consortium; Anttila, V.; de Vries, B.; Malik, R.; Kallela, M.; Terwindt, G.M.; Pozo-Rosich, P.; Winsvold, B.; Nyholt, D.R.; et al. Genome-wide association analysis identifies susceptibility loci for migraine without aura. *Nat. Genet.* **2012**, *44*, 777–782. [CrossRef]
80. Choquet, H.; Yin, J.; Jacobson, A.S.; Horton, B.H.; Hoffmann, T.J.; Jorgenson, E.; Avins, A.L.; Pressman, A.R. New and sex-specific migraine susceptibility loci identified from a multiethnic genome-wide meta-analysis. *Commun. Biol.* **2021**, *4*, 864. [CrossRef]
81. Hautakangas, H.; Winsvold, B.S.; Ruotsalainen, S.E.; Bjornsdottir, G.; Harder, A.V.E.; Kogelman, L.J.A.; Thomas, L.F.; Noordam, R.; Benner, C.; Gormley, P.; et al. Genome-wide analysis of 102,084 migraine cases identifies 123 risk loci and subtype-specific risk alleles. *Nat. Genet.* **2022**, *54*, 152–160. [CrossRef]
82. Cutrer, F.M.; Black, D.F. Imaging Findings of Migraine. *Headache J. Head Face Pain* **2006**, *46*, 1095–1107. [CrossRef] [PubMed]
83. Del Zompo, M.; Cherchi, A.; Palmas, M.A.; Ponti, M.; Bocchetta, A.; Gessa, G.L.; Piccardi, M.P. Association between dopamine receptor genes and migraine without aura in a Sardinian sample. *Neurology* **1998**, *51*, 781–786. [CrossRef] [PubMed]
84. Moskowitz, M.A.; Cutrer, F.M. Sumatriptan: A Receptor-Targeted Treatment for Migraine. *Annu. Rev. Med.* **1993**, *44*, 145–154. [CrossRef]
85. Bolay, H.; Reuter, U.; Dunn, A.K.; Huang, Z.; Boas, D.A.; Moskowitz, M.A. Intrinsic brain activity triggers trigeminal meningeal afferents in a migraine model. *Nat. Med.* **2002**, *8*, 136–142. [CrossRef] [PubMed]
86. Dimtriadou, V.; Buzzi, M.; Moskowitz, M.; Theoharides, T. Trigeminal sensory fiber stimulation induces morphological changes reflecting secretion in rat dura mater mast cells. *Neuroscience* **1991**, *44*, 97–112. [CrossRef]
87. Peroutka, S.J. Neurogenic inflammation and migraine: Implications for the therapeutics. *Mol. Interv.* **2005**, *5*, 304–311. [CrossRef]
88. Goadsby, P.J. Pathophysiology of migraine. *Ann. Indian Acad. Neurol.* **2012**, *15*, 15. [CrossRef]
89. Do, T.P.; Deligianni, C.; Amirguliyev, S.; Snellman, J.; Lopez, C.L.; Al-Karagholi, M.A.-M.; Guo, S.; Ashina, M. Second messenger signaling bypasses CGRP receptor blockade to provoke migraine attacks in humans. *Brain* **2023**, awad261. [CrossRef]
90. Amin, F.M.; Schytz, H.W. Transport of the pituitary adenylate cyclase-activating polypeptide across the blood-brain barrier: Implications for migraine. *J. Headache Pain* **2018**, *19*, 35. [CrossRef]
91. Grände, G.; Nilsson, E.; Edvinsson, L. Comparison of responses to vasoactive drugs in human and rat cerebral arteries using myography and pressurized cerebral artery method. *Cephalalgia* **2012**, *33*, 152–159. [CrossRef]
92. Iannetti, G.D.; Zambreanu, L.; Wise, R.G.; Buchanan, T.J.; Huggins, J.P.; Smart, T.S.; Vennart, W.; Tracey, I. Pharmacological modulation of pain-related brain activity during normal and central sensitization states in humans. *Proc. Natl. Acad. Sci. USA* **2005**, *102*, 18195–18200. [CrossRef] [PubMed]
93. Birk, S.; Sitarz, J.T.; Petersen, K.A.; Oturai, P.S.; Kruuse, C.; Fahrenkrug, J.; Olesen, J. The effect of intravenous PACAP38 on cerebral hemodynamics in healthy volunteers. *Regul. Pept.* **2007**, *140*, 185–191. [CrossRef] [PubMed]
94. Olesen, J.; Burstein, R.; Ashina, M.; Tfelt-Hansen, P. Origin of pain in migraine: Evidence for peripheral sensitisation. *Lancet Neurol.* **2009**, *8*, 679–690. [CrossRef] [PubMed]

95. Ghanizada, H.; Al-Karagholi, M.A.-M.; Arngrim, N.; Mørch-Rasmussen, M.; Walker, C.S.; Hay, D.L.; Ashina, M. Effect of Adrenomedullin on Migraine-like Attacks in Patients 2ith Migraine: A Randomized Crossover Study. *Neurology* **2021**, *96*, e2488–e2499. [CrossRef]
96. Hinson, J.P.; Kapas, S.; Smith, D.M. Adrenomedullin, a Multifunctional Regulatory Peptide. *Endocr. Rev.* **2000**, *21*, 138–167. [CrossRef] [PubMed]
97. Bhakta, M.; Vuong, T.; Taura, T.; Wilson, D.S.; Stratton, J.R.; Mackenzie, K.D. Migraine therapeutics differentially modulate the CGRP pathway. *Cephalalgia* **2021**, *41*, 499–514. [CrossRef]
98. Carlsson, A.; Forsgren, L.; Nylander, P.-O.; Hellman, U.; Forsman-Semb, K.; Holmgren, G.; Holmberg, D.; Holmberg, M. Identification of a susceptibility locus for migraine with and without aura on 6p12.2-p21.1. *Neurology* **2002**, *59*, 1804–1807. [CrossRef]
99. Oterino, A.; Toriello, M.; Valle, N.; Castillo, J.; Alonso-Arranz, A.; Bravo, Y.; Ruiz-Alegria, C.; Quintela, E.; Pascual, J. The Relationship Between Homocysteine and Genes of Folate-Related Enzymes in Migraine Patients. *Headache J. Head Face Pain* **2010**, *50*, 99–168. [CrossRef]
100. Perini, F.; D'Andrea, G.; Galloni, E.; Pignatelli, F.; Billo, G.; Alba, S.; Bussone, G.; Toso, V. Plasma Cytokine Levels in Migraineurs and Controls. *Headache J. Head Face Pain* **2005**, *45*, 926–931. [CrossRef]
101. Schwedt, T.J.; Dodick, D.W. Advanced neuroimaging of migraine. *Lancet Neurol.* **2009**, *8*, 560–568. [CrossRef]
102. Burstein, R.; Yamamura, H.; Malick, A.; Strassman, A.M.; Goadsby, P.J.; Holland, P.R.; Martins-Oliveira, M.; Hoffmann, J.; Schankin, C.; Akerman, S.; et al. Chemical Stimulation of the Intracranial Dura Induces Enhanced Responses to Facial Stimulation in Brain Stem Trigeminal Neurons. *J. Neurophysiol.* **1998**, *79*, 964–982. [CrossRef]
103. Burstein, R.; Yarnitsky, D.; Goor-Aryeh, I.; Ransil, B.J.; Bajwa, Z.H. An association between migraine and cutaneous allodynia. *Ann. Neurol.* **2000**, *47*, 614–624. [CrossRef] [PubMed]
104. Jakubowski, M.; Silberstein, S.; Ashkenazi, A.; Burstein, R. Can allodynic migraine patients be identified interictally using a questionnaire. *Neurology* **2005**, *65*, 1419–1422. [CrossRef] [PubMed]
105. Bigal, M.E.; Ashina, S.; Burstein, R.; Reed, M.L.; Buse, D.; Serrano, D.; Lipton, R.B.; On behalf of the AMPP Group. Prevalence and characteristics of allodynia in headache sufferers: A population study. *Neurology* **2008**, *70*, 1525–1533. [CrossRef] [PubMed]
106. Zambreanu, L.; Wise, R.G.; Brooks, J.C.; Iannetti, G.D.; Tracey, I. A role for the brainstem in central sensitisation in humans. Evidence from functional magnetic resonance imaging. *Pain* **2005**, *114*, 397–407. [CrossRef]
107. Lee, M.C.; Zambreanu, L.; Menon, D.K.; Tracey, I. Identifying Brain Activity Specifically Related to the Maintenance and Perceptual Consequence of Central Sensitization in Humans. *J. Neurosci.* **2008**, *28*, 11642–11649. [CrossRef] [PubMed]
108. Schulte, L.H.; Mehnert, J.; May, A. Longitudinal Neuroimaging over 30 Days: Temporal Characteristics of Migraine. *Ann. Neurol.* **2020**, *87*, 646–651. [CrossRef]
109. Gross, E.C.; Lisicki, M.; Fischer, D.; Sándor, P.S.; Schoenen, J. The metabolic face of migraine—From pathophysiology to treatment. *Nat. Rev. Neurol.* **2019**, *15*, 627–643. [CrossRef]
110. Ingram, E.E.; Bocklud, B.E.; Corley, S.C.; Granier, M.A.; Neuchat, E.E.; Ahmadzadeh, S.; Shekoohi, S.; Kaye, A.D. Non-CGRP Antagonist/Non-Triptan Options for Migraine Disease Treatment: Clinical Considerations. *Curr. Pain Headache Rep.* **2023**, 1–6. [CrossRef]
111. Goadsby, P.J.; Hoskin, K.L. The distribution of trigeminovascular afferents in the nonhuman primate brain Macaca nemestrina: A c-fos immunocytochemical study. *J. Anat.* **1997**, *190*, 367–375. [CrossRef]
112. Bartsch, T.; Goadsby, P.J. Stimulation of the greater occipital nerve induces increased central excitability of dural afferent input. *Brain* **2002**, *125*, 1496–1509. [CrossRef] [PubMed]
113. Shepheard, S.; Edvinsson, L.; Cumberbatch, M.; Williamson, D.; Mason, G.; Webb, J.; Boyce, S.; Hill, R.; Hargreaves, R. Possible Antimigraine Mechanisms of Action of the 5HT$_{1F}$ Receptor Agonist LY334370. *Cephalalgia* **1999**, *19*, 851–858. [CrossRef]
114. Andreou, A.P.; Goadsby, P.J. Therapeutic potential of novel glutamate receptor antagonists in migraine. *Expert Opin. Investig. Drugs* **2009**, *18*, 789–803. [CrossRef] [PubMed]
115. Weiss, B.; Alt, A.; Ogden, A.M.; Gates, M.; Dieckman, D.K.; Clemens-Smith, A.; Ho, K.H.; Jarvie, K.; Rizkalla, G.; Wright, R.A.; et al. Pharmacological Characterization of the Competitive GLU$_{K5}$ Receptor Antagonist Decahydroisoquinoline LY466195 in Vitro and in Vivo. *J. Pharmacol. Exp. Ther.* **2006**, *318*, 772–781. [CrossRef] [PubMed]
116. Coppola, G.; Vandenheede, M.; Di Clemente, L.; Ambrosini, A.; Fumal, A.; De Pasqua, V.; Schoenen, J. Somatosensory evoked high-frequency oscillations reflecting thalamo-cortical activity are decreased in migraine patients between attacks. *Brain* **2004**, *128*, 98–103. [CrossRef]
117. de Tommaso, M.; Ambrosini, A.; Brighina, F.; Coppola, G.; Perrotta, A.; Pierelli, F.; Sandrini, G.; Valeriani, M.; Marinazzo, D.; Stramaglia, S.; et al. Altered processing of sensory stimuli in patients with migraine. *Nat. Rev. Neurol.* **2014**, *10*, 144–155. [CrossRef]
118. Wang, W.; Timsit-Berthier, M.; Schoenen, J. Intensity dependence of auditory evoked potentials is pronounced in migraine: An indication of cortical potentiation and low serotonergic neurotransmission. *Neurology* **1996**, *46*, 1404. [CrossRef]
119. Judit, Á.; Sándor, P.; Schoenen, J. Habituation of Visual and Intensity Dependence of Auditory Evoked Cortical Potentials Tends to Normalize Just Before and During the Migraine Attack. *Cephalalgia* **2000**, *20*, 714–719. [CrossRef]

120. Proietti-Cecchini, A.; Áfra, J.; Schoenen, J. Intensity Dependence of the Cortical Auditory Evoked Potentials as A Surrogate Marker of Central Nervous System Serotonin Transmission in Man: Demonstration of A Central Effect for the $5Ht_{1B/1D}$ Agonist Zolmitriptan (311C90, Zomig®). *Cephalalgia* **1997**, *17*, 849–854. [CrossRef]
121. Goadsby, P.J.; Holland, P.R.; Martins-Oliveira, M.; Hoffmann, J.; Schankin, C.; Akerman, S. Pathophysiology of Migraine: A Disorder of Sensory Processing. *Physiol. Rev.* **2017**, *97*, 553–622. [CrossRef]
122. Valfrè, W.; Rainero, I.; Bergui, M.; Pinessi, L. Voxel-Based Morphometry Reveals Gray Matter Abnormalities in Migraine. *Headache J. Head Face Pain* **2007**, *48*, 109–117. [CrossRef]
123. Maleki, N.; Becerra, L.; Nutile, L.; Pendse, G.; Brawn, J.; Bigal, M.; Burstein, R.; Borsook, D. Migraine Attacks the Basal Ganglia. *Mol. Pain* **2011**, *7*, 71. [CrossRef] [PubMed]
124. DaSilva, A.F.; Granziera, C.; Tuch, D.S.; Snyder, J.; Vincent, M.; Hadjikhani, N. Interictal alterations of the trigeminal somatosensory pathway and periaqueductal gray matter in migraine. *NeuroReport* **2007**, *18*, 301–305. [CrossRef] [PubMed]
125. Coppola, G.; Tinelli, E.; Lepre, C.; Iacovelli, E.; Di Lorenzo, C.; Di Lorenzo, G.; Serrao, M.; Pauri, F.; Fiermonte, G.; Bianco, F.; et al. Dynamic changes in thalamic microstructure of migraine without aura patients: A diffusion tensor magnetic resonance imaging study. *Eur. J. Neurol.* **2013**, *21*, 287-e13. [CrossRef] [PubMed]
126. Kim, J.; Kim, S.; Suh, S.-I.; Koh, S.-B.; Park, K.-W.; Oh, K. Interictal Metabolic Changes in Episodic Migraine: A Voxel-Based FDG-PET Study. *Cephalalgia* **2009**, *30*, 53–61. [CrossRef] [PubMed]
127. Vanagaite, J.; Pareja, J.; St⊘Ren, O.; White, L.; Sanc, T.; Stovner, L. Light-Induced Discomfort and Pain in Migraine. *Cephalalgia* **1997**, *17*, 733–741. [CrossRef] [PubMed]
128. Demarquay, G.; Royet, J.; Mick, G.; Ryvlin, P. Olfactory Hypersensitivity in Migraineurs: A $H_2^{15}O$-PET Study. *Cephalalgia* **2008**, *28*, 1069–1080. [CrossRef]
129. Stankewitz, A.; May, A. The phenomenon of changes in cortical excitability in migraine is not migraine-specific–A unifying thesis. *Pain* **2009**, *145*, 14–17. [CrossRef]
130. Mainero, C.; Bs, J.B.; Hadjikhani, N. Altered functional magnetic resonance imaging resting-state connectivity in periaqueductal gray networks in migraine. *Ann. Neurol.* **2011**, *70*, 838–845. [CrossRef]
131. Schwedt, T.J.; Berisha, V.; Chong, C.D. Temporal Lobe Cortical Thickness Correlations Differentiate the Migraine Brain from the Healthy Brain. *PLoS ONE* **2015**, *10*, e0116687. [CrossRef]
132. Chong, C.D.; Gaw, N.; Fu, Y.; Li, J.; Wu, T.; Schwedt, T.J. Migraine classification using magnetic resonance imaging resting-state functional connectivity data. *Cephalalgia* **2016**, *37*, 828–844. [CrossRef] [PubMed]
133. Tessitore, A.; Russo, A.; Giordano, A.; Conte, F.; Corbo, D.; De Stefano, M.; Cirillo, S.; Cirillo, M.; Esposito, F.; Tedeschi, G. Disrupted default mode network connectivity in migraine without aura. *J. Headache Pain* **2013**, *14*, 89. [CrossRef] [PubMed]
134. Schoenen, J.; Jacquy, J.; Lenaerts, M. Effectiveness of high-dose riboflavin in migraine prophylaxis A randomized controlled trial. *Neurology* **1998**, *50*, 466–470. [CrossRef] [PubMed]
135. Welch, K.; Levine, S.R.; D'Andrea, G.; Schultz, L.R.; Helpern, J.A. Preliminary observations on brain energy metabolism in migraine studied by in vivo phosphorus 31 NMR spectroscopy. *Neurology* **1989**, *39*, 538. [CrossRef] [PubMed]
136. Montagna, P.; Cortelli, P.; Monari, L.; Pierangeli, G.; Parchi, P.; Lodi, R.; Iotti, S.; Frassineti, C.; Zaniol, P.; Lugaresi, E.; et al. ^{31}P-Magnetic resonance spectroscopy in migraine without aura. *Neurology* **1994**, *44*, 666. [CrossRef]
137. Reyngoudt, H.; Paemeleire, K.; Descamps, B.; De Deene, Y.; Achten, E. 31P-MRS demonstrates a reduction in high-energy phosphates in the occipital lobe of migraine without aura patients. *Cephalalgia Int. J. Headache* **2011**, *31*, 1243–1253. [CrossRef]
138. Stankewitz, A.; Aderjan, D.; Eippert, F.; May, A. Trigeminal Nociceptive Transmission in Migraineurs Predicts Migraine Attacks. *J. Neurosci.* **2011**, *31*, 1937–1943. [CrossRef]
139. Krowicki, Z.K.; Kapusta, D.R. Microinjection of Glycine into the Hypothalamic Paraventricular Nucleus Produces Diuresis, Natriuresis, and Inhibition of Central Sympathetic Outflow. *J. Pharmacol. Exp. Ther.* **2011**, *337*, 247–255. [CrossRef]
140. Maniyar, F.H.; Sprenger, T.; Monteith, T.; Schankin, C.; Goadsby, P.J. Brain activations in the premonitory phase of nitroglycerin-triggered migraine attacks. *Brain* **2013**, *137*, 232–241. [CrossRef]
141. Schulte, L.H.; May, A. The migraine generator revisited: Continuous scanning of the migraine cycle over 30 days and three spontaneous attacks. *Brain* **2016**, *139*, 1987–1993. [CrossRef]
142. Denuelle, M.; Fabre, N.; Payoux, P.; Chollet, F.; Geraud, G. Hypothalamic Activation in Spontaneous Migraine Attacks. *Headache: J. Head Face Pain* **2007**, *47*, 1418–1426. [CrossRef]
143. Lashley, K.S. Patterns of cerebral integration indicated by the scotomas of migraine. *Arch. Neurol. Psychiatry* **1941**, *46*, 331. [CrossRef]
144. Leo, A.A.P.; Morison, R.S. Propagation of spreading cortical depression. *J. Neurophysiol.* **1945**, *8*, 33–45. [CrossRef]
145. Lauritzen, M.; Dreier, J.P.; Fabricius, M.; Hartings, A.J.; Graf, R.; Strong, A.J. Clinical Relevance of Cortical Spreading Depression in Neurological Disorders: Migraine, Malignant Stroke, Subarachnoid and Intracranial Hemorrhage, and Traumatic Brain Injury. *J. Cereb. Blood Flow Metab.* **2010**, *31*, 17–35. [CrossRef] [PubMed]
146. Olesen, J.; Larsen, B.; Lauritzen, M. Focal hyperemia followed by spreading oligemia and impaired activation of rcbf in classic migraine. *Ann. Neurol.* **1981**, *9*, 344–352. [CrossRef] [PubMed]
147. Leao, A.A.P.; de Baaij, J.H.F.; Hoenderop, J.G.J.; Bindels, R.J.M.; Funke, F.; Kron, M.; Dutschmann, M.; Müller, M.; Goadsby, P.J.; Mayevsky, A.; et al. Spreading depression of activity in the cerebral cortex. *J. Neurophysiol.* **1944**, *7*, 359–390. [CrossRef]

148. Hadjikhani, N.; del Rio, M.S.; Wu, O.; Schwartz, D.; Bakker, D.; Fischl, B.; Kwong, K.K.; Cutrer, F.M.; Rosen, B.R.; Tootell, R.B.H.; et al. Mechanisms of migraine aura revealed by functional MRI in human visual cortex. *Proc. Natl. Acad. Sci. USA* **2001**, *98*, 4687–4692. [CrossRef]
149. Headache Classification Committee of the International Headache Society (IHS). The International Classification of Headache Disorders, 3rd edition (beta version). *Cephalalgia* **2013**, *33*, 629–808. [CrossRef]
150. May, A.; Kaube, H.; Büchel, C.; Eichten, C.; Rijntjes, M.; Jüptner, M.; Weiller, C.; Diener, C.H. Experimental cranial pain elicited by capsaicin: A PET study. *Pain* **1998**, *74*, 61–66. [CrossRef]
151. Russell, F.A.; King, R.; Smillie, S.-J.; Kodji, X.; Brain, S.D.; Pressly, J.D.; Soni, H.; Jiang, S.; Wei, J.; Liu, R.; et al. Calcitonin Gene-Related Peptide: Physiology and Pathophysiology. *Physiol. Rev.* **2014**, *94*, 1099–1142. [CrossRef]
152. Stoker, K.; Baker, D.E. Erenumab-aooe. *Hosp. Pharm.* **2018**, *53*, 363–368. [CrossRef] [PubMed]
153. MacGregor, E.A. Migraine. *Ann. Intern. Med.* **2017**, *166*, ITC49–ITC64. [CrossRef] [PubMed]
154. Roy, A.; Adinoff, B.; DeJong, J.; Linnoila, M. Cerebrospinal fluid variables among alcoholics lack seasonal variation. *Acta Psychiatr. Scand.* **1991**, *84*, 579–582. [CrossRef] [PubMed]
155. Rashid, A.; Manghi, A. Calcitonin Gene-Related Peptide Receptor. In *StatPearls*; StatPearls Publishing: Treasure Island, FL, USA, 2023. Available online: http://www.ncbi.nlm.nih.gov/books/NBK560648/ (accessed on 24 July 2023).
156. Messlinger, K.; Russo, A.F. Current understanding of trigeminal ganglion structure and function in headache. *Cephalalgia* **2018**, *39*, 1661–1674. [CrossRef]
157. Edvinsson, J.C.A.; Warfvinge, K.; Krause, D.N.; Blixt, F.W.; Sheykhzade, M.; Edvinsson, L.; Haanes, K.A. C-fibers may modulate adjacent Aδ-fibers through axon-axon CGRP signaling at nodes of Ranvier in the trigeminal system. *J. Headache Pain* **2019**, *20*, 105. [CrossRef]
158. Sacco, S.; Kurth, T. Migraine and the Risk for Stroke and Cardiovascular Disease. *Curr. Cardiol. Rep.* **2014**, *16*, 524. [CrossRef]
159. Negro, A.; Martelletti, P. Gepants for the treatment of migraine. *Expert Opin. Investig. Drugs* **2019**, *28*, 555–567. [CrossRef]
160. Marcus, R.; Goadsby, P.J.; Dodick, D.; Stock, D.; Manos, G.; Fischer, T.Z. BMS-927711 for the acute treatment of migraine: A double-blind, randomized, placebo controlled, dose-ranging trial. *Cephalalgia* **2013**, *34*, 114–125. [CrossRef]
161. Becker, W.J. Acute Migraine Treatment in Adults. *Headache J. Head Face Pain* **2015**, *55*, 778–793. [CrossRef]
162. Smith, H.S. Potential analgesic mechanisms of acetaminophen. *Pain Physician* **2009**, *12*, 269–280. [CrossRef]
163. Taylor, F.R.; Kaniecki, R.G. Symptomatic Treatment of Migraine: When to Use NSAIDs, Triptans, or Opiates. *Curr. Treat. Options Neurol.* **2010**, *13*, 15–27. [CrossRef] [PubMed]
164. Colman, I.; Brown, M.D.; Innes, G.D.; Grafstein, E.; Roberts, T.E.; Rowe, B.H. Parenteral Dihydroergotamine for Acute Migraine Headache: A Systematic Review of the Literature. *Ann. Emerg. Med.* **2005**, *45*, 393–401. [CrossRef] [PubMed]
165. Silberstein, S.D.; McCrory, D.C.; Silberstein, F.S.D. Ergotamine and Dihydroergotamine: History, Pharmacology, and Efficacy. *Headache J. Head Face Pain* **2003**, *43*, 144–166. [CrossRef] [PubMed]
166. Sprenger, T.; Viana, M.; Tassorelli, C. Current Prophylactic Medications for Migraine and Their Potential Mechanisms of Action. *Neurotherapeutics* **2018**, *15*, 313–323. [CrossRef]
167. Lambru, G.; Andreou, A.P.; Guglielmetti, M.; Martelletti, P. Emerging drugs for migraine treatment: An update. *Expert Opin. Emerg. Drugs* **2018**, *23*, 301–318. [CrossRef]
168. Assas, M.B. Anti-migraine agents from an immunological point of view. *J. Transl. Med.* **2021**, *19*, 23. [CrossRef]
169. Mathew, R.; Andreou, A.P.; Chami, L.; Bergerot, A.; van den Maagdenberg, A.M.; Ferrari, M.D.; Goadsby, P.J. Immunohistochemical characterization of calcitonin gene-related peptide in the trigeminal system of the familial hemiplegic migraine 1 knock-in mouse. *Cephalalgia* **2011**, *31*, 1368–1380. [CrossRef]
170. Biella, G.; Panara, C.; Pecile, A.; Sotgiu, M. Facilitatory role of calcitonin gene-related peptide (CGRP) on excitation induced by substance P (SP) and noxious stimuli in rat spinal dorsal horn neurons. An iontophoretic study in vivo. *Brain Res.* **1991**, *559*, 352–356. [CrossRef]
171. Olesen, J.; Diener, H.-C.; Husstedt, I.W.; Goadsby, P.J.; Hall, D.; Meier, U.; Pollentier, S.; Lesko, L.M. Calcitonin Gene–Related Peptide Receptor Antagonist BIBN 4096 BS for the Acute Treatment of Migraine. *N. Engl. J. Med.* **2004**, *350*, 1104–1110. [CrossRef]
172. Ho, T.W.; Connor, K.M.; Zhang, Y.; Pearlman, E.; Koppenhaver, J.; Fan, X.; Lines, C.; Edvinsson, L.; Goadsby, P.J.; Michelson, D. Randomized controlled trial of the CGRP receptor antagonist telcagepant for migraine prevention. *Neurology* **2014**, *83*, 958–966. [CrossRef]
173. Diener, H.-C.; Barbanti, P.; Dahlöf, C.; Reuter, U.; Habeck, J.; Podhorna, J. BI 44370 TA, an oral CGRP antagonist for the treatment of acute migraine attacks: Results from a phase II study. *Cephalalgia* **2010**, *31*, 573–584. [CrossRef] [PubMed]
174. Voss, T.; Lipton, R.B.; Dodick, D.W.; Dupre, N.; Ge, J.Y.; Bachman, R.; Assaid, C.; Aurora, S.K.; Michelson, D. A phase IIb randomized, double-blind, placebo-controlled trial of ubrogepant for the acute treatment of migraine. *Cephalalgia* **2016**, *36*, 887–898. [CrossRef] [PubMed]
175. Goadsby, P.J.; Reuter, U.; Hallström, Y.; Broessner, G.; Bonner, J.H.; Zhang, F.; Sapra, S.; Picard, H.; Mikol, D.D.; Lenz, R.A. A Controlled Trial of Erenumab for Episodic Migraine. *N. Engl. J. Med.* **2017**, *377*, 2123–2132. [CrossRef] [PubMed]
176. Ashina, M.; Dodick, D.; Goadsby, P.J.; Reuter, U.; Silberstein, S.; Zhang, F.; Gage, J.R.; Cheng, S.; Mikol, D.D.; Lenz, R.A. Erenumab (AMG 334) in episodic migraine: Interim analysis of an ongoing open-label study. *Neurology* **2017**, *89*, 1237–1243. [CrossRef]

177. Tepper, S.; Ashina, M.; Reuter, U.; Brandes, J.L.; Doležil, D.; Silberstein, S.; Winner, P.; Leonardi, D.; Mikol, D.; Lenz, R. Safety and efficacy of erenumab for preventive treatment of chronic migraine: A randomised, double-blind, placebo-controlled phase 2 trial. *Lancet Neurol.* **2017**, *16*, 425–434. [CrossRef]
178. Dodick, D.W.; Goadsby, P.J.; Spierings, E.L.H.; Scherer, J.C.; Sweeney, S.P.; Grayzel, D.S. Safety and efficacy of LY2951742, a monoclonal antibody to calcitonin gene-related peptide, for the prevention of migraine: A phase 2, randomised, double-blind, placebo-controlled study. *Lancet Neurol.* **2014**, *13*, 885–892. [CrossRef]
179. Skljarevski, V.; Oakes, T.M.; Zhang, Q.; Ferguson, M.B.; Martinez, J.; Camporeale, A.; Johnson, K.W.; Shan, Q.; Carter, J.; Schacht, A.; et al. Effect of Different Doses of Galcanezumab vs Placebo for Episodic Migraine Prevention: A Randomized Clinical Trial. *JAMA Neurol.* **2018**, *75*, 187–193. [CrossRef]
180. Skljarevski, V.; Matharu, M.; Millen, B.A.; Ossipov, M.H.; Kim, B.-K.; Yang, J.Y. Efficacy and safety of galcanezumab for the prevention of episodic migraine: Results of the EVOLVE-2 Phase 3 randomized controlled clinical trial. *Cephalalgia* **2018**, *38*, 1442–1454. [CrossRef]
181. Bigal, M.E.; Dodick, D.W.; Rapoport, A.M.; Silberstein, S.D.; Ma, Y.; Yang, R.; Loupe, P.S.; Burstein, R.; Newman, L.C.; Lipton, R.B. Safety, tolerability, and efficacy of TEV-48125 for preventive treatment of high-frequency episodic migraine: A multicentre, randomised, double-blind, placebo-controlled, phase 2b study. *Lancet Neurol.* **2015**, *14*, 1081–1090. [CrossRef]
182. Dodick, D.W.; Silberstein, S.D.; Bigal, M.E.; Yeung, P.P.; Goadsby, P.J.; Blankenbiller, T.; Grozinski-Wolff, M.; Yang, R.; Ma, Y.; Aycardi, E. Effect of Fremanezumab Compared with Placebo for Prevention of Episodic Migraine. *JAMA* **2018**, *319*, 1999–2008. [CrossRef]
183. Bigal, M.E.; Dodick, D.W.; Krymchantowski, A.V.; VanderPluym, J.H.; Tepper, S.J.; Aycardi, E.; Loupe, P.S.; Ma, Y.; Goadsby, P.J. TEV-48125 for the preventive treatment of chronic migraine: Efficacy at early time points. *Neurology* **2016**, *87*, 41–48. [CrossRef]
184. Silberstein, S.D.; Dodick, D.W.; Bigal, M.E.; Yeung, P.P.; Goadsby, P.J.; Blankenbiller, T.; Grozinski-Wolff, M.; Yang, R.; Ma, Y.; Aycardi, E. Fremanezumab for the Preventive Treatment of Chronic Migraine. *N. Engl. J. Med.* **2017**, *377*, 2113–2122. [CrossRef] [PubMed]
185. Dodick, D.W.; Goadsby, P.J.; Silberstein, S.D.; Lipton, R.B.; Olesen, J.; Ashina, M.; Wilks, K.; Kudrow, D.; Kroll, R.; Kohrman, B.; et al. Safety and efficacy of ALD403, an antibody to calcitonin gene-related peptide, for the prevention of frequent episodic migraine: A randomised, double-blind, placebo-controlled, exploratory phase 2 trial. *Lancet Neurol.* **2014**, *13*, 1100–1107. [CrossRef] [PubMed]
186. Hasselmo, M.E. Neuromodulation: Acetylcholine and memory consolidation. *Trends Cogn. Sci.* **1999**, *3*, 351–359. [CrossRef]
187. Tiwari, V.; Agrawal, S. Migraine and Neuromodulation: A Literature Review. *Cureus* **2022**, *14*, e31223. [CrossRef]
188. Barloese, M.; Lambru, G. Methodological Difficulties in Clinical Trials Assessing Neuromodulation Devices in the Headache Field. In *Neuromodulation in Headache and Facial Pain Management*; Lambru, G., Lanteri-Minet, M., Eds.; Springer International Publishing: Cham, Switzerland, 2020; pp. 227–239. [CrossRef]
189. Oshinsky, M.L.; Murphy, A.L.; Hekierski, H.; Cooper, M.; Simon, B.J. Noninvasive vagus nerve stimulation as treatment for trigeminal allodynia. *Pain* **2014**, *155*, 1037–1042. [CrossRef]
190. Puledda, F.; Shields, K. Non-Pharmacological Approaches for Migraine. *Neurotherapeutics* **2018**, *15*, 336–345. [CrossRef]
191. Reuter, U.; McClure, C.; Liebler, E.; Pozo-Rosich, P. Non-invasive neuromodulation for migraine and cluster headache: A systematic review of clinical trials. *J. Neurol. Neurosurg. Psychiatry* **2019**, *90*, 796–804. [CrossRef]
192. Yuan, H.; Chuang, T.-Y. Update of Neuromodulation in Chronic Migraine. *Curr. Pain Headache Rep.* **2021**, *25*, 71. [CrossRef]
193. Schoenen, J.; Vandersmissen, B.; Jeangette, S.; Herroelen, L.; Vandenheede, M.; Gérard, P.; Magis, D. Migraine prevention with a supraorbital transcutaneous stimulator: A randomized controlled trial. *Neurology* **2013**, *80*, 697–704. [CrossRef]
194. E Chou, D.; Yugrakh, M.S.; Winegarner, D.; Rowe, V.; Kuruvilla, D.; Schoenen, J. Acute migraine therapy with external trigeminal neurostimulation (ACME): A randomized controlled trial. *Cephalalgia* **2018**, *39*, 3–14. [CrossRef]
195. Miller, S.; Watkins, L.; Matharu, M. Long-term outcomes of occipital nerve stimulation for chronic migraine: A cohort of 53 patients. *J. Headache Pain* **2016**, *17*, 68. [CrossRef]
196. Garcia-Ortega Rn, R.; Rn, T.E.; Moir, L.; Aziz, T.Z.; Green, A.L.; Fitzgerald, J.J. Burst Occipital Nerve Stimulation for Chronic Migraine and Chronic Cluster Headache. *Neuromodul. Technol. Neural Interface* **2018**, *22*, 638–644. [CrossRef]
197. Ashkan, K.; Sokratous, G.; Göbel, H.; Mehta, V.; Gendolla, A.; Dowson, A.; Wodehouse, T.; Heinze, A.; Gaul, C. Peripheral nerve stimulation registry for intractable migraine headache (RELIEF): A real-life perspective on the utility of occipital nerve stimulation for chronic migraine. *Acta Neurochir.* **2020**, *162*, 3201–3211. [CrossRef]
198. De Agostino, R.; Federspiel, B.; Cesnulis, E.; Sandor, P.S. High-Cervical Spinal Cord Stimulation for Medically Intractable Chronic Migraine. *Neuromodul. Technol. Neural Interface* **2015**, *18*, 289–296. [CrossRef]
199. Tassorelli, C.; Diener, H.-C.; Silberstein, S.D.; Dodick, D.W.; Goadsby, P.J.; Jensen, R.H.; Magis, D.; Pozo-Rosich, P.; Yuan, H.; Martinelli, D.; et al. Guidelines of the International Headache Society for clinical trials with neuromodulation devices for the treatment of migraine. *Cephalalgia* **2021**, *41*, 1135–1151. [CrossRef]
200. Dodick, D.W. A Phase-by-Phase Review of Migraine Pathophysiology. *Headache J. Head Face Pain* **2018**, *58*, 4–16. [CrossRef]
201. Blom, R.M.; Figee, M.; Vulink, N.; Denys, D. Update on repetitive transcranial magnetic stimulation in obsessive-compulsive disorder: Different targets. *Curr. Psychiatry Rep.* **2011**, *13*, 289–294. [CrossRef]
202. Lan, L.; Zhang, X.; Li, X.; Rong, X.; Peng, Y. The efficacy of transcranial magnetic stimulation on migraine: A meta-analysis of randomized controlled trails. *J. Headache Pain.* **2017**, *18*, 1–7. [CrossRef] [PubMed]

203. Shehata, H.S.; Esmail, E.H.; Abdelalim, A.; El-Jaafary, S.; Elmazny, A.; Sabbah, A.; Shalaby, N.M. Repetitive transcranial magnetic stimulation versus botulinum toxin injection in chronic migraine prophylaxis: A pilot randomized trial. *J. Pain Res.* **2016**, *9*, 771–777. [CrossRef]
204. Kalita, J.; Laskar, S.; Bhoi, S.K.; Misra, U.K. Efficacy of single versus three sessions of high rate repetitive transcranial magnetic stimulation in chronic migraine and tension-type headache. *J. Neurol.* **2016**, *263*, 2238–2246. [CrossRef] [PubMed]
205. Granato, A.; Fantini, J.; Monti, F.; Furlanis, G.; Musho Ilbeh, S.; Semenic, M.; Manganotti, P. Dramatic placebo effect of high frequency repetitive TMS in treatment of chronic migraine and medication overuse headache. *J. Clin. Neurosci.* **2019**, *60*, 96–100. [CrossRef] [PubMed]

Disclaimer/Publisher's Note: The statements, opinions and data contained in all publications are solely those of the individual author(s) and contributor(s) and not of MDPI and/or the editor(s). MDPI and/or the editor(s) disclaim responsibility for any injury to people or property resulting from any ideas, methods, instructions or products referred to in the content.

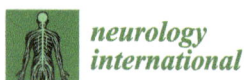

Review

All Roads Lead to the Gut: The Importance of the Microbiota and Diet in Migraine

Eleonóra Spekker [1,*] and Gábor Nagy-Grócz [2,3,4]

1. Pharmacoidea Ltd., H-6726 Szeged, Hungary
2. Department of Neurology, Albert Szent-Györgyi Medical School, University of Szeged, H-6725 Szeged, Hungary; nagy-grocz.gabor@szte.hu
3. Faculty of Health Sciences and Social Studies, University of Szeged, H-6726 Szeged, Hungary
4. Preventive Health Sciences Research Group, Incubation Competence Centre of the Centre of Excellence for Interdisciplinary Research, Development and Innovation of the University of Szeged, H-6720 Szeged, Hungary
* Correspondence: spekker.eleonora@gmail.com

Abstract: Migraine, a prevalent neurological condition and the third most common disease globally, places a significant economic burden on society. Despite extensive research efforts, the precise underlying mechanism of the disease remains incompletely comprehended. Nevertheless, it is established that the activation and sensitization of the trigeminal system are crucial during migraine attacks, and specific substances have been recognized for their distinct involvement in the pathomechanism of migraine. Recently, an expanding body of data indicates that migraine attacks can be prevented and treated through dietary means. It is important to highlight that the various diets available pose risks for patients without professional guidance. This comprehensive overview explores the connection between migraine, the gut microbiome, and gastrointestinal disorders. It provides insight into migraine-triggering foods, and discusses potential diets to help reduce the frequency and severity of migraine attacks. Additionally, it delves into the benefits of using pre- and probiotics as adjunctive therapy in migraine treatment.

Keywords: migraine; headache; gut microbiome; gut-bran axis; nutrition; dietary triggers; diets; prebiotics; probiotics

1. Migraine

Migraine ranks among the most prevalent neurological conditions, is a major cause of socio-economic and health problems worldwide, and affects approximately 12% of the population [1–3]. Repeated migraine attacks can make sufferers physically, mentally, and socially incapacitated for several days [4].

Four distinct phases of the clinical course of migraine have been identified: the premonitory (prodrome) phase, a possible aura, the headache, and recovery (postdrome) phase, and their occurrence is not necessarily linear [2]. The premonitory phase occurs hours or days before the headache and is characterized by, among other things, irritability, fatigue, concentration difficulties, neck stiffness [5]. Behavioral changes that affect mood, appetite, and energy indicate the involvement of the hypothalamus [6]. This belief is substantiated by the participation of several hypothalamic neurotransmitters in migraine, including orexin, dopamine, somatostatin, melatonin, cholecystokinin, and antidiuretic hormone [7,8]. In 25% of migraine sufferers, the aura occurs, which is a reversible neurological phenomenon. It most often manifests itself in the form of visual disturbances, but it can also cause other sensory, language, and motor dysfunctions [2,9]. The clinical occurrence known as migraine aura is thought to be a temporary wave of depolarization among cortical neurons, referred to as cortical spreading depression (CSD) [5]. The headache phase is characterized by attacks of a moderate-to-severe unilateral headache (lasting for 4–72 h) accompanied by a variety of other symptoms, such as sensitivity to light, sounds, and odors, cranial allodynia, and some gastrointestinal (GI) symptoms including nausea, vomiting, diarrhea, or constipation. Furthermore, physical activity can contribute to worsening pain [1–3]. The postdrome phase is the last stage of a migraine attack, and can include many symptoms such as neck stiffness, difficulty concentrating, fatigue, restlessness, and irritability [10] (Figure 1).

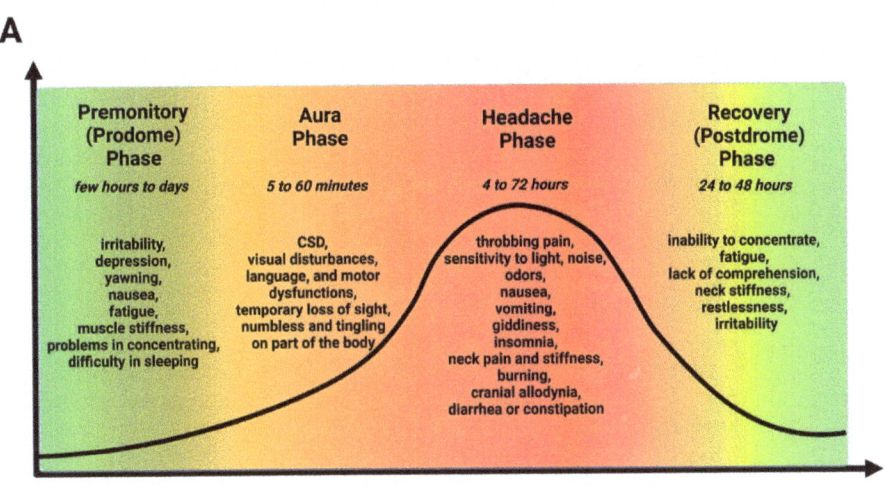

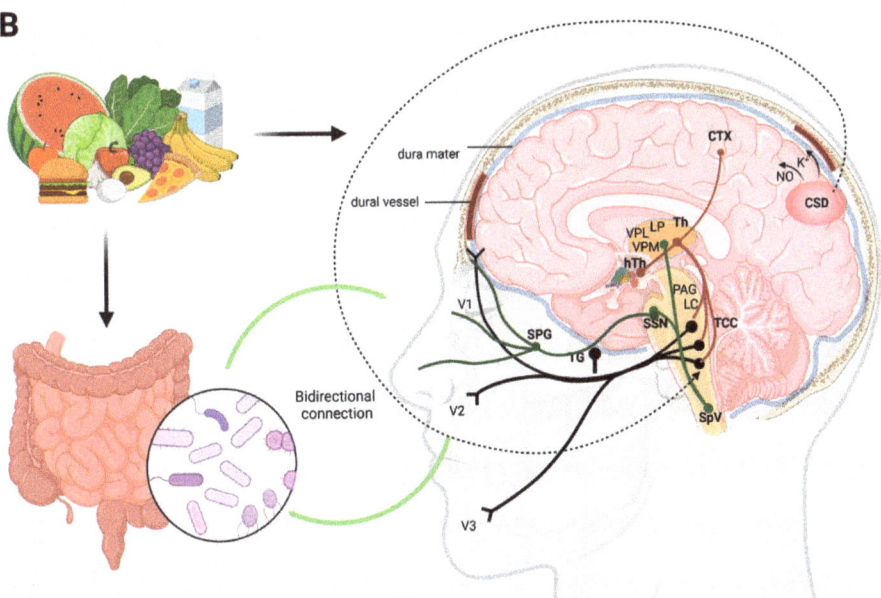

Figure 1. Migraine's phases and the factors assumed to be involved in its pathomechanism. (**A**) The four phases of migraine: the premonitory (prodome) phase, a possible aura, the headache, and recovery (post-drome). (**B**) Vascular dysfunction, CSD, activation of the trigeminovascular pathway, and inflammatory and oxidative conditions may play a fundamental role in the development of migraine pain. Moreover, nutrition and the composition and function of the gut microbiome influence

the development of migraine attacks. The trigeminal ganglion (TG) originates pseudo-unipolar trigeminal primary sensory neurons that establish connections with both intra- and extracranial structures, including blood vessels, as well as the spinal cord's trigeminocervical complex (TCC) (black line). Second-order neurons arising from the TCC ascend via the trigeminothalamic tract, where they form synapses with third-order thalamocortical neurons. There are also direct and indirect ascending projections to the locus coeruleus (LC), periaqueductal gray (PAG), and hypothalamus. Subsequently, these third-order thalamocortical neurons synapse within an extensive network of cortical regions (red line). There is also activation of the parasympathetic reflex through the outflow from the superior salivatory nucleus (SSN) via the facial nerve, predominantly involving the sphenopalatine ganglion (SPG), which acts to dilate blood vessels and activate trigeminal nerve endings (green line). CTX, cortex; NO, nitric oxide; CSD, cortical spreading depression; Th, thalamus; hTh, hypothalamus; LP, lateral posterior nucleus; VPM, ventral posteromedial nucleus; VPL, ventral posterolateral nucleus; PAG, periaqueductal grey matter; LC, locus coeruleus; TCC, trigeminocervical complex; SSN, superior salivatory nucleus; SpV, spinal trigeminal nucleus caudalis; TG, trigeminal ganglion; SPG, sphenopalatine ganglion; V1, ophthalmic nerve; V2, maxillary nerve; V3, mandibular nerve.

Despite intensive research, the pathogenesis of migraine disease remains poorly understood. At the same time, vascular dysfunction, CSD, activation of the trigeminovascular pathway, and inflammatory and oxidative conditions may play a fundamental role in the development of migraine pain [11–15]. During the activation of the trigeminal system, neurotransmitters, such as calcitonin gene-related peptide (CGRP), substance P (SP), pituitary adenylate cyclase-activating polypeptide (PACAP), and neurokinin A (NKA), are released from the primary sensory neurons and induce mast cell degranulation and plasma extravasation, which can eventually lead to the development of neurogenic inflammation [14,16].

Numerous endogenous (such as gene variants and hormones) and exogenous (such as diet and drugs) factors contribute to the severity and frequency of migraine [17,18]. The most common migraine triggers are stress, fatigue, fasting, lack of sleep, and the weather. In addition, about 20% of migraine sufferers report food as a migraine trigger [19,20].

In the gut, inflammatory mediators act as sensitizers of afferent endings. In addition, pro-inflammatory cytokines such as interleukin (IL)-1β, IL-6, IL-8, and tumor necrosis factor-α (TNF-α) are increased during migraine attacks [21,22]. Furthermore, CGRP, SP, vasoactive intestinal peptide (VIP), and neuropeptide Y (NPY), are thought to have an antimicrobial impact on a variety of gut bacterial strains; thus, they can be involved in the bidirectional gut–brain communication [23]. Another fundamental factor contributing to this relationship is altered serotonergic signaling, which can activate the trigeminovascular system and lead to the development of gastric symptoms, including nausea, vomiting, and delayed gastric emptying, which occur in both GI disorders and migraine [24,25]. A growing number of GI disorders are associated with migraines, suggesting that gut microbiota may play a key role in this disease [26]. Moreover, several recently published studies have suggested that diet plays a significant role in migraine, so dietary changes may be useful in headache prevention and treatment [18,25,27] (Figure 1).

Although the number of studies on the effects of gut microbiota composition and diet on migraine is not yet large, the present review summarizes the available evidence.

2. Gut Microbiota and Brain

The gut microbiota consists of bacteria, viruses, protozoa, and fungi present in the GI tract. These microorganisms have a tremendous impact on our physiology, both in health and in disease; among other things, they contribute to metabolic functions, influence brain–gut communication, provide protection against pathogens, and affect the immune system [28]. The human metabolism greatly benefits from the involvement of the gut microbiome in producing enzymes, as well as synthesizing essential vitamins like biotin, thiamine, cobalamin, riboflavin, nicotine, and pantothenic acids, along with branched-chain amino acids, phenols, and indoles [29]. In addition, they can metabolize indigestible carbohydrates such as cellulose, starch, and pectin into short-chain fatty acids (SCFAs) [30].

Numerous studies have demonstrated that there is a complex and diverse interaction between the gut microbiome and the central nervous system (CNS). This specific connection is known as the "gut–brain axis", a bidirectional relationship between the two, which includes afferent and efferent neural, endocrine, nutrient, and immunological signals [31] (Figure 2). The gut–brain axis serves as a coordination system for gut functions and maintenance, linking the emotional centers of the brain with peripheral intestinal mechanisms, including enteric reflexes, intestinal permeability, immune responses, and entero-endocrine signaling [32].

The composition of the gut microbiota plays an important role in the gut–brain axis. Gut microbiota can affect the CNS through two mechanisms: microbiota-derived neurotransmitters, inflammatory molecules, and hormones; and through a direct connection with the stimulating end terminals of the vagus nerve [25]. At the same time, the CNS can modulate the gut microbiota through the sympathetic and parasympathetic systems and the release of neuroendocrine peptides [23] (Figure 2).

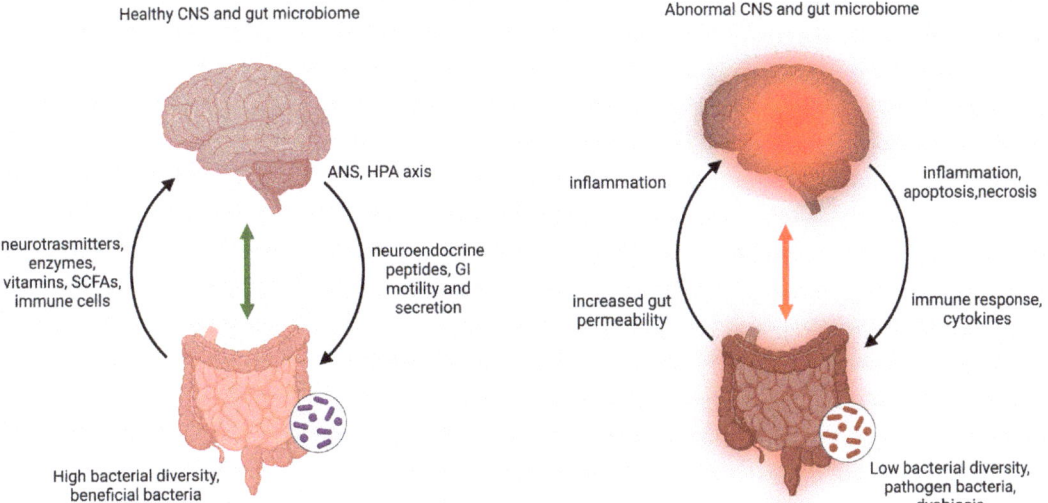

Figure 2. Bidirectional connection between the brain and the gut microbiome in both a healthy and abnormal state. CNS, central nervous system; ANS, autonomic nervous system; HPA, hypothalamic–pituitary–adrenal; SCFAs, short-chain fatty acids; GI, gastrointestinal.

Several diseases are now thought to be influenced by processes in the gut microbiome. Those include cancer, autoimmune disorders, cardiovascular diseases, and various neurological and psychiatric disorders [33]. The gut–brain axis has shown signs of dysfunction in various neurological disorders, including multiple sclerosis, Alzheimer's disease, and migraine [34] (Figure 2).

As the gut microbiota plays a crucial role in host health, manipulation of the gut microbiome, such as diets and pre- and probiotic supplementation to restore the balance of disturbed gut microbiota, may offer opportunities for disease prevention and mitigation [35,36].

3. Migraine, the Microbiome, and GI Disorders

The gut–brain axis can trigger a migraine attack in many ways, e.g., through the composition of the gut microbiome, neuropeptides, stress hormones and nutrients. Different stressors (physical or psychological) can lead to dysbiosis (an imbalance or disruption in the composition and function of the microbial communities), which causes an increase in the secretion of CGRP, which correlates with the symptoms observed during migraine attacks [25,37]. In addition, increased secretion of serum cytokines (ILs, TNF-α)—an important regulator of inflammatory responsiveness—has been observed during migraine attacks [38].

Many neurotransmitters are involved in pain perception; the most specific of these are glutamate and gamma-aminobutyric acid (GABA), which are widely distributed in the body [39]. These neurotransmitters in the gut are involved in several signaling pathways that, in addition to modulating pain, regulate the release of pro-inflammatory cytokines [40]. Research has verified that various bacterial strains, including those found in the environment or employed in food fermentation, are capable of generating glutamate [41]. Since glutamate can exert a stimulating effect on nociceptive neurons along the trigeminovascular pathway, it may be crucial in the pathophysiology of migraine headaches and migraine-related central sensitization. This theory is further proven by the fact that elevated blood levels of glutamate have been recorded in migraine patients both interictally and ictally. In addition, there is evidence that glutamate plays a major role in CSD, which is hypothesized to be the physiological substrate of migraine aura [42]. Based on these, glutamatergic neurotransmission may be a link between migraine and the microbiome.

An imbalance in the gut microbiota has been demonstrated to play a role in the development of migraine [40]. Nitrates have been identified as a prevalent migraine trigger. Higher levels of bacterial species capable of reducing nitrates, nitrites, and nitric oxide, such as Haemophilus sp. and Rothia sp., were observed in the oral and fecal samples of individuals with migraines compared to those without the condition [43]. It was also observed that in migraineurs, the species diversity and metabolic functions of gut microbiota decreased, and the number of Clostridium species (e.g., *Cl. asparagiforme, Cl. clostridioforme, Cl. bolteae, Cl. citroniae, Cl. hathewayi, Cl. ramosum, Cl. spiroforme, Cl. symbiosum*) increased, as opposed to beneficial species, which is more common in non-migraine subjects [44].

Since the microbiome contributes to other neurological disorders, it is not surprising that a connection between migraine and gastrointestinal (GI) disorders has been noted, with the frequency of GI complaints rising in tandem with the frequency of headaches [45] (Figure 3). There is evidence that migraine and GI disorders share a common pathophysiology, which is thought to occur through the interaction of several factors, including inflammatory mediators, gut microbiota, neuropeptides, and the serotonin (5-HT) pathway [25,46].

An increased inflammatory immune response has been observed in both inflammatory diseases and migraines. During migraine attacks, increased levels of pro-inflammatory cytokines such as TNF-α and IL-1β have been detected in the serum [47,48]. The main trigger of pro-inflammatory immune responses is the entry of lipopolysaccharides (LPS) into the circulation as a result of increased gut permeability. Consequently, inflammatory responses may manifest in various body regions, such as the activation of nociceptors on the trigeminal nerve in the context of migraine [48].

Furthermore, an increasing body of research indicates a heightened occurrence of migraines in individuals diagnosed with irritable bowel syndrome (IBS) and inflammatory bowel disease (IBD) [49–51]. Both are severe intestinal diseases associated with increased gut permeability and inflammation caused by microbes. Moreover, central, visceral, and thermal cutaneous hypersensitization are common among IBS and migraine [49]. Migraine patients with long-standing and more frequent headaches were more likely to be diagnosed with IBS [52].

In gastroparesis, gastric emptying time was observed to be significantly correlated with the severity of headache, nausea, and sensitivity to light in patients with migraine attacks [53]. Domperidone, a dopamine receptor antagonist, can be used to treat gastroparesis and has been shown to prevent most migraine attacks when administered early in higher doses [54,55]. Another dopamine receptor antagonist, metoclopramide, can be used to treat gastroparesis and nausea, and is effective as an acute intravenous treatment for migraine [56,57].

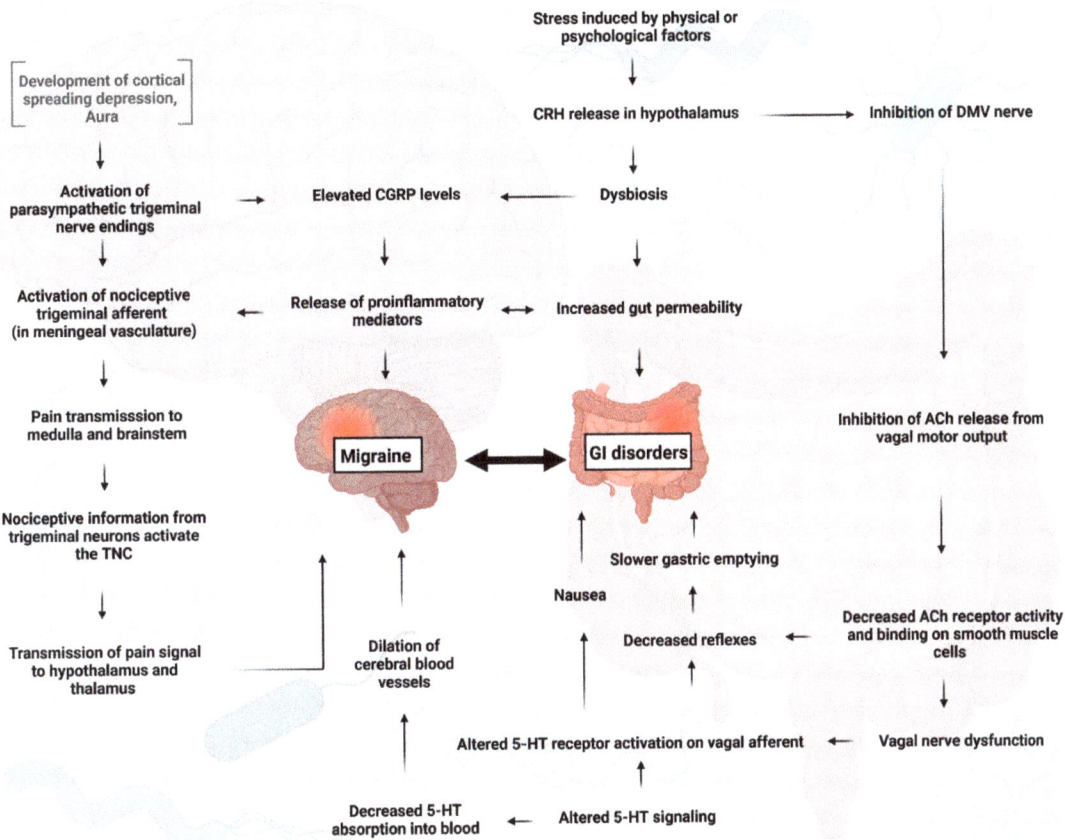

Figure 3. The relationship between migraine, gastrointestinal disorders and microbiota. Changes in sympathetic and parasympathetic activity and the gut microbiota profile—mediated by different cytokines, hormones and neurotransmitters—contribute to the development of migraine and GI diseases [46]. CGRP, calcitonin gene-related peptide; CRH, corticotrophin-releasing hormone; ACh, acetylcholine; 5-HT, serotonin; TNC, trigeminal nucleus caudalis; DMV, dorsal motor nucleus of the vagus; GI; gastrointestinal.

Individuals diagnosed with celiac disease (CD), an autoimmune disorder triggered by gluten peptides, exhibit a higher occurrence of migraines in comparison to those without the condition, and conversely, individuals with migraines have a higher prevalence of CD [50,58,59]. The link between migraines and CD can be attributed to several simultaneous mechanisms, encompassing the activation of pro-inflammatory cytokines due to gluten, deficiencies in vital vitamins and essential elements, disturbances in vascular tone, and an increased sensitivity of the nervous system [26,60].

Unfortunately, the exact mechanisms behind the involvement of the gut microbiota in migraine are unknown.

4. Migraine and Diets

4.1. Nutrition and Dietary Triggers

Nutrition and dietary triggers may be an important factor in migraine prevention, since we know that migraine attacks can be triggered by certain dietary compounds [18]. It is well known that in the treatment of several disorders, e.g., obesity [61] and metabolic syndrome [62], personalized or precision nutrition (PN) is used. PN establishes dynamic and comprehensive nutritional guidance based on personal differences, including genetics, metabolic profile, microbiome, physical activity, health status, food environment, dietary pattern, and socioeconomic and psychosocial features. The pathomechanism of migraine can be linked to metabolic endocrine disorders and metabolic processes [63,64], so PN may work as a promising supplementary therapy for migraine in the future.

Potential Dietary Triggers in Migraine

Many dietary compounds are known as potential migraine triggers, which can influence the frequency of attacks depending on the individual (Figure 4) [65,66].

The reaction of patients to these above-mentioned ingredients depends on genetic factors, quantity, and time of exposure [65], with most experiment findings concerning monosodium glutamate, caffeine, and alcohol.

Monosodium glutamate is a flavor enhancer and can be found in canned and frozen foods, salad dressings, soups, snack foods, ketchup, and barbecue sauces [67]. Based on literature data, monosodium glutamate might be a migraine trigger in high concentrations and dissolved in liquids, but not as a component of solid foods [68], which proves that it is not possible to generalize and say that one ingredient can provoke migraine attacks in every form and in every patient.

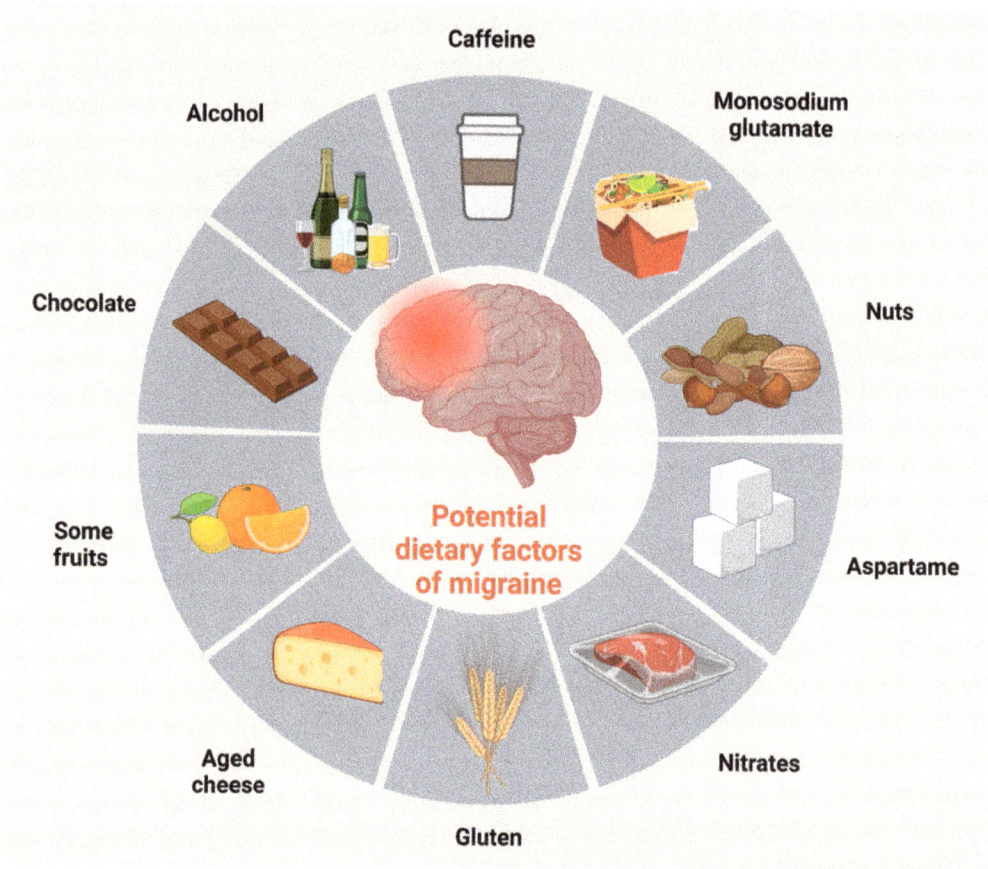

Figure 4. Potential dietary factors of migraine. Scientific evidence suggests that certain foods can trigger migraine attacks. Common migraine-triggering foods include chocolate, coffee, and red wine.

The other often-mentioned compound in association with migraine is caffeine, known for its ability to eliminate or provoke attacks. In combination with aspirin and acetaminophen, caffeine is a highly efficient pain killer. On the other hand, it is well known that caffeine withdrawal can initiate migraine attacks in caffeine users [69]. Regarding caffeine, people must pay attention to their dosage, as we know that low amounts of caffeine (~200 mg per day) have no unsafe effects contribute to decreasing the symptoms of depression [70]. Based on the literature data, we have inconclusive results concerning the connection between caffeine and migraine frequency. Some research data show that different headaches, migraine, and chronic daily headaches are more common in caffeine users than in people who do not consume this substance [71]. In contrast, other observations indicate that there is no association between headache, migraine frequency, and caffeine consumption [72].

Another substance that is the focus of attention when it comes to migraine prevention is alcohol. Ethanol can stimulate meningeal nociceptors in the trigeminal ganglion, triggering pain signals that are then transmitted in the spinal trigeminal nucleus to the thalamic nuclei, and finally to the somatosensory cortex [73]. Other mechanisms may also be involved, e.g., the vasodilator effect, dehydration, toxicity, etc. [74]. In addition to alcohol, alcoholic beverages also contain certain compounds (the byproducts of alcohol fermentation) that can trigger migraine attacks [73]. Hindiyeh and her colleagues have shown in an exceptional systematic review that alcohol consumption is one of the most common causes of migraine attacks, and the most frequently mentioned alcoholic drink is red wine [27].

Numerous studies have proposed an association between chocolate consumption and headaches, yet the precise physiological mechanisms responsible remain unclear [20,75]. One possible explanation for why chocolate triggers migraine attacks may be that the flavanols in it stimulate endothelial nitric oxide synthase (eNOS) activity, which can lead to vasodilation through increased nitric oxide (NO) production [76]. However, the results are contradictory [77,78]. Another possible cause is 5-HT. It is well known, that the concentration of 5-HT increases during a migraine attack. Moreover, 5-HT and its precursor tryptophan were found in chocolate. It is possible that by increasing 5-HT levels, chocolate consumption can trigger a migraine attack. However, there are many studies that support the beneficial effects of chocolate [78–81]. Chocolate contains many vitamins and minerals (for example, magnesium and riboflavin) that are recommended for migraine prevention [81]. Furthermore, Cady and colleagues discovered that a diet enriched with cocoa prevented inflammatory reactions in trigeminal ganglion neurons by suppressing the expression of CGRP [77].

Tyramine, an amine compound derived from the amino acid tyrosine, is present in various food items, including aged cheeses, cured meats, smoked fish, beer, fermented foods, and yeast extract, among others [82]. Tyramine has the potential to trigger headaches by promoting the release of norepinephrine and exerting an agonistic influence on α-adrenergic receptors [83].

Aspartame is an artificial sweetener. Several studies suggest that it causes various neurological or behavioral symptoms; in addition, its use can cause headaches, especially in people who consume moderate or high doses (900–3000 mg/day) for a long time [84–86].

Based on the above, recognizing and avoiding dietary migraine triggers is essential, as it can help reduce the frequency of migraines, allowing migraineurs to gain control over a condition that leaves them feeling exhausted and helpless.

4.2. Diets

4.2.1. Elimination Diets

As we discussed earlier, patients are also different in what compounds can trigger an attack in them. Based on this fact, they can avoid ingredients that have provoked migraine for them already. This process is called an elimination diet. Randomized crossover studies and double-blind, randomized, crossover trials have found that elimination diets can reduce attack frequency, duration, severity, and the amount of medication required to counter these attacks [87,88]. Using this method is not guaranteed to resolve migraines, because migraine attacks are almost always multi-triggered; thus, eliminating or identifying one compound is not a failsafe way to avoid migraine. Electronic diaries and artificial intelligence might help us use big data from patients and identify headache-associated ingredients [18,87].

4.2.2. Migraine and Other Targeted Diets

Researchers have developed targeted migraine diets [18] that influence many "migraine-specific" areas and mechanisms of the body, namely brain mitochondrial function, neuroinflammation, NO, CGRP, or neuronal excitability [89].

Among these diets, the ketogenic diet has increasingly come into focus in the treatment of neurological disorders, including migraine, which balances severe restriction of carbohydrates with higher intakes of lipids and proteins. Ketogenic diets increase the number of ketone bodies, which has a beneficial effect on migraine prevention. Ketogenic diets and ketone bodies have roles in enhancing neuroprotection, acting against serotonergic dysfunctions, repairing mitochondrial function, suppressing neuroinflammation, and reducing CGRP levels in patients [89]. Thus, enhancing ketone bodies might have a positive effect on migraine prevention [90]. In a 2016 study, adherence to the ketogenic diet for 1 month was found to be able to decrease the frequency and duration of migraine attacks in a small group of patients [91].

Besides ketogenic diets, patients should also know about the benefits of consuming omega-3 and omega-6 fatty acids. Balancing these acids is not only important in migraine prevention and treatment, but it is also crucial in preventing other disorders, e.g., atherosclerosis, as well. Decreasing omega-6 and enhancing omega-3 fatty acids in the body might have a positive effect in trying to reduce migraine attacks [90].

Increased blood sugar stability may benefit migraineurs [92]. In an experiment run in 2018, a low-glycemic-index diet was able to decrease attack frequency in the first month after beginning this diet [93].

Relatively recent epigenetic diets aim to influence the mechanisms of cellular structures, e.g., mitochondria or some molecules, e.g., DNA, using specific dietary ingredients. Their name came from Hardy and Tollefsboll, who have shown the possibility of dietary ingredients influencing the epigenetic system of patients with certain disorders, and that many ingredients might have a role in preventing diseases [94]. In migraine prevention and treatment, we should focus on compounds that can inhibit certain mechanisms that have a role in migraine's pathomechanism or can boost prevention. In this regard, one of the most promising ingredients is folate or vitamin B9, which has a role in DNA methylation. A previous study has found that abnormal mitochondrial DNA methylation occurs in migraine patients [95]; thus, folate will be a target of future studies in this field. Besides folate, riboflavin, or vitamin B2, is another compound that influences mitochondrial mechanisms. In migraine patients, riboflavin intake can inhibit the development of attacks [96–99] and their duration [100], which confirms the neuroprotective effect of riboflavin. On the other hand, besides mitochondrial DNA methylation, we should focus on histone modification in chromatin, as it can influence protein and RNA production, which can be adjusted by introducing certain dietary compounds into a patient's diet. A histone deacetylase inhibitor drug, namely valproate, is usually an effective treatment option in epilepsy and in different types of migraine [101,102], and is considered an epigenetic drug [103]; it is another future treatment option and an alternative to epigenetic diets. In addition to this, an experimental cortical CSD model has shown that CSD can induce chromatin modification in rats [104], which proves a link between migraine and histone modification. The usage of epigenetic diets requires further research, possibly with the epigenetic profiles of patients defined prior to introduction [105].

Other much-researched diets are Dietary Approaches to Stop Hypertension (DASH), the Mediterranean Diet, and the Mediterranean-DASH Intervention for Neurodegenerative Delay (MIND) Diet, which have not been exclusively examined in the context of migraine. The DASH diet was originally developed to counter hypertension, and focuses on the consumption of fruits, vegetables, and whole grains while refraining from sodium, sweets, or saturated fats [92]. There are few data on migraine and the DASH diet, but what we do have are positive; the diet decreases the Migraine Index, which measures the frequency and severity of the attacks, it reduces the Headache Diary Result, which shows the frequency and duration of migraine pain, and also cuts back the Migraine Headache Index Score, which surveys the frequency, the duration and the severity of attacks in women [92]. The Mediterranean Diet, which focuses on vegetables, legumes, fruits, nuts, olive oil, and limited animal-based meat consumption, yields similar results. The MIND Diet was originally developed for the prevention of Alzheimer's disease [106], and has very little effect on migraine pain in women [107]. Relatively new data have also shown that tryptophan-rich nutrition (flaxseed, salami, lentils, turkey, nuts, and eggs) in a healthy diet can decrease the odds of migraine attacks in migraineurs [79,108].

Tryptophan has a distinguished role in migraine's pathomechanism, since it is also a precursor of serotonin and kynurenines. Migraine patients have attenuated levels of serotonin and tryptophan during interictal periods, and show enhanced levels of serotonin and tryptophan under ictal periods [109,110]. Besides serotonin, the other pathway produced by tryptophan is the kynurenine pathway. Abnormal concentrations of kynurenines have been described in chronic migraine patients [111] and in a nitroglycerin model of migraine in rats [112]; thus, tryptophan-rich diets might have a role in the prevention and treatment of migraine. However, this requires further investigation, as acute and chronic intake of tryptophan has produced contradictory results [113,114].

4.3. Pre- and Probiotics

Plenty of research data have shown that there is pivotal crosstalk between the brain and gut, as we have discussed earlier. The modification of gut microflora can prevent or even treat certain disorders.

Prebiotics are fermentable food ingredients that have a beneficial effect on the health of their host [115,116], and these substances serve as food for probiotics, which are usually bacteria. Usage of probiotics might be effective in neurological disorders, e.g., Parkinson's disease [117]. Currently, there is a lack of information about the possible positive roles of pre- or probiotics and the gut–brain axis in migraine's pathomechanism, but we have enough data to justify further research in this field. We know that enhanced intestinal permeability and pro-inflammatory items can be found in many intestinal disorders, and these conditions might influence the trigeminovascular system, thus provoking migraine attacks [118]. The fact that some other disorders, namely allergies and asthma, are connected to migraine proves the hypothesis that inflammatory processes can contribute to migraine pathomechanism [119,120]. Adequate fiber and low-glycemic-index diets generate the production of normal gut flora and have a role in migraine prevention [25], as well. Nowadays, we have only little human data on the application of pre-and probiotics in migraine patients. In an experiment, female patients took a mixture of different strains of Lactobacillus, Bifidobacterium, and Streptococcus for 12 weeks, and the frequency and the applied numbers of painkillers were reduced, but the severity and duration of attacks did not change [121]. Another study has shown that application of a mixture of Bacillus, Bifidobacterium, Lactobacillus and Streptococcus strains for 8–10 weeks can decrease the severity and frequency of attacks in episodic migraine patients, and reduce the frequency, severity, duration, and the number of drugs taken per day in chronic migraine patients [122]. In one other experiment, researchers could not detect any change in migraine frequency, and drug usage after a 12-week application of a mixture of different Bifidobacterium and Lactobacillus strains [123]. On the other hand, we should note that some Lactic acid bacteria can produce biogenic amines (e.g., histamine, tyramine), which can cause an increase or decrease in blood pressure, thus contributing to triggering headache in people [65].

To summarize, we must acknowledge that we do not have enough data concerning the usage of pre- or probiotics in migraine prevention and treatment yet. Despite all of this, some bacteria, such as *Bacillus subtilis*, *Lactobacillus casei*, *Lactobacillus acidophilus*,

Lactobacillus gasseri, Lactobacillus bulgaricus, Lactobacillus helveticus, Lactobacillus plantarum, Lactobacillus rhamnosus, Bifidobacterium lactis, Bifidobacterium longum, Bifidobacterium breve, Bifidobacterium bifidum, and *Streptococcus thermophilus* require further study, but might prove to be a good alternative treatment in the future (Figure 5).

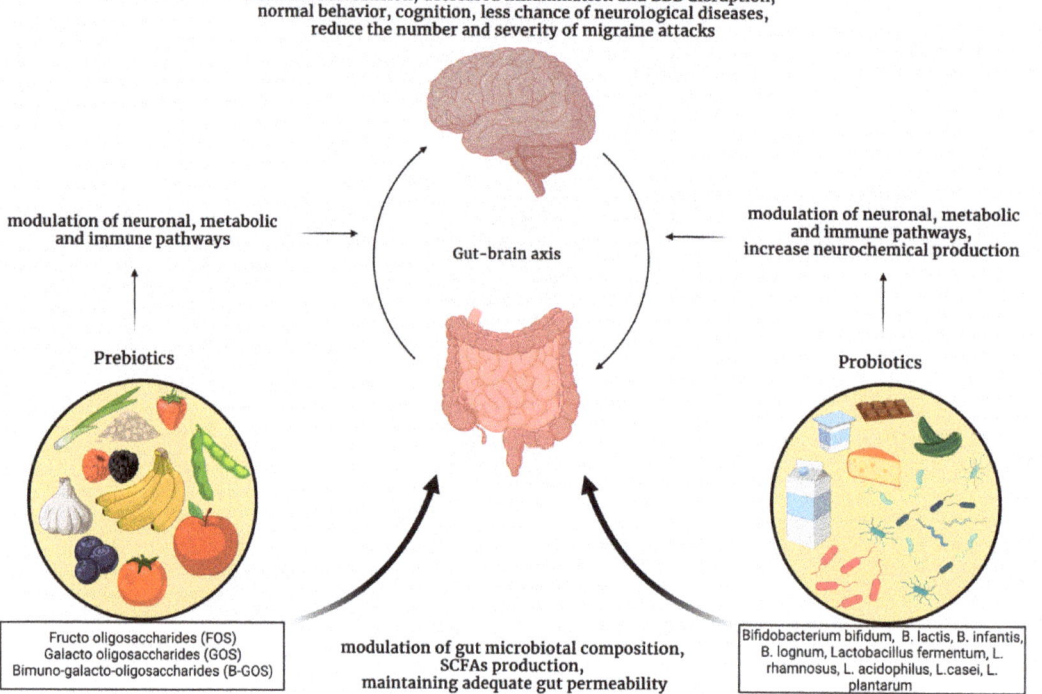

Figure 5. The beneficial effect of pre- and probiotics. Recently, pre-and probiotics have become the focus of migraine treatment, as the gut microbiota can influence the function of the CNS through various mechanisms. Taking pre- and probiotics can help restore and maintain a healthy gut microbiome, and can thus affect the frequency and severity of migraines. SCFAs, short-chain fatty acids, BBB, blood–brain barrier.

5. Conclusions

Migraine is a prevalent, recurrent, and multifactorial disorder of the CNS, and it seems gut microbiota dysbiosis contributes to this disease; thus, preserving the species richness and composition of the microbiome and improving the stability of the micro-ecosystem can improve the quality of life of migraine patients, and reduce the risk of migraine headaches and the various GI diseases comorbid with migraine.

Taken together, we can summarize that there are many possibilities for migraine treatment and prevention in the context of nutrition, and combinations of these diets might serve as good additional therapy in migraine management. In addition to this, it is important to note that patients should consult a dietician in this regard. Generally, we can recommend that patients with migraine should pay attention to meal regularity and weight loss, because healthier diets and a normal body mass index (BMI) can decrease the probability of migraine.

Author Contributions: Conceptualization, E.S. and G.N.-G.; writing—original draft preparation, E.S. and G.N.-G.; writing—review and editing, G.N.-G.; visualization, E.S. All authors have read and agreed to the published version of the manuscript.

Funding: The research was supported by the Incubation Competence Centre of the Centre of Excellence for Interdisciplinary Research, Development and Innovation of the University of Szeged. G.N-G. is a member of the Preventive Health Sciences Research Group.

Institutional Review Board Statement: Not applicable.

Informed Consent Statement: Not applicable.

Data Availability Statement: Not applicable.

Acknowledgments: All figures were created using BioRender.com (accessed on 23 June 2023).

Conflicts of Interest: We cannot identify any commercial or financial relationships that could be construed as potential conflict of interest.

Abbreviations

5-HT	serotonin
Ach	acetylcholine
BMI	body mass index
CD	celiac disease
CGRP	calcitonin gene-related peptide
CNS	central nervous system
CRH	corticotrophin-releasing hormone
CTX	cortex
CSD	cortical spreading depression
DASH	Dietary Approaches to Stop Hypertension
DMV	dorsal motor nucleus of the vagus
eNOS	endothelial nitric oxide synthase
GABA	gamma-aminobutyric acid
GI	gastrointestinal
hTh	hypothalamus
IBD	inflammatory bowel disease
IBS	irritable bowel syndrome
IL	interleukin
LC	locus coeruleus
LP	lateral posterior nucleus
LPS	lipopolysaccharides
MIND	Mediterranean-DASH Intervention for Neurodegenerative Delay
NKA	neurokinin A
NO	nitric-oxide
NPY	neuropeptide Y
PACAP	pituitary adenylate cyclase-activating polypeptide
PAG	periaqueductal grey matter
PN	personalized or precision nutrition
SCFAs	short-chain fatty acids
SP	substance P
SPG	sphenopalatine ganglion
SpV	spinal trigeminal nucleus caudalis
SSN	superior salivatory nucleus
TCC	trigeminocervical complex
TG	trigeminal ganglion
Th	thalamus
TNC	trigeminal nucleus caudalis
TNF-α	tumor necrosis factor-α
V1	ophthalmic nerve

V2	maxillary nerve
V3	mandibular nerve
VIP	vasoactive intestinal peptide
VPL	ventral posterolateral nucleus
VPM	ventral posteromedial nucleus

References

1. Lipton, R.B.; Bigal, M.E.; Steiner, T.J.; Silberstein, S.D.; Olesen, J. Classification of primary headaches. *Neurology* **2004**, *63*, 427–435. [CrossRef] [PubMed]
2. Headache Classification Committee of the International Headache Society (IHS). The International Classification of Headache Disorders, 3rd edition, (beta version). *Cephalalgia* **2013**, *33*, 629–808. [CrossRef] [PubMed]
3. GBD 2016 Disease and Injury Incidence and Prevalence Collaborators. Global, regional, and national incidence, prevalence, and years lived with disability for 328 diseases and injuries for 195 countries, 1990–2016: A systematic analysis for the Global Burden of Disease Study 2016. *Lancet* **2017**, *390*, 1211–1259. [CrossRef] [PubMed]
4. Al Ghadeer, H.A.; AlSalman, S.A.; Albaqshi, F.M.; Alsuliman, S.R.; Alsowailem, F.A.; Albusror, H.A.; AlAbdi, Z.I.; Alwabari, E.M.; Alturaifi, Z.A.; AlHajji, A.M. Quality of Life and Disability Among Migraine Patients: A Single-Center Study in AlAhsa, Saudi Arabia. *Cureus* **2021**, *13*, e19210. [CrossRef] [PubMed]
5. Goadsby, P.J.; Holland, P.R.; Martins-Oliveira, M.; Hoffmann, J.; Schankin, C.; Akerman, S. Pathophysiology of Migraine: A Disorder of Sensory Processing. *Physiol. Rev.* **2017**, *97*, 553–622. [CrossRef] [PubMed]
6. Schulte, L.H.; May, A. The migraine generator revisited: Continuous scanning of the migraine cycle over 30 days and three spontaneous attacks. *Brain* **2016**, *139 Pt 7*, 1987–1993. [CrossRef]
7. Karsan, N.; Bose, P.; Goadsby, P.J. The Migraine Premonitory Phase. *Contin. Lifelong Learn. Neurol.* **2018**, *24*, 996–1008. [CrossRef]
8. Lai, J.; Dilli, E. Migraine Aura: Updates in Pathophysiology and Management. *Curr. Neurol. Neurosci. Rep.* **2020**, *20*, 17. [CrossRef]
9. Chen, P.K.; Wang, S.J. Non-headache symptoms in migraine patients. *F1000Research* **2018**, *7*, 188. [CrossRef]
10. Qubty, W.; Patniyot, I. Migraine Pathophysiology. *Pediatr. Neurol.* **2020**, *107*, 1–6. [CrossRef]
11. Moskowitz, M.A.; Reinhard, J.F., Jr.; Romero, J.; Melamed, E.; Pettibone, D.J. Neurotransmitters and the fifth cranial nerve: Is there a relation to the headache phase of migraine? *Lancet* **1979**, *2*, 883–885. [CrossRef] [PubMed]
12. Zhang, X.; Levy, D.; Kainz, V.; Noseda, R.; Jakubowski, M.; Burstein, R. Activation of central trigeminovascular neurons by cortical spreading depression. *Ann. Neurol.* **2011**, *69*, 855–865. [CrossRef] [PubMed]
13. Bernstein, C.; Burstein, R. Sensitization of the trigeminovascular pathway: Perspective and implications to migraine pathophysiology. *J. Clin. Neurol.* **2012**, *8*, 89–99. [CrossRef] [PubMed]
14. Spekker, E.; Tanaka, M.; Szabó, Á.; Vécsei, L. Neurogenic Inflammation: The Participant in Migraine and Recent Advancements in Translational Research. *Biomedicines* **2021**, *10*, 76. [CrossRef] [PubMed]
15. Borkum, J.M. Brain Energy Deficit as a Source of Oxidative Stress in Migraine: A Molecular Basis for Migraine Susceptibility. *Neurochem. Res.* **2021**, *46*, 1913–1932. [CrossRef]
16. Edvinsson, L. Role of CGRP in Migraine. *Handb. Exp. Pharmacol.* **2019**, *255*, 121–130. [CrossRef]
17. Robblee, J.; Starling, A.J. SEEDS for success: Lifestyle management in migraine. *Cleve Clin. J. Med.* **2019**, *86*, 741–749. [CrossRef]
18. Gazerani, P. Migraine and Diet. *Nutrients* **2020**, *12*, 1658. [CrossRef]
19. Peroutka, S.J. What turns on a migraine? A systematic review of migraine precipitating factors. *Curr. Pain Headache Rep.* **2014**, *18*, 454. [CrossRef]
20. Nowaczewska, M.; Wiciński, M.; Kaźmierczak, W.; Kaźmierczak, H. To Eat or Not to Eat: A Review of the Relationship between Chocolate and Migraines. *Nutrients* **2020**, *12*, 608. [CrossRef]
21. Theoharides, T.C.; Donelan, J.; Kandere-Grzybowska, K.; Konstantinidou, A. The role of mast cells in migraine pathophysiology. *Brain Res. Rev.* **2005**, *49*, 65–76. [CrossRef] [PubMed]
22. Ramachandran, R. Neurogenic inflammation and its role in migraine. *Semin. Immunopathol.* **2018**, *40*, 301–314. [CrossRef] [PubMed]
23. Holzer, P.; Farzi, A. Neuropeptides and the microbiota-gut-brain axis. *Adv. Exp. Med. Biol.* **2014**, *817*, 195–219. [CrossRef] [PubMed]
24. Kohler, D.R.; Goldspiel, B.R. Ondansetron: A serotonin receptor (5-HT3) antagonist for antineoplastic chemotherapy-induced nausea and vomiting. *DICP* **1991**, *25*, 367–380. [CrossRef] [PubMed]
25. Arzani, M.; Jahromi, S.R.; Ghorbani, Z.; Vahabizad, F.; Martelletti, P.; Ghaemi, A.; Sacco, S.; Togha, M.; School of Advanced Studies of the European Headache Federation (EHF-SAS). Gut-brain Axis and migraine headache: A comprehensive review. *J. Headache Pain* **2020**, *21*, 15. [CrossRef]
26. Cámara-Lemarroy, C.R.; Rodriguez-Gutierrez, R.; Monreal-Robles, R.; Marfil-Rivera, A. Gastrointestinal disorders associated with migraine: A comprehensive review. *World J. Gastroenterol.* **2016**, *22*, 8149–8160. [CrossRef]
27. Hindiyeh, N.A.; Zhang, N.; Farrar, M.; Banerjee, P.; Lombard, L.; Aurora, S.K. The Role of Diet and Nutrition in Migraine Triggers and Treatment: A Systematic Literature Review. *Headache* **2020**, *60*, 1300–1316. [CrossRef]
28. Thursby, E.; Juge, N. Introduction to the human gut microbiota. *Biochem. J.* **2017**, *474*, 1823–1836. [CrossRef]

29. Rowland, I.; Gibson, G.; Heinken, A.; Scott, K.; Swann, J.; Thiele, I.; Tuohy, K. Gut microbiota functions: Metabolism of nutrients and other food components. *Eur. J. Nutr.* **2018**, *57*, 1–24. [CrossRef]
30. Lin, L.; Zhang, J. Role of intestinal microbiota and metabolites on gut homeostasis and human diseases. *BMC Immunol.* **2017**, *18*, 2. [CrossRef]
31. Romijn, J.A.; Corssmit, E.P.; Havekes, L.M.; Pijl, H. Gut-brain axis. *Curr. Opin. Clin. Nutr. Metab. Care* **2008**, *11*, 518–521. [CrossRef] [PubMed]
32. Wang, Y.; Kasper, L.H. The role of microbiome in central nervous system disorders. *Brain Behav. Immun.* **2014**, *38*, 1–12. [CrossRef] [PubMed]
33. Zang, Y.; Lai, X.; Li, C.; Ding, D.; Wang, Y.; Zhu, Y. The Role of Gut Microbiota in Various Neurological and Psychiatric Disorders-An Evidence Mapping Based on Quantified Evidence. *Mediat. Inflamm.* **2023**, *2023*, 5127157. [CrossRef] [PubMed]
34. Mayer, E.A.; Tillisch, K.; Gupta, A. Gut/brain axis and the microbiota. *J. Clin. Investig.* **2015**, *125*, 926–938. [CrossRef]
35. Shreiner, A.B.; Kao, J.Y.; Young, V.B. The gut microbiome in health and in disease. *Curr. Opin. Gastroenterol.* **2015**, *31*, 69–75. [CrossRef]
36. Gomaa, E.Z. Human gut microbiota/microbiome in health and diseases: A review. *Antonie Van Leeuwenhoek* **2020**, *113*, 2019–2040. [CrossRef]
37. Ustianowska, K.; Ustianowski, Ł.; Machaj, F.; Gorący, A.; Rosik, J.; Szostak, B.; Szostak, J.; Pawlik, A. The Role of the Human Microbiome in the Pathogenesis of Pain. *Int. J. Mol. Sci.* **2022**, *23*, 13267. [CrossRef]
38. Amaral, F.A.; Sachs, D.; Costa, V.V.; Fagundes, C.T.; Cisalpino, D.; Cunha, T.M.; Ferreira, S.H.; Cunha, F.Q.; Silva, T.A.; Nicoli, J.R.; et al. Commensal microbiota is fundamental for the development of inflammatory pain. *Proc. Natl. Acad. Sci. USA* **2008**, *105*, 2193–2197. [CrossRef]
39. Strandwitz, P.; Kim, K.H.; Terekhova, D.; Liu, J.K.; Sharma, A.; Levering, J.; McDonald, D.; Dietrich, D.; Ramadhar, T.R.; Lekbua, A.; et al. GABA-modulating bacteria of the human gut microbiota. *Nat. Microbiol.* **2019**, *4*, 396–403. [CrossRef]
40. Cryan, J.F.; O'Riordan, K.J.; Sandhu, K.; Peterson, V.; Dinan, T.G. The gut microbiome in neurological disorders. *Lancet Neurol.* **2020**, *19*, 179–194. [CrossRef]
41. Baj, A.; Moro, E.; Bistoletti, M.; Orlandi, V.; Crema, F.; Giaroni, C. Glutamatergic Signaling Along the Microbiota-Gut-Brain Axis. *Int. J. Mol. Sci.* **2019**, *20*, 1482. [CrossRef] [PubMed]
42. Hoffmann, J.; Charles, A. Glutamate and Its Receptors as Therapeutic Targets for Migraine. *Neurotherapeutics* **2018**, *15*, 361–370. [CrossRef]
43. Gonzalez, A.; Hyde, E.; Sangwan, N.; Gilbert, J.A.; Viirre, E.; Knight, R. Migraines Are Correlated with Higher Levels of Nitrate-, Nitrite-, and Nitric Oxide-Reducing Oral Microbes in the American Gut Project Cohort. *mSystems* **2016**, *1*, e00105-16. [CrossRef] [PubMed]
44. Chen, J.; Wang, Q.; Wang, A.; Lin, Z. Structural and Functional Characterization of the Gut Microbiota in Elderly Women with Migraine. *Front. Cell. Infect. Microbiol.* **2020**, *9*, 470. [CrossRef] [PubMed]
45. Aamodt, A.H.; Stovner, L.J.; Hagen, K.; Zwart, J.A. Comorbidity of headache and gastrointestinal complaints. The Head-HUNT Study. *Cephalalgia* **2008**, *28*, 144–151. [CrossRef]
46. Aurora, S.K.; Shrewsbury, S.B.; Ray, S.; Hindiyeh, N.; Nguyen, L. A link between gastrointestinal disorders and migraine: Insights into the gut-brain connection. *Headache* **2021**, *61*, 576–589. [CrossRef]
47. Schuppan, D.; Junker, Y.; Barisani, D. Celiac disease: From pathogenesis to novel therapies. *Gastroenterology* **2009**, *137*, 1912–1933. [CrossRef]
48. Van Hemert, S.; Breedveld, A.C.; Rovers, J.M.; Vermeiden, J.P.; Witteman, B.J.; Smits, M.G.; de Roos, N.M. Migraine associated with gastrointestinal disorders: Review of the literature and clinical implications. *Front. Neurol.* **2014**, *5*, 241. [CrossRef]
49. Chang, F.Y.; Lu, C.L. Irritable bowel syndrome and migraine: Bystanders or partners? *J. Neurogastroenterol. Motil.* **2013**, *19*, 301–311. [CrossRef]
50. Dimitrova, A.K.; Ungaro, R.C.; Lebwohl, B.; Lewis, S.K.; Tennyson, C.A.; Green, M.W.; Babyatsky, M.W.; Green, P.H. Prevalence of migraine in patients with celiac disease and inflammatory bowel disease. *Headache* **2013**, *53*, 344–355. [CrossRef]
51. Crawford, J.; Liu, S.; Tao, F. Gut microbiota and migraine. *Neurobiol. Pain* **2022**, *11*, 100090. [CrossRef]
52. Li, C.; Yu, S.; Li, H.; Zhou, J.; Liu, J.; Tang, W.; Zhang, L. Clinical features and risk factors for irritable bowel syndrome in Migraine patients. *Pak. J. Med. Sci.* **2017**, *33*, 720–725. [CrossRef]
53. Boyle, R.; Behan, P.O.; Sutton, J.A. A correlation between severity of migraine and delayed gastric emptying measured by an epigastric impedance method. *Br. J. Clin. Pharmacol.* **1990**, *30*, 405–409. [CrossRef]
54. Waelkens, J. Dopamine blockade with domperidone: Bridge between prophylactic and abortive treatment of migraine? A dose-finding study. *Cephalalgia* **1984**, *4*, 85–90. [CrossRef] [PubMed]
55. Acosta, A.; Camilleri, M. Prokinetics in gastroparesis. *Gastroenterol. Clin. N. Am.* **2015**, *44*, 97–111. [CrossRef] [PubMed]
56. Friedman, B.W.; Mulvey, L.; Esses, D.; Solorzano, C.; Paternoster, J.; Lipton, R.B.; Gallagher, E.J. Metoclopramide for acute migraine: A dose-finding randomized clinical trial. *Ann. Emerg. Med.* **2011**, *57*, 475–482.e1. [CrossRef] [PubMed]
57. Shakhatreh, M.; Jehangir, A.; Malik, Z.; Parkman, H.P. Metoclopramide for the treatment of diabetic gastroparesis. *Expert. Rev. Gastroenterol. Hepatol.* **2019**, *13*, 711–721. [CrossRef] [PubMed]
58. Kopishinskaya, S.V.; Gustov, A.V. Gluten migraine. *Zhurnal Nevrologii Psikhiatrii Imeni SS Korsakova* **2015**, *115*, 13–17. [CrossRef]

59. Zis, P.; Julian, T.; Hadjivassiliou, M. Headache Associated with Coeliac Disease: A Systematic Review and Meta-Analysis. *Nutrients* **2018**, *6*, 1445. [CrossRef]
60. Mormile, R. Celiac disease and migraine: Is there a common backstage? *Int. J. Color. Dis.* **2014**, *29*, 1571. [CrossRef]
61. Voruganti, V.S. Precision Nutrition: Recent Advances in Obesity. *Physiology* **2023**, *38*, 42–50. [CrossRef] [PubMed]
62. Muniesa, G.; Martinez, J.A.; González-Muniesa, P. Precision Nutrition and Metabolic Syndrome Management. *Nutrients* **2019**, *11*, 2411. [CrossRef] [PubMed]
63. Kokavec, A. Migraine: A disorder of metabolism? *Med. Hypotheses* **2016**, *97*, 117–130. [CrossRef] [PubMed]
64. Rainero, I.; Govone, F.; Gai, A.; Vacca, A.; Rubino, E. Is Migraine Primarily a Metaboloendocrine Disorder? *Curr. Pain Headache Rep.* **2018**, *22*, 36. [CrossRef]
65. Martin, V.T.; Vij, B. Diet and Headache: Part 1. *Headache J. Head Face Pain* **2016**, *56*, 1543–1552. [CrossRef]
66. Cairns, B.E. Influence of pro-algesic foods on chronic pain conditions. *Expert. Rev. Neurother.* **2016**, *16*, 415–423. [CrossRef]
67. Scopp, A.L. MSG and hydrolyzed vegetable protein induced headache: Review and case studies. *Headache* **1991**, *31*, 107–110. [CrossRef]
68. Shimada, A.; Cairns, B.E.; Vad, N.; Ulriksen, K.; Pedersen Lynge, A.M.; Svensson, P.; Baad-Hansen, L. Headache and mechanical sensitization of human pericranial muscles after repeated intake of monosodium glutamate (MSG). *J. Headache Pain* **2013**, *14*, 2. [CrossRef]
69. Juliano, L.M.; Griffiths, R.R. A critical review of caffeine withdrawal: Empirical validation of symptoms and signs, incidence, severity, and associated features. *Psychopharmacology* **2004**, *176*, 1–29. [CrossRef]
70. Nehlig, A. Effects of coffee/caffeine on brain health and disease: What should I tell my patients? *Pract. Neurol.* **2016**, *16*, 89–95. [CrossRef]
71. Shapiro, R.E. Caffeine and headaches. *Curr. Pain Headache Rep.* **2008**, *12*, 311–315. [CrossRef] [PubMed]
72. Boardman, H.F.; Thomas, E.; Millson, D.S.; Croft, P.R. Psychological, sleep, lifestyle, and comorbid associations with headache. *Headache* **2005**, *45*, 657–669. [CrossRef] [PubMed]
73. Zhu, H.; Xing, Y.; Akan, O.D.; Yang, T. Alcohol-Induced Headache with Neuroinflammation: Recent Progress. *Fermentation* **2023**, *9*, 184. [CrossRef]
74. Panconesi, A. Alcohol and migraine: Trigger factor, consumption, mechanisms. A review. *J. Headache Pain* **2008**, *9*, 19–27. [CrossRef] [PubMed]
75. Lippi, G.; Mattiuzzi, C.; Cervellin, G. Chocolate and migraine: The history of an ambiguous association. *Acta Biomed.* **2014**, *85*, 216–221. [PubMed]
76. Ellam, S.; Williamson, G. Cocoa and human health. *Annu. Rev. Nutr.* **2013**, *33*, 105–128. [CrossRef] [PubMed]
77. Cady, R.J.; Durham, P.L. Cocoa-enriched diets enhance expression of phosphatases and decrease expression of inflammatory molecules in trigeminal ganglion neurons. *Brain Res.* **2010**, *1323*, 18–32. [CrossRef]
78. Magrone, T.; Russo, M.A.; Jirillo, E. Cocoa and Dark Chocolate Polyphenols: From Biology to Clinical Applications. *Front. Immunol.* **2017**, *8*, 677. [CrossRef]
79. Razeghi Jahromi, S.; Togha, M.; Ghorbani, Z.; Hekmatdoost, A.; Khorsha, F.; Rafiee, P.; Shirani, P.; Nourmohammadi, M.; Ansari, H. The association between dietary tryptophan intake and migraine. *Neurol. Sci.* **2019**, *40*, 2349–2355. [CrossRef]
80. Abbey, M.J.; Patil, V.V.; Vause, C.V.; Durham, P.L. Repression of calcitonin gene-related peptide expression in trigeminal neurons by a Theobroma cacao extract. *J. Ethnopharmacol.* **2008**, *115*, 238–248. [CrossRef]
81. Nattagh-Eshtivani, E.; Sani, M.A.; Dahri, M.; Ghalichi, F.; Ghavami, A.; Arjang, P.; Tarighat-Esfanjani, A. The role of nutrients in the pathogenesis and treatment of migraine headaches: Review. *Biomed. Pharmacother.* **2018**, *102*, 317–325. [CrossRef] [PubMed]
82. Sun-Edelstein, C.; Mauskop, A. Foods and supplements in the management of migraine headaches. *Clin. J. Pain* **2009**, *25*, 446–452. [CrossRef] [PubMed]
83. Martin, V.T.; Behbehani, M.M. Toward a rational understanding of migraine trigger factors. *Med. Clin. N. Am.* **2001**, *85*, 911–941. [CrossRef]
84. Council of Scientific Affairs. Aspartame: Review of safety issues. *JAMA* **1985**, *254*, 400–402. [CrossRef]
85. Van den Eeden, S.K.; Koepsell, T.D.; Longstreth, W.T., Jr.; van Belle, G.; Daling, J.R.; McKnight, B. Aspartame ingestion and headaches: A randomized crossover trial. *Neurology* **1994**, *44*, 1787–1793. [CrossRef]
86. Loehler, S.M.; Glaros, A. The effect of aspartame on migraine headache. *Headache* **1988**, *28*, 10–14. [CrossRef]
87. Ozon, A.O.; Karadas, O.; Ozge, A. Efficacy of diet restriction on migraines. *Arch. Neuropsychiatry* **2018**, *55*, 233–237. [CrossRef]
88. Aydinla, E.I.; Dikmen, P.Y.; Tiftikci, A.; Saruc, M.; Aksu, M.; Gunsoy, H.G.; Tozun, N. IgG-based elimination diet in migraine plus irritable bowel syndrome. *Headache* **2013**, *53*, 514–525. [CrossRef]
89. Jahromi, S.R.; Ghorbani, Z.; Martelletti, P.; Lampl, C.; Togha, M.; On behalf of the School of Advanced Studies of the European Headache Federation (EHF-SAS). Association of diet and headache. *J. Headache Pain* **2019**, *20*, 106–111. [CrossRef]
90. Gross, E.C.; Klement, R.J.; Schoenen, J.; D'Agostino, D.P.; Fischer, D. Potential Protective Mechanisms of Ketone Bodies in Migraine Prevention. *Nutrients* **2019**, *11*, 811. [CrossRef]
91. Di Lorenzo, C.; Coppola, G.; Bracaglia, M.; Di Lenola, D.; Evangelista, M.; Sirianni, G.; Rossi, P.; Di Lorenzo, G.; Serrao, M.; Parisi, V.; et al. Cortical functional correlates of responsiveness to short-lasting preventive intervention with ketogenic diet in migraine: A multimodal evoked potentials study. *J. Headache Pain* **2016**, *17*, 58. [CrossRef] [PubMed]

92. Moskatel, L.S.; Zhang, N. Migraine and Diet: Updates in Understanding. *Curr. Neurol. Neurosci. Rep.* **2022**, *22*, 327–334. [CrossRef] [PubMed]
93. Evcili, G.; Utku, U.; Ogun, M.N.; Ozdemir, G. Early and long period follow-up results of low glycemic index diet for migraine prophylaxis. *J. Turk. Soc. Algol.* **2018**, *30*, 8–11. [CrossRef] [PubMed]
94. Hardy, T.M.; Tollefsbol, T.O. Epigenetic diet: Impact on the epigenome and cancer. *Epigenomics* **2011**, *3*, 503–518. [CrossRef] [PubMed]
95. Fila, M.; Pawłowska, E.; Blasiak, J. Mitochondria in migraine pathophysiology—Does epigenetics play a role? *Arch. Med. Sci.* **2019**, *15*, 944–956. [CrossRef]
96. Thompson, D.F.; Saluja, H.S. Prophylaxis of migraine headaches with riboflavin: A systematic review. *J. Clin. Pharm. Ther.* **2017**, *42*, 394–403. [CrossRef]
97. Daniel, O.; Mauskop, A. Nutraceuticals in acute and prophylactic treatment of migraine. *Curr. Treat. Options Neurol.* **2016**, *18*, 14. [CrossRef]
98. Marashly, E.T.; Bohlega, S.A. Riboflavin has neuroprotective potential: Focus on Parkinson's disease and migraine. *Front. Neurol.* **2017**, *8*, 333. [CrossRef]
99. Namazi, N.; Heshmati, J.; Tarighat-Esfanjani, A. Supplementation with riboflavin (Vitamin B2) for migraine prophylaxis in adults and children: A review. *Int. J. Vitam. Nutr. Res.* **2015**, *85*, 79–87. [CrossRef]
100. Schoenen, J.; Jacquy, J.; Lenaerts, M. Effectiveness of high-dose riboflavin in migraine prophylaxis. A randomized controlled trial. *Neurology* **1998**, *50*, 466–470. [CrossRef]
101. Karimi, N.; Tavakoli, M.; Charati, J.Y.; Shamsizade, M. Single-dose intravenous sodium valproate (Depakine) versus dexamethasone for the treatment of acute migraine headache: A double-blind randomized clinical trial. *Clin. Exp. Emerg. Med.* **2017**, *4*, 138–145. [CrossRef] [PubMed]
102. Liu, F.; Ma, T.; Che, X.; Wang, Q.; Yu, S. The efficacy of venlafaxine, flunarizine, and valproic acid in the prophylaxis of vestibular migraine. *Front. Neurol.* **2017**, *8*, 524. [CrossRef] [PubMed]
103. Ganesan, A.; Arimondo, P.B.; Rots, M.G.; Jeronimo, C.; Berdasco, M. The timeline of epigenetic drug discovery: From reality to dreams. *Clin. Epigenet.* **2019**, *11*, 17. [CrossRef]
104. Passaro, D.; Rana, G.; Piscopo, M.; Viggiano, E.; De Luca, B.; Fucci, L. Epigenetic chromatin modifications in the cortical spreading depression. *Brain Res.* **2010**, *1329*, 1–9. [CrossRef] [PubMed]
105. Gazerani, P. Current Evidence on the Role of Epigenetic Mechanisms in Migraine: The Way Forward to Precision Medicine. *OBM Genet.* **2018**, *2*, 1. [CrossRef]
106. Morris, M.C.; Tangney, C.C.; Wang, Y.; Sacks, F.M.; Barnes, L.L.; Bennett, D.A.; Aggarwal, N.T. MIND diet slows cognitive decline with aging. *Alzheimers Dement.* **2015**, *11*, 1015–1022. [CrossRef]
107. Askarpour, M.; Yarizadeh, H.; Sheikhi, A.; Khorsha, F.; Mirzaei, K. Associations between adherence to MIND diet and severity, duration and frequency of migraine headaches among migraine patients. *BMC Res. Notes* **2020**, *13*, 341. [CrossRef] [PubMed]
108. Escott-Stump, S. *Nutrition and Diagnosis-Related Care*; Lippincott Williams & Wilkins: Philadelphia, PA, USA, 2011.
109. Deen, M.; Christensen, C.E.; Hougaard, A.; Hansen, H.D.; Knudsen, G.M.; Ashina, M. Serotonergic mechanisms in the migraine brain—A systematic review. *Cephalalgia* **2017**, *37*, 251–264. [CrossRef]
110. Gasparini, C.F.; Smith, R.A.; Griffiths, L.R. Genetic and biochemical changes of the serotonergic system in migraine pathobiology. *J. Headache Pain* **2017**, *18*, 20. [CrossRef]
111. Curto, M.; Lionetto, L.; Fazio, F.; Mitsikostas, D.D.; Martelletti, P. Fathoming the kynurenine pathway in migraine: Why understanding the enzymatic cascades is still critically important. *Intern. Emerg. Med.* **2015**, *10*, 413–421. [CrossRef]
112. Nagy-Grócz, G.; Laborc, K.F.; Veres, G.; Bajtai, A.; Bohár, Z.; Zádori, D.; Fejes-Szabó, A.; Spekker, E.; Vécsei, L.; Párdutz, Á. The Effect of Systemic Nitroglycerin Administration on the Kynurenine Pathway in the Rat. *Front. Neurol.* **2017**, *8*, 278. [CrossRef] [PubMed]
113. Sicuteri, F. The ingestion of serotonin precursors (L-5-hydroxytryptophan and L-tryptophan) improves migraine headache. *Headache* **1973**, *13*, 19–22. [CrossRef] [PubMed]
114. Gedye, A. Hypothesized treatment for migraines using low doses of tryptophan, niacin, calcium, caffeine, and acetylsalicylic acid. *Med. Hypotheses* **2001**, *56*, 91–94. [CrossRef]
115. Roberfroid, M. Prebiotics: The concept revisited. *J. Nutr.* **2007**, *137* (Suppl. 2), 830S–837S. [CrossRef] [PubMed]
116. Gibson, G.R.; Hutkins, R.; Sanders, M.E.; Prescott, S.L.; Reimer, R.A.; Salminen, S.J.; Scott, K.; Stanton, C.; Swanson, K.S.; Cani, P.D.; et al. Expert consensus document: The International Scientific Association for Probiotics and Prebiotics (ISAPP) consensus statement on the definition and scope of prebiotics. *Nat. Rev. Gastroenterol. Hepatol.* **2017**, *14*, 491–502. [CrossRef] [PubMed]
117. Gazerani, P. Probiotics for Parkinson's Disease. *Int. J. Mol. Sci.* **2019**, *20*, 4121. [CrossRef]
118. Galland, L. The Gut Microbiome and the Brain. *J. Med. Food* **2014**, *17*, 1261–1272. [CrossRef]
119. Saberi, A.; Nemati, S.; Shakib, R.J.; Kazemnejad, E.; Maleki, M. Association between allergic rhinitis and migraine. *J. Res. Med. Sci.* **2012**, *17*, 508–512.
120. Kim, S.Y.; Min, C.; Oh, D.J.; Lim, J.-S.; Choi, H.-G. Bidirectional association between asthma and migraines in adults: Two longitudinal follow-up studies. *Sci. Rep.* **2019**, *9*, 18343–18349. [CrossRef]

121. Ghavami, A.; Khorvash, F.; Heidari, Z.; Khalesi, S.; Askari, G. Effect of synbiotic supplementation on migraine characteristics and inflammatory biomarkers in women with migraine: Results of a randomized controlled trial. *Pharmacol. Res.* **2021**, *169*, 105668. [CrossRef]
122. Martami, F.; Togha, M.; Seifishahpar, M.; Ghorbani, Z.; Ansari, H.; Karimi, T.; Jahromi, S.R. The effects of a multispecies probiotic supplement on inflammatory markers and episodic and chronic migraine characteristics: A randomized double-blind controlled trial. *Cephalalgia* **2019**, *39*, 841–853. [CrossRef] [PubMed]
123. De Roos, N.M.; van Hemert, S.; Rovers, J.M.P.; Smits, M.G.; Witteman, B.J.M. The effects of a multispecies probiotic on migraine and markers of intestinal permeability—Results of a randomized placebo-controlled study. *Eur. J. Clin. Nutr.* **2017**, *71*, 1455–1462. [CrossRef] [PubMed]

Disclaimer/Publisher's Note: The statements, opinions and data contained in all publications are solely those of the individual author(s) and contributor(s) and not of MDPI and/or the editor(s). MDPI and/or the editor(s) disclaim responsibility for any injury to people or property resulting from any ideas, methods, instructions or products referred to in the content.

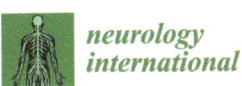

Article

Genetic Variability in Vitamin D Receptor and Migraine Susceptibility: A Southeastern European Case-Control Study

Maria Papasavva [1,*], Michail Vikelis [2], Vasileios Siokas [3], Martha-Spyridoula Katsarou [1], Emmanouil V. Dermitzakis [4], Athanasios Raptis [1], Efthimios Dardiotis [3] and Nikolaos Drakoulis [1,*]

1 Research Group of Clinical Pharmacology and Pharmacogenomics, Faculty of Pharmacy, School of Health Sciences, National and Kapodistrian University of Athens, 157 71 Athens, Greece
2 Headache Clinic, Mediterraneo Hospital, 166 75 Glifada, Greece
3 Laboratory of Neurogenetics, Department of Neurology, University Hospital of Larissa, Faculty of Medicine, School of Health Sciences, University of Thessaly, 411 00 Larissa, Greece
4 Euromedica General Clinic, 546 45 Thessaloniki, Greece
* Correspondence: mariapapa@pharm.uoa.gr (M.P.); drakoulis@pharm.uoa.gr (N.D.)

Abstract: Migraine is a common primary headache disorder with both environmental and genetic inputs. Cumulative evidence indicates an association between vitamin D and headache. Unravelling the precise role of vitamin D and its receptor in the pathophysiology of migraine can eventually contribute to more efficient prevention and management of this headache disorder. The aim of the study was to investigate the relation of the three most studied *VDR* variants, i.e., *FokI* (rs2228570), *TaqI* (rs731236) and *BsmI* (rs1544410), with migraine susceptibility and distinct clinical phenotypes in a Southeastern European case-control population residing in Greece. DNA was extracted from 191 unrelated patients diagnosed with migraine and 265 headache-free controls and genotyped using real-time PCR (LightSNiP assays) followed by melting curve analysis. Genotype frequency distribution analysis of the *TaqI* and *BsmI* variants showed a statistically significant difference between migraine cases and controls. In addition, subgroup analyses revealed a significant association between all three studied *VDR* variants, particularly with a migraine without aura subtype. Therefore, the current study provides supporting evidence for a possible association of *VDR* variants with migraines, particularly migraine without aura susceptibility in Southeastern Europeans residing in Greece, further reinforcing the emerging role of vitamin D and its receptor in migraines.

Keywords: VDR; precision medicine; single nucleotide variants (SNVs); primary headaches; migraine genetics; *FokI*; *TaqI*; *BsmI*

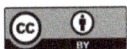

1. Introduction

Migraine is a common primary headache disorder with a high disability burden and considerable detrimental effects on public health [1]. According to the Global Burden of Disease Study 2019 (GBD2019), migraine ranks second among the causes of global years lived with disability (YLDs), being responsible for 4.8% (0.8–10.1) of total YLDs and comprising 88.2% (60.7–97.7) of the burden of headache disorders in 2019. The highest burden, i.e., 7.3% (1.1–15.1), was observed in the age group 15–49 years, the most productive years of life in both genders [2]. Although the pathophysiology of the disease has not been fully elucidated, among the proposed mechanisms being implicated are the activation of trigeminovascular system, cortical spreading depression, inflammation and vascular dysfunction [3]. Besides environmental factors, migraine is largely affected by genetic factors, with several genetic variants, each having a minor effect contributing to its liability [4–6].

In the last decades, vitamin D, a fat-soluble hormone belonging to the secosteroid family, has received enormous attention due to its large spectrum of musculoskeletal and non-skeletal biological functions, including regulation of cellular proliferation and differentiation, hormone secretion, control of immune function and metabolism [7]. A two-step sequentially metabolism of vitamin D occurs to attain its biological effects; the first step is the metabolism in the liver by the enzyme D-25-hydroxylase (CYP2R1) into 25-hydroxyvitamin D (25(OH)D), the major circulating form, followed by hydroxylation into 1α,25-dihydroxyvitamin D (1,25(OH)$_2$D) by 1-alpha-hydroxylase (CYP27B1) located in target organs, e.g., the kidney, skin, brain, lungs, eyes, and breasts. 1,25(OH)$_2$D, the biologically active metabolite of vitamin D, exerts its responses through the vitamin D receptor (VDR) via genomic and non-genomic functions [8–10]. VDR occurs ubiquitously in almost all cells and tissues, and approximately 3% of the human genome is regulated by VDR-1,25(OH)$_2$D [11]. The activity of VDR and its ligand do not fully overlap. VDR can also bind its low-affinity nutritional ligands, such as curcumin and polyunsaturated fatty acids, while alternative molecules, e.g., resveratrol, can promote the nuclear VDR signalling [12,13]. Single nucleotide variants (SNVs) in the VDR gene, which is located in chromosome 12 (12q13.11), can likely modify VDR expression and function [14,15]. Among the most studied *VDR* SNPs are *FokI* (rs2228570), *TaqI* (rs731236) and *BsmI* (rs1544410). The *FokI* (rs2228570) polymorphic variant is a T (or *f* allele) to C (or *F* allele) substitution at the *VDR* translation start site. The presence of the C allele eliminates the translation start site in exon 2, resulting in a shortened protein by three amino acids, which exerts higher transcriptional activity [14,16–18]. In a longitudinal population-based study, the T allele was associated with a higher 25(OH)D level [16]. The *BsmI* (rs1544410) variant, a G (or b allele) to A (or B allele) substitution in intron 8 and the *TaqI* (rs731236) variant, a T (or T allele) to C (or t allele) substitution in exon 9, both located at the 3' end of the *VDR*, may modify transcript stability [14,19,20].

A review by Prakash et al. provided evidence for a positive association between prevalence rates of both migraine and tension-type headache (TTH) and higher latitudes. In addition, the review pointed out that headache attacks are more frequent during autumn and winter and less prevalent during summer. Since the aforementioned observations are in accordance with regional and seasonal alterations in serum vitamin D levels, the increasing prevalence of these headache disorders seems to be related to vitamin D deficiency [21]. Likewise, a study by Mitsikostas et al. in Greece indicated that daily headache prevalence might be affected by both latitude and low mean temperature [22]. Several published scientific articles addressed the relationship between vitamin D and headache, with most of them indicating an inverse association between migraine and serum vitamin D levels [23–40]. In addition, serum VDR levels were found to be lower in migraine patients compared to controls [35]. Further to the wide expression of vitamin D receptor (VDR) and vitamin D key metabolic enzymes, including 25-hydroxylase, 1-alpha-hydroxylase (CYP27B1) and CYP24A1 in Central Nervous System (CNS) regions, vitamin D seems to be involved in various physiological brain processes, i.e., brain development, synaptic plasticity, neurotransmission, and cell death prevention [25,41–43]. SNVs in the vitamin D pathway genes, including *VDR*, *CYP2R1*, *CYP24A1* and *CYP27B1*, were associated with vitamin D serum levels [44–46]. Although the exact role of vitamin D in migraine remains obscure, vitamin D might be implicated via a variety of proposed mechanisms in the complex pathways involved in the pathophysiology of migraine [47–50].

While several prophylactic medications and pharmacological treatments alleviating migraine acute attacks are available [51], the quality of life of a great percentage of migraine patients is still declining due to improper diagnosis and/or therapeutic treatment. Thus, new diagnostic and therapeutic treatment strategies are needed to establish precision-medicine approaches, prevent migraine progression, attenuate disabilities related to the disorder and improve patient's quality of life. Since VDR has a central role in exerting the majority of 1,25(OH)$_2$D biological responses, and it occurs in various CNS regions, VDR could represent a candidate gene for migraine. The implication of VDR genetic variants in migraine pathogenesis has not been previously investigated in the Southeastern European population residing in Greece, although a study in an Iranian population provided evidence for an association between *VDR* polymorphisms and migraine susceptibility [52]. Hence, the aim of the current study was to investigate the possible association of three variants in the gene encoding for vitamin D receptor (*VDR*), namely rs2228570 (*FokI*), rs731236 (*TaqI*) and rs1544410 (*BsmI*), with migraine susceptibility and clinical phenotypes, in a Southeastern European case-control population residing in Greece. The findings of the current study may eventually shed more light on the relationship between vitamin D and migraine and contribute to the identification of molecules involved in disease pathophysiology, the discovery of new therapeutic targets, the establishment of migraine-specific biomarkers for precision medicine strategies, and to overcome the barriers in the treatment of migraine.

2. Subjects and Methods

2.1. Study Population

A total of 191 migraine subjects (33 males and 158 females) aged between 18 to 72 years (mean ± standard deviation 42.0 ± 11.5 years) were prospectively recruited in specialised headache clinics located in Glyfada and Thessaloniki, Greece, from September 2019 to July 2021 as a case group. The migraine diagnosis was made by experienced headache specialists according to the International Classification of Headache Disorders 3rd edition (ICHD-3) guidelines. Key inclusion criteria included age ≥ 18 years; clinically diagnosed migraine [1.1 migraine without aura (MwoA); 1.2 migraine with aura (MwA); or 1.3 chronic migraine (CM)]; and Southeastern European origin. A group of 265 headache-free subjects (133 males and 132 females), aged between 21 to 85 years (mean ± standard deviation 57.7 ± 12.8 years), was recruited from the Neurology Department, University Hospital of Larissa, Greece and served as a control group.

A written informed consent was provided by all study subjects. The study was approved by the appropriate Ethics Committees (Mediterraneo Hospital, Glyfada, Greece, and University Hospital of Larissa) and conducted according to the principles outlined in the Declaration of Helsinki.

2.2. DNA Extraction and Genotyping

Epithelial cell samples were collected from the oral cavity of each subject. Sterile buccal swabs were used for the collection. For the DNA extraction, a commercial nucleic acid isolation kit (Nucleospin Tissue; Macherey-Nagel GmbH & Co., KG, Düren, Germany) was used, according to the manufacturer's protocol. All extracted DNA samples were stored at −20 °C until further analysis. Genotyping of the three investigated *VDR* variants i.e., *FokI* (rs2228570), *TaqI* (rs731236), and *BsmI* (rs1544410), was carried out by real-time Polymerase Chain Reaction (LightCycler® 480; Roche) using simple probes for each SNP (LightSNiP Assays; TIBMOLBIOL, Berlin, Germany) according to the manufacturer's instructions. DNA samples (50 ng) were amplified using the respective LightSNiP Assay and LightCycler FastStart DNA Master HybProbe Mix (Roche, Germany). The following PCR protocol was applied: initial denaturation at 95 °C for 10 min, followed by 45 cycles of denaturation at 95 °C for 10 s, annealing at 60 °C for 10 s and elongation at 72 °C for 15 s. Melting curve analysis was performed to determine homozygosity for the wild-type alleles, heterozygosity, and homozygosity for the variant alleles.

2.3. Statistical Analysis

Categorical data are presented as frequencies (n) and percentages (%), and continuous data as mean ± standard deviation (SD). Differences in genotypic and allelic frequency distribution between case and control subjects and between case subgroups were evaluated using chi-square (χ^2) (Pearson or Fischer's exact) tests. Crude odds ratios (OR) with their corresponding 95% confidence intervals (95% CI) were calculated to investigate the association of the selected *VDR* variants with migraine susceptibility and clinical aspects under co-dominant, dominant, recessive, over-dominant genotypic and allelic inheritance models. To exclude any bias introduced by the differences in age and sex ratio between the study groups, adjustment for potential confounding factors, including age and sex, as well as Body Mass Index (BMI) and smoking status, was performed using logistic regression analysis. Kolmogorov–Smirnov and Shapiro–Wilks tests were used to examine the distribution of the continuous variables. Non-parametric test. i.e., Kruskal–Wallis was used to investigate the association of the three *VDR* variants with disease-specific clinical characteristics in the case subjects (disease age at onset and frequency of migraine attacks), while chi-square test and logistic regression analysis were used to assess the association of the variants with typical duration of migraine attacks (≤24 h vs. >24 h). All statistical tests were two-sided, and a *p*-value less than 0.05 was considered statistically significant. Statistical analyses were carried out using IBM SPSS Statistics software (version 28.0 for Windows). The consistency with Hardy–Weinberg Equilibrium (HWE) for *FokI* (rs2228570), *TaqI* (rs731236) and *BsmI* (rs1544410) variants in the control group was verified ($p > 0.05$) using the web-based Online Encyclopedia for Genetic Epidemiology studies software [53]. Haplotype analysis was performed using the SHEsis web-based platform (http://analysis.bio-x.cn/myAnalysis.php, accessed on 4 June 2023) [54,55]. An a posteriori power analysis was performed using G-Power software [56], which resulted in a 0.999 power for the chi-square test (degrees of freedom = 2). Thus, it confirms that the study results/conclusions were reliable and robust.

3. Results

3.1. Demographic and Clinical Characteristics

The population of the current prospective, case-control study consisted of 456 non-related subjects (191 migraine patients and 265 headache-free controls) of Southeast European origin residing in the geographical area of Greece. Detailed information on demographics and clinical disease-specific characteristics was obtained for each case subject via predesigned questionnaires. One hundred and nine (109) case subjects met the diagnostic criteria for MwoA (57.1%), 24 for MwA (12.6%) and 58 for CM (30.4%). The mean ± SD age of disease onset was 20.0 ± 8.4 years, ranging from 5 to 52 years. Positive family history was reported for 137 migraine patients (71.7%). Data collected from control subjects included only age and sex (Table 1).

Table 1. Demographic and clinical characteristics of the study population.

	Migraine Patients (N = 191)		Headache-Free Controls (N = 265)	
Age (years) *	42.0 ± 11.5 ranged from 18 to 72		57.7 ± 12.8 ranged from 21 to 85	
Sex, *n (%)*				
Male	33	(17.3)	133	(50.2)
Female	158	(82.7)	132	(49.8)
BMI (kg/m^2) *	24.6 ± 4.2		-	
Smoking, *n (%)*				
Never	116	(60.7)		-
Former	23	(12.1)		-
Ever	52	(27.2)		-
Age of onset (years) *	20.0 ± 8.4 ranged from 5 to 52		-	
Positive family history, *n (%)*	137	(71.7)		
Type of Migraine, *n (%)*				
1.1 MwoA	109	(57.1)		-
1.2 MwA	24	(12.6)		-
1.3 CM	58	(30.4)		-

* Values are presented as mean ± SD, BMI, body mass index; MwoA, Migraine without Aura; MwA, Migraine with Aura; CM, Chronic Migraine.

3.2. Associations between VDR SNVs and Migraine Phenotypes

As presented in Table 2, the genotype frequency distribution for the *TaqI* (rs731236) and *BsmI* (rs1544410) variants differed significantly between migraine and control subjects. Heterozygosity for both *TaqI* [TC vs. TT + CC: OR$_{adj}$ (95%CI) = 1.697 (1.053–2.733), p_{adj} = 0.030] and *BsmI* [GA vs. GG + AA: OR$_{adj}$ (95%CI) = 1.611 (1.002–2.592), p_{adj} = 0.049] variants was significantly more prevalent in migraine subjects compared to controls and remained significant after adjustment for age and sex. Regarding the *FokI* variant, no statistically significant differences were observed between case and control subjects in any of the genetic inheritance models assessed ($p > 0.05$) (Table 2).

Table 2. Genotypic and allelic frequency distribution analysis of the *VDR* SNPs between migraine cases and controls.

	Migraine Cases (N = 191)		Controls (N = 265)		OR (95%CI)	p	OR$_{adj}$ (95%CI) *	p_{adj} *
	n	(%)	n	(%)				
				FokI rs2228570				
CC	80	(41.9)	123	(46.4)	1.0 (reference)	-	-	-
CT	95	(49.7)	110	(41.5)	0.753 (0.508–1.116)	0.157	0.891 (0.540–1.470)	0.651
TT	16	(8.4)	32	(12.1)	1.301 (0.670–2.524)	0.436	0.988 (0.400–2.443)	0.980
CT + TT	111	(58.1)	142	(53.6)	0.832 (0.572–1.211)	0.337	0.899 (0.559–1.445)	0.659
TT	16	(8.4)	32	(12.1)	1.0 (reference)	-	-	-
CT	95	(49.7)	110	(41.5)	0.579 (0.299–1.120)	0.102	0.839 (0.362–1.942)	0.682
CT + CC	175	(91.6)	233	(87.9)	0.666 (0.354–1.252)	0.204	0.934 (0.404–2.157)	0.872
CT	95	(49.7)	110	(41.5)	1.0 (reference)	-	-	-
TT + CC	96	(50.3)	155	(58.5)	1.394 (0.959–2.028)	0.081	1.138 (0.707–1.832)	0.593
C	255	(66.8)	356	(67.2)	1.0 (reference)	-	-	-
T	127	(33.2)	174	(32.8)	0.981 (0.742–1.298)	0.895	-	-
				TaqI rs731236				
TT	65	(34.0)	102	(38.5)	1.0 (reference)	-	-	-
TC	102	(53.4)	113	(42.6)	0.706 (0.468–1.064)	0.096	0.645 (0.381–1.094)	0.104
CC	24	(12.6)	50	(18.9)	1.328 (0.745–2.366)	0.336	1.356 (0.647–2.839)	0.420
TC + CC	126	(66.0)	163	(61.5)	0.824 (0.559–1.216)	0.329	0.778 (0.475–1.274)	0.319
CC	24	(12.6)	50	(18.9)	1.0 (reference)	-	-	-
TC	102	(53.4)	113	(42.6)	0.532 (0.305–0.927)	**0.025**	0.481 (0.241–0.959)	**0.038**
TC + TT	167	(87.4)	215	(81.1)	0.618 (0.365–1.047)	0.072	0.570 (0.293–1.107)	0.097
TC	102	(53.4)	113	(42.6)	1.0 (reference)	-	-	-
CC + TT	89	(46.6)	152	(57.4)	1.542 (1.060–2.241)	**0.023**	1.697 (1.053–2.733)	**0.030**
T	232	(60.7)	317	(59.8)	1.0 (reference)	-	-	-
C	150	(39.3)	213	(40.2)	1.039 (0.794–1.360)	0.779	-	-
				BsmI rs1544410				
GG	59	(30.9)	90	(34.0)	1.0 (reference)	-	-	-
GA	109	(57.1)	119	(44.9)	0.716 (0.471–1.088)	0.117	0.713 (0.418–1.218)	0.216
AA	23	(12.0)	56	(21.1)	1.596 (0.888–2.868)	0.117	1.481 (0.705–3.115)	0.300
GA + AA	132	(69.1)	175	(66.0)	0.869 (0.583–1.295)	0.490	0.851 (0.513–1.411)	0.531
AA	23	(12.0)	56	(21.1)	1.0 (reference)	-	-	-
GA	109	(57.1)	119	(44.9)	0.448 (0.259–0.778)	**0.004**	0.473 (0.239–0.936)	**0.032**
GA + GG	168	(88.0)	209	(78.9)	0.511 (0.302–0.865)	**0.011**	0.536 (0.277–1.036)	0.064
GA	109	(57.1)	119	(44.9)	1.0 (reference)	-	-	-
AA + GG	82	(42.9)	146	(55.1)	1.631 (1.121–2.373)	**0.010**	1.611 (1.002–2.592)	**0.049**
G	227	(59.4)	299	(56.4)	1.0 (reference)	-	-	-
A	155	(40.6)	231	(43.6)	1.131 (0.866–1.477)	0.364	-	-

OR, Odds Ratio; CI, Confidence Interval * Adjusted for age and sex. Bold values indicate statistical significance.

Genotype frequency distribution analysis between migraine subtypes and control subjects revealed significant associations for all three investigated *VDR* variants with MwoA susceptibility. Homozygosity for the less common alleles of the *TaqI* [CC vs. TC + TT: OR$_{adj}$ (95%CI) = 0.427 (0.183–0.997), p_{adj} = 0.049; CC vs. TC: OR$_{adj}$ (95%CI) = 0.378 (0.157–0.908),

p_{adj} = 0.030] and *BsmI* [AA vs. GA + GG: OR_{adj} (95%CI) = 0.399 (0.170–0.934), p_{adj} = 0.034; AA vs. GA: OR_{adj} (95%CI) = 0.374 (0.156–0.898), p_{adj} = 0.028] variants was significantly less prevalent in MwoA case subjects compared to control subjects after adjusting for age and sex. Concerning the *FokI* variant, χ^2 test showed a significant difference between MwoA and controls [CT vs. CC + TT: OR (95%CI) = 1.663 (1.061–2.605), p = 0.026; CC vs. CT: OR (95%CI) = 0.621 (0.387–0.999), p = 0.049], and the significance remained after adjusting for sex, while disappeared when adjusting for both age and sex (Table 3). No significant differences in the genotype and allele frequency distributions were observed between MwA patients versus controls, CM patients versus controls or MwoA versus MwA patients (p > 0.05).

Table 3. Genotypic and allelic frequency distribution analysis of the *VDR* SNPs between Migraine without Aura (MwoA) cases and controls.

	MwoA (N = 109)		Controls (N = 265)		OR (95%CI)	p	OR_{adj} (95%CI) *	p_{adj} *
	n	(%)	n	(%)				
				FokI rs2228570				
CC	41	(37.6)	123	(46.4)	1.0 (reference)	-	-	-
CT	59	(54.1)	110	(41.5)	0.621 (0.387–0.999)	**0.049**	0.894 (0.491–1.627)	0.714
TT	9	(8.3)	32	(12.1)	1.185 (0.522–2.690)	0.684	1.291 (0.436–3.822)	0.645
CT + TT	68	(62.4)	142	(53.6)	0.696 (0.441–1.099)	0.119	0.929 (0.523–1.648)	0.800
TT	9	(8.3)	32	(12.1)	1.0 (reference)	-	-	-
CT	59	(54.1)	110	(41.5)	0.524 (0.235–1.172)	0.112	0.683 (0.238–1.963)	0.479
CT + CC	100	(91.7)	233	(87.9)	0.655 (0.302–1.423)	0.283	0.718 (0.256–2.018)	0.530
CT	59	(54.1)	110	(41.5)	1.0 (reference)	-	-	-
TT + CC	50	(45.9)	155	(58.5)	1.663 (1.061–2.605)	**0.026**	1.193 (0.676–2.105)	0.543
C	141	(64.7)	356	(67.2)	1.0 (reference)	-	-	-
T	77	(35.3)	174	(32.8)	0.895 (0.642–1.247)	0.512	-	-
				TaqI rs731236				
TT	39	(35.8)	102	(38.5)	1.0 (reference)	-	-	-
TC	59	(54.1)	113	(42.6)	0.732 (0.451–1.189)	0.207	0.731 (0.395–1.354)	0.319
CC	11	(10.1)	50	(18.9)	1.738 (0.821–3.679)	0.146	1.935 (0.759–4.932)	0.167
TC + CC	70	(64.2)	163	(61.5)	0.890 (0.560–1.415)	0.623	0.916 (0.513–1.635)	0.767
CC	11	(10.1)	50	(18.9)	1.0 (reference)	-	-	-
TC	59	(54.1)	113	(42.6)	0.421 (0.204–0.870)	**0.017**	0.378 (0.157–0.908)	**0.030**
TC + TT	98	(89.9)	215	(81.1)	0.483 (0.241–0.967)	**0.037**	0.427 (0.183–0.997)	**0.049**
TC	59	(54.1)	113	(42.6)	1.0 (reference)	-	-	-
CC + TT	50	(45.9)	152	(57.4)	1.587 (1.014–2.486)	**0.043**	1.652 (0.938–2.907)	0.082
T	137	(62.8)	317	(59.8)	1.0 (reference)	-	-	-
C	81	(37.2)	213	(40.2)	1.136 (0.821–1.573)	0.440	-	-
				BsmI rs1544410				
GG	37	(33.9)	90	(34.0)	1.0 (reference)	-	-	-
GA	62	(56.9)	119	(44.9)	0.789 (0.483–1.289)	0.344	0.853 (0.457–1.591)	0.617
AA	10	(9.2)	56	(21.1)	2.302 (1.062–4.993)	**0.032**	2.154 (0.836–5.555)	0.112
GA + AA	72	(66.1)	175	(66.0)	0.999 (0.624–1.600)	0.997	1.049 (0.581–1.893)	0.874
AA	10	(9.2)	56	(21.1)	1.0 (reference)	-	-	-
GA	62	(56.9)	119	(44.9)	0.343 (0.164–0.718)	**0.003**	0.374 (0.156–0.898)	**0.028**
GA + GG	99	(90.8)	209	(78.9)	0.377 (0.185–0.770)	**0.006**	0.399 (0.170–0.934)	**0.034**
GA	62	(56.9)	119	(44.9)	1.0 (reference)	-	-	-
AA + GG	47	(43.1)	146	(55.1)	1.618 (1.032–2.538)	**0.035**	1.511 (0.860–2.654)	0.151
G	136	(62.4)	299	(56.4)	1.0 (reference)	-	-	-
A	82	(37.6)	231	(43.6)	1.281 (0.927–1.771)	0.133	-	-

OR, Odds Ratio; CI, Confidence Interval * Adjusted for age and sex. Bold values indicate statistical significance.

The frequency distribution analysis of the *VDR* haplotypes in migraine patients versus the control group (Table 4) and MwoA patients versus controls (Table 5) did not reveal any significant associations.

Furthermore, frequency distribution analysis of the three investigated variants in subsets of migraineurs according to migraine attack duration (≤24 h vs. >24 h) indicated no significant differences. Finally, no significant association was shown for any of the *VDR* variants studied with disease-specific clinical features, i.e., age at onset and attack frequency in the study cohort ($p > 0.05$) (Table 6).

Table 4. Frequency distribution analysis of the 3 *VDR* SNPs haplotypes in migraine patients and controls.

Haplotypes				Case Frequency n (%)		Control Frequency n (%)		OR (95% CI)	*p*-Value
	FokI	TaqI	BsmI						
H1	C	T	G	151.29	(0.396)	216.90	(0.409)	0.929 (0.708–1.218)	0.592
H2	C	C	A	94.70	(0.248)	131.74	(0.249)	0.982 (0.723–1.334)	0.909
H3	T	T	G	73.68	(0.193)	82.10	(0.155)	1.289 (0.911–1.825)	0.151
H4	T	C	A	53.26	(0.139)	81.26	(0.153)	0.883 (0.607–1.285)	0.516

Table 5. Frequency distribution analysis of the 3 *VDR* SNPs haplotypes in migraine without aura (MwoA) patients and controls.

Haplotypes				MwoA Frequency n (%)		Control Frequency n (%)		OR (95% CI)	*p*-Value
	FokI	TaqI	BsmI						
H1	C	T	G	90.05	(0.413)	216.90	(0.409)	0.997 (0.721–1.378)	0.985
H2	C	C	A	45.90	(0.211)	131.74	(0.249)	0.793 (0.541–1.162)	0.234
H3	T	T	G	43.92	(0.201)	82.10	(0.155)	1.361 (0.906–2.045)	0.137
H4	T	C	A	33.07	(0.152)	81.26	(0.153)	0.975 (0.628–1.513)	0.909

Table 6. Analysis of the association of the three VDR variants with clinical features in migraineurs.

FokI rs2228570	CC	CT	TT	*p*
Migraineurs subjects (N = 191)	80	95	16	-
Age at onset (years)	20.73 ± 8.85 19 (7–52)	19.34 ± 8.40 17 (5–47)	20.19 ± 5.37 20 (5–29)	0.179
Attack frequency (days/month)	11.09 ± 8.60 8 (0.25–30)	10.81 ± 9.02 8 (1–30)	12.18 ± 8.89 10 (0.25–25)	0.773
TaqI rs731236	**TT**	**TC**	**CC**	***p***
Migraineurs subjects (N = 191)	65	102	24	-
Age at onset (years)	21.12 ± 9.27 19 (9–52)	19.34 ± 7.68 18 (5–47)	19.67 ± 8.73 18 (6–40)	0.698
Attack frequency (days/month)	11.32 ± 9.31 7 (1–30)	10.47 ± 8.33 8 (0.25–30)	12.71 ± 9.41 11 (1–30)	0.598
BsmI rs1544410	**GG**	**GA**	**AA**	***p***
Migraineurs subjects (N = 191)	59	109	23	-
Age at onset (years)	22.25 ± 9.94 19 (12–52)	18.78 ± 7.10 17 (5–45)	19.91 ± 8.84 18 (6–40)	0.200
Attack frequency (days/month)	10.81 ± 8.95 7 (1–30)	10.92 ± 8.68 8 (0.25–30)	12.17 ± 9.24 10 (1–30)	0.766

Data are presented as mean ± SD and median (min–max).

4. Discussion

To the best of the author's knowledge, the current case-control study is the first investigating the association of the three most intensively studied SNVs in *VDR*, namely *FokI* (rs222857, also known as rs10735810), *TaqI* (rs731236), and *BsmI* (rs1544410), with the susceptibility to develop migraine and diverse clinical phenotypes and features in a Southeastern European population residing in Greece. According to the genotypic and allelic frequency distribution analysis, although no significant association for the *FokI* variant with the occurrence and development of migraine was revealed in the study cohort, heterozygous TC (p_{adj} = 0.030) and GA (p_{adj} = 0.049) genotypes for the *TaqI* and *BsmI* variants, respectively, were significantly more prevalent in migraine cases compared to control subjects. Additionally, subgroup analysis revealed an association between all studied *VDR* variants and the MwoA subtype. Consequently, variability in the *VDR* gene may serve as a genetic susceptibility factor for migraine and MwoA subtype in Southeastern Europeans.

Scientific data point toward a key role of vitamin D in brain health maintenance. VDR and vitamin D metabolising enzymes are present in various brain regions, indicating the distinctive functioning of vitamin D and particularly VDR in the CNS. In addition, evidence indicates that vitamin D plays a crucial role in brain development, acts as a neuroprotective factor by controlling neurotrophic factor production, influences the release of several neurotransmitters, such as serotonin and dopamine, and serves as a potent antioxidant agent [50]. Migraine is a complex brain disorder with metabolic, hormonal, and genetic components. While multiple lines of evidence highlight a link between migraine headaches and vitamin D, with various studies denoting vitamin D deficiency or insufficiency in a great percentage of migraine sufferers, the precise relation between migraine and vitamin D deficiency remains enigmatic [38,57].

Variability in the *VDR* gene may modify VDR expression, structure, or function and, therefore, influence vitamin D signalling pathways [58]. To date, only two studies have investigated the association between *VDR* SNVs and migraine susceptibility in diverse populations. A previous study by Motaghi et al. indicated an association of *TaqI* and *FokI* SNVs with MwoA in an Iranian case-control population. Heterozygous genotypes for both *FokI* (33.9% vs. 15%, p = 0.001) and *TaqI* (50.4% vs. 36%, p = 0.018) variants were statistically more prevalent in MwoA patients compared to control subjects [52]. In accordance, the heterozygosity for *FokI* (54.1% vs. 41.5%, p = 0.026) and *TaqI* (54.1% vs. 42.6%, p = 0.043) SNVs were also more frequent in MwoA patients compared to headache-free controls in the population of the current study. On the contrary, a study by Schürks et al. investigating the relationship between 77 SNVs and migraine in a Caucasian female population with self-reported migraine found no significant association of the *VDR FokI* and *BsmI* variants with migraine [59]. A major difference between the current study and the study by Schürks et al. is the population selection; Schürks et al. included only female U.S. Caucasian health professionals aged ≥ 45 years participating in the Women's Health Study with self-reported migraine and migraine aura status, whereas the current study included both male and female migraine patients residing in Greece, diagnosed by experienced headache specialists according to the International Classification of Headache Disorders 3rd edition (ICHD-3) guidelines.

The study has certain potential limitations that should be considered when interpreting the current findings. Firstly, a limitation of the study is the relatively small sample size, which has insufficient power to detect associations with small effect size genetic variants; migraine is mainly a polygenic disorder with several genetic variants, each having a small effect size. Hence, genetic variants with small effect sizes do occur. Although adjustment for sex, age and other confounding factors was performed, the difference in sex ratio between cases and controls and the small number of male subjects in the case group due to the female preponderance of the disorder may serve as a potential limitation of the study. Moreover, investigation of other variants in the *VDR* gene and in further genes encoding for proteins implicated in vitamin D signalling systems, such as CYP2R1, CYP27B1, and

CYP24A1, was not conducted, restricting the acquisition of additional genetic information. Finally, other confounding factors, including gene–gene or gene–environment interactions, were not assessed. Therefore, larger-scale studies from diverse ethnic populations are required to obtain more definite results.

5. Conclusions

In conclusion, the findings of the current study further support a possible association of SNVs in *VDR* with the susceptibility to develop migraine and MwoA subtype. Heterozygosity for the *VDR TaqI* (TC) and *BsmI* (GA) variants may serve as a risk factor for migraine and MwoA susceptibility in the studied Southeastern European population. Despite the abovementioned limitations, the current study provides a reference for further investigations among the Southeastern European population to translate genetically derived data into clinical applications for the precision management of migraines.

Author Contributions: M.P. conceptualised the study, performed the research and data analysis, and wrote the manuscript; M.P. and M.-S.K. designed the experiments; N.D. supervised the study; M.V., V.S., E.V.D. and E.D. contributed to clinical data and specimen collection; M.P. analysed the specimens; N.D., V.S. and E.D. revised the study; A.R. revised the data analysis. All authors have read and agreed to the published version of the manuscript.

Funding: No funding was received for conducting this study.

Institutional Review Board Statement: The study was performed in accordance with the principles outlined in the Declaration of Helsinki. Approval was received by the Ethics Committee of Mediterraneo Hospital, Glyfada, Greece (protocol code: 3918/1-8-2019) and by the University Hospital of Larissa Ethics Committee.

Informed Consent Statement: All participants included in the study signed a written informed consent.

Data Availability Statement: Available upon reasonable request.

Conflicts of Interest: The authors declare that they have no conflict of interest.

References

1. Steiner, T.J.; Stovner, L.J.; Vos, T.; Jensen, R.; Katsarava, Z. Migraine Is First Cause of Disability in under 50s: Will Health Politicians Now Take Notice? *J. Headache Pain* **2018**, *19*, 17. [CrossRef]
2. Steiner, T.J.; Stovner, L.J.; Jensen, R.; Uluduz, D.; Katsarava, Z. Migraine Remains Second among the World's Causes of Disability, and First among Young Women: Findings from GBD2019. *J. Headache Pain* **2020**, *21*, 137. [CrossRef]
3. Dodick, D.W. A Phase-by-Phase Review of Migraine Pathophysiology. *Headache J. Head Face Pain* **2018**, *58*, 4–16. [CrossRef]
4. Ducros, A. Genetics of Migraine. *Rev. Neurol.* **2021**, *177*, 801–808. [CrossRef]
5. Dias, A.; Mariz, T.; Sousa, A.; Lemos, C.; Alves-Ferreira, M. A Review of Migraine Genetics: Gathering Genomic and Transcriptomic Factors. *Hum. Genet.* **2021**, *141*, 1–14. [CrossRef]
6. Papasavva, M.; Vikelis, M.; Siokas, V.; Katsarou, M.S.; Dermitzakis, E.V.; Raptis, A.; Kalliantasi, A.; Dardiotis, E.; Drakoulis, N. Variability in Oxidative Stress-Related Genes (SOD2, CAT, GPX1, GSTP1, NOS3, NFE2L2, and UCP2) and Susceptibility to Migraine Clinical Phenotypes and Features. *Front. Neurol.* **2023**, *13*, 1054333. [CrossRef]
7. Carlberg, C.; Campbell, M.J.; Park, R. Vitamin D Receptor Signaling Mecahnisms: Integrated Actions of a Well-Defined Transcription Factor. *Steroids* **2015**, *78*, 127–136. [CrossRef]
8. Christakos, S.; Dhawan, P.; Verstuyf, A.; Verlinden, L.; Carmeliet, G. Vitamin D: Metabolism, Molecular Mechanism of Action, and Pleiotropic Effects. *Physiol. Rev.* **2016**, *96*, 365–408. [CrossRef]
9. Plantone, D.; Primiano, G.; Manco, C.; Locci, S.; Servidei, S.; De Stefano, N. Vitamin D in Neurological Diseases. *Int. J. Mol. Sci.* **2022**, *24*, 87. [CrossRef]
10. Xenos, K.; Papasavva, M.; Raptis, A.; Katsarou, M.-S.; Drakoulis, N. Vitamin D Supplementation and Genetic Polymorphisms Impact on Weight Loss Diet Outcomes in Caucasians: A Randomized Double-Blind Placebo-Controlled Clinical Study. *Front. Med.* **2022**, *9*, 811326. [CrossRef]

11. Bouillon, R.; Carmeliet, G.; Verlinden, L.; van Etten, E.; Verstuyf, A.; Luderer, H.F.; Lieben, L.; Mathieu, C.; Demay, M. Vitamin D and Human Health: Lessons from Vitamin D Receptor Null Mice. *Endocr. Rev.* **2008**, *29*, 726–776. [CrossRef] [PubMed]
12. Lasoń, W.; Jantas, D.; Leśkiewicz, M.; Regulska, M.; Basta-Kaim, A. The Vitamin D Receptor as a Potential Target for the Treatment of Age-Related Neurodegenerative Diseases Such as Alzheimer's and Parkinson's Diseases: A Narrative Review. *Cells* **2023**, *12*, 660. [CrossRef]
13. Gil, Á.; Plaza-Diaz, J.; Mesa, M.D. Vitamin D: Classic and Novel Actions. *Ann. Nutr. Metab.* **2018**, *72*, 87–95. [CrossRef]
14. Poon, A.H.; Gong, L.; Brasch-Andersen, C.; Litonjua, A.A.; Raby, B.A.; Hamid, Q.; Laprise, C.; Weiss, S.T.; Altman, R.B.; Klein, T.E. Very Important Pharmacogene Summary for VDR. *Pharmacogenet. Genom.* **2012**, *22*, 758–763. [CrossRef]
15. Alhawari, H.; Jarrar, Y.; Abulebdah, D.; Abaalkhail, S.J.; Alkhalili, M.; Alkhalili, S.; Alhawari, H.; Momani, M.; Obeidat, M.N.; Fram, R.K.; et al. Effects of Vitamin D Receptor Genotype on Lipid Profiles and Retinopathy Risk in Type 2 Diabetes Patients: A Pilot Study. *J. Pers. Med.* **2022**, *12*, 1488. [CrossRef] [PubMed]
16. Dastani, Z.; Li, R.; Richards, B. Genetic Regulation of Vitamin D Levels. *Calcif. Tissue Int.* **2013**, *92*, 106–117. [CrossRef]
17. Uitterlinden, A.G.; Fang, Y.; van Meurs, J.B.J.; Pols, H.A.P.; van Leeuwen, J.P.T.M. Genetics and Biology of Vitamin D Receptor Polymorphisms. *Gene* **2004**, *338*, 143–156. [CrossRef]
18. Awasthi, R.; Manger, P.T.; Khare, R.K. Fok I and Bsm I Gene Polymorphism of Vitamin D Receptor and Essential Hypertension: A Mechanistic Link. *Clin. Hypertens.* **2023**, *29*, 5. [CrossRef]
19. Bienertová-Vašků, J.; Zlámal, F.; Pohořalá, A.; Mikeš, O.; Goldbergová-Pávková, M.; Novák, J.; Šplíchal, Z.; Pikhart, H. Allelic Variants in Vitamin D Receptor Gene Are Associated with Adiposity Measures in the Central-European Population. *BMC Med. Genet.* **2017**, *18*, 90. [CrossRef] [PubMed]
20. Saccone, D.; Asani, F.; Bornman, L. Regulation of the Vitamin D Receptor Gene by Environment, Genetics and Epigenetics. *Gene* **2015**, *561*, 171–180. [CrossRef]
21. Prakash, S.; Mehta, N.C.; Dabhi, A.S.; Lakhani, O.; Khilari, M.; Shah, N.D. The Prevalence of Headache May Be Related with the Latitude: A Possible Role of Vitamin D Insufficiency? *J. Headache Pain* **2010**, *11*, 301–307. [CrossRef] [PubMed]
22. Mitsikostas, D.D.; Tsaklakidou, D.; Athanasiadis, N.; Thomas, A. The Prevalence of Headache in Greece: Correlations to Latitude and Climatological Factors. *Headache* **1996**, *36*, 168–173. [CrossRef] [PubMed]
23. Lippi, G.; Cervellin, G.; Mattiuzzi, C. No Evidence for an Association of Vitamin D Deficiency and Migraine: A Systematic Review of the Literature. *BioMed Res. Int.* **2014**, *2014*, 827635. [CrossRef]
24. Martin, V.T.; Vij, B. Diet and Headache: Part 2. *Headache* **2016**, *56*, 1553–1562. [CrossRef]
25. Orr, S.L. The Evidence for the Role of Nutraceuticals in the Management of Pediatric Migraine: A Review. *Curr. Pain Headache Rep.* **2018**, *22*, 37. [CrossRef]
26. Wu, Z.; Malihi, Z.; Stewart, A.W.; Lawes, C.M.; Scragg, R. The Association between Vitamin D Concentration and Pain: A Systematic Review and Meta-Analysis. *Vic. Lit. Cult.* **2018**, *21*, 2022–2037. [CrossRef] [PubMed]
27. Nattagh-Eshtivani, E.; Sani, M.A.; Dahri, M.; Ghalichi, F.; Ghavami, A.; Arjang, P.; Tarighat-Esfanjani, A. The Role of Nutrients in the Pathogenesis and Treatment of Migraine Headaches: Review. *Biomed. Pharmacother.* **2018**, *102*, 317–325. [CrossRef]
28. Hancı, F.; Kabakuş, N.; Türay, S.; Bala, K.A.; Dilek, M. The Role of Obesity and Vitamin D Deficiency in Primary Headaches in Childhood. *Acta Neurol. Belg.* **2020**, *120*, 1123–1131. [CrossRef]
29. Togha, M.; Razeghi Jahromi, S.; Ghorbani, Z.; Martami, F.; Seifishahpar, M. Serum Vitamin D Status in a Group of Migraine Patients Compared with Healthy Controls: A Case–Control Study. *Headache J. Head Face Pain* **2018**, *58*, 1530–1540. [CrossRef]
30. Song, T.-J.; Chu, M.-K.; Sohn, J.-H.; Ahn, H.-Y.; Lee, S.H.; Cho, S.-J. Effect of Vitamin D Deficiency on the Frequency of Headaches in Migraine. *J. Clin. Neurol.* **2018**, *14*, 366–373. [CrossRef]
31. Donmez, A.; Orun, E.; Sonmez, F.M. Vitamin D Status in Children with Headache: A Case-Control Study. *Clin. Nutr. ESPEN* **2018**, *23*, 222–227. [CrossRef]
32. Rapisarda, L.; Mazza, M.R.; Tosto, F.; Gambardella, A.; Bono, F.; Sarica, A. Relationship between Severity of Migraine and Vitamin D Deficiency: A Case-Control Study. *Neurol. Sci.* **2018**, *39*, 167–168. [CrossRef]
33. Gazerani, P.; Fuglsang, R.; Pedersen, J.G.; Sørensen, J.; Kjeldsen, J.L.; Yassin, H.; Nedergaard, B.S. A Randomized, Double-Blinded, Placebo-Controlled, Parallel Trial of Vitamin D3 Supplementation in Adult Patients with Migraine. *Curr. Med. Res. Opin.* **2019**, *35*, 715–723. [CrossRef] [PubMed]
34. Iannacchero, R.; Costa, A.; Squillace, A.; Gallelli, L.; Cannistrà, U.; De Sarro, G. P060. Vitamin D Deficiency in Episodic Migraine, Chronic Migraine and Medication-Overuse Headache Patients. *J. Headache Pain* **2015**, *16*, A184. [CrossRef]
35. Celikbilek, A.; Gocmen, A.Y.; Zararsız, G.; Tanik, N.; Ak, H.; Borekci, E.; Delibas, N. Serum Levels of Vitamin D, Vitamin D-Binding Protein and Vitamin D Receptor in Migraine Patients from Central Anatolia Region. *Int. J. Clin. Pract.* **2014**, *68*, 1272–1277. [CrossRef] [PubMed]
36. Zandifar, A.; Masjedi, S.S.; Banihashemi, M.; Asgari, F.; Manouchehri, N.; Ebrahimi, H.; Haghdoost, F.; Saadatnia, M. Vitamin D Status in Migraine Patients: A Case-Control Study. *BioMed Res. Int.* **2014**, *2014*, 514782. [CrossRef]

37. Rebecchi, V.; Gallo, D.; Princiotta Cariddi, L.; Piantanida, E.; Tabaee Damavandi, P.; Carimati, F.; Gallazzi, M.; Clemenzi, A.; Banfi, P.; Candeloro, E.; et al. Vitamin D, Chronic Migraine, and Extracranial Pain: Is There a Link? Data from an Observational Study. *Front. Neurol.* **2021**, *12*, 651750. [CrossRef] [PubMed]
38. Ghorbani, Z.; Togha, M.; Rafiee, P.; Ahmadi, Z.S.; Rasekh Magham, R.; Haghighi, S.; Razeghi Jahromi, S.; Mahmoudi, M. Vitamin D in Migraine Headache: A Comprehensive Review on Literature. *Neurol. Sci.* **2019**, *40*, 2459–2477. [CrossRef]
39. Elsayed, D.A.; Amin, K.S.; Elsayed, I.A.; Hashim, N.A. Elucidation of the Levels of Vitamin D, Calcium, and Magnesium in the Serum of Egyptian Migraine Patients: A Case-Control Study. *Egypt. J. Neurol. Psychiatry Neurosurg.* **2020**, *56*, 43. [CrossRef]
40. Gallelli, L.; Michniewicz, A.; Cione, E.; Squillace, A.; Colosimo, M.; Pelaia, C.; Fazio, A.; Zampogna, S.; Peltrone, F.; Iannacchero, R.; et al. 25-Hydroxy Vitamin D Detection Using Different Analytic Methods in Patients with Migraine. *J. Clin. Med.* **2019**, *8*, 895. [CrossRef]
41. Eyles, D.W.; Smith, S.; Kinobe, R.; Hewison, M.; McGrath, J.J. Distribution of the Vitamin D Receptor and 1α-Hydroxylase in Human Brain. *J. Chem. Neuroanat.* **2005**, *29*, 21–30. [CrossRef]
42. Jirikowski, G.F.; Kauntzer, U.W.; Dief, A.E.E.; Caldwell, J.D. Distribution of Vitamin D Binding Protein Expressing Neurons in the Rat Hypothalamus. *Histochem. Cell Biol.* **2009**, *131*, 365–370. [CrossRef] [PubMed]
43. Cui, X.; Gooch, H.; Petty, A.; McGrath, J.J.; Eyles, D. Vitamin D and the Brain: Genomic and Non-Genomic Actions. *Mol. Cell. Endocrinol.* **2017**, *453*, 131–143. [CrossRef] [PubMed]
44. Wang, M.; Zhang, R.; Wang, M.; Zhang, L.; Ding, Y.; Tang, Z.; Wang, H.; Zhang, W.; Chen, Y.; Wang, J. Genetic Polymorphism of Vitamin D Family Genes CYP2R1, CYP24A1, and CYP27B1 Are Associated with a High Risk of Non-Alcoholic Fatty Liver Disease: A Case-Control Study. *Front. Genet.* **2021**, *12*, 717533. [CrossRef] [PubMed]
45. Galvão, A.A.; de Araújo Sena, F.; de Andrade Belitardo, E.M.M.; de Santana, M.B.R.; de Oliveira Costa, G.N.; Cruz, Á.A.; Barreto, M.L.; Costa, R.D.S.; Alcantara-Neves, N.M.; Figueiredo, C.A. Genetic Polymorphisms in Vitamin D Pathway Influence 25(OH)D Levels and Are Associated with Atopy and Asthma. *Allergy Asthma Clin. Immunol.* **2020**, *16*, 62. [CrossRef]
46. Zhou, W.; Wang, P.; Bai, Y.; Zhang, Y.; Shu, J.; Liu, Y. Vitamin D Metabolic Pathway Genes Polymorphisms and Vitamin D Levels in Association with Neonatal Hyperbilirubinemia in China: A Single-Center Retrospective Cohort Study. *BMC Pediatr.* **2023**, *23*, 275. [CrossRef]
47. Di Somma, C.; Scarano, E.; Barrea, L.; Zhukouskaya, V.; Savastano, S.; Mele, C.; Scacchi, M.; Aimaretti, G.; Colao, A.; Marzullo, P. Vitamin D and Neurological Diseases: An Endocrine View. *Int. J. Mol. Sci.* **2017**, *18*, 2482. [CrossRef]
48. Moretti, R.; Morelli, M.E.; Caruso, P. Vitamin D in Neurological Diseases: A Rationale for a Pathogenic Impact. *Int. J. Mol. Sci.* **2018**, *19*, 2245. [CrossRef]
49. Liampas, I.; Siokas, V.; Brotis, A.; Dardiotis, E. Vitamin D Serum Levels in Patients with Migraine: A Meta-Analysis. *Rev. Neurol.* **2020**, *176*, 560–570. [CrossRef]
50. Nowaczewska, M.; Wiciński, M.; Osiński, S.; Kaźmierczak, H. The Role of Vitamin D in Primary Headache–from Potential Mechanism to Treatment. *Nutrients* **2020**, *12*, 243. [CrossRef]
51. Khan, J.; Al Asoom, L.I.; Al Sunni, A.; Rafique, N.; Latif, R.; Al Saif, S.; Almandil, N.B.; Almohazey, D.; AbdulAzeez, S.; Borgio, J.F. Genetics, Pathophysiology, Diagnosis, Treatment, Management, and Prevention of Migraine. *Biomed. Pharmacother.* **2021**, *139*, 111557. [CrossRef]
52. Motaghi, M.; Haghjooy Javanmard, S.; Haghdoost, F.; Tajadini, M.; Saadatnia, M.; Rafiee, L.; Zandifar, A. Relationship between Vitamin D Receptor Gene Polymorphisms and Migraine without Aura in an Iranian Population. *BioMed Res. Int.* **2013**, *2013*, 351942. [CrossRef]
53. Rodriguez, S.; Gaunt, T.R.; Day, I.N.M. Hardy-Weinberg Equilibrium Testing of Biological Ascertainment for Mendelian Randomization Studies. *Am. J. Epidemiol.* **2009**, *169*, 505–514. [CrossRef]
54. Shi, Y.Y.; He, L. SHEsis, a Powerful Software Platform for Analyses of Linkage Disequilibrium, Haplotype Construction, and Genetic Association at Polymorphism Loci. *Cell Res.* **2005**, *15*, 97–98. [CrossRef]
55. Li, Z.; Zhang, Z.; He, Z.; Tang, W.; Li, T.; Zeng, Z.; He, L.; Shi, Y. A Partition-Ligation-Combination-Subdivision EM Algorithm for Haplotype Inference with Multiallelic Markers: Update of the SHEsis (Http://Analysis.Bio-x.Cn). *Cell Res.* **2009**, *19*, 519–523. [CrossRef]
56. Faul, F.; Erdfelder, E.; Buchner, A.; Lang, A.-G. Statistical Power Analyses Using G*Power 3.1: Tests for Correlation and Regression Analyses. *Behav. Res. Methods* **2009**, *41*, 1149–1160. [CrossRef]
57. Hussein, M.; Fathy, W.; Abd Elkareem, R.M. The Potential Role of Serum Vitamin D Level in Migraine Headache: A Case-Control Study. *J. Pain Res.* **2019**, *12*, 2529–2536. [CrossRef] [PubMed]

58. Papasavva, M.; Vikelis, M.; Siokas, V.; Katsarou, M.-S.; Dermitzakis, E.; Raptis, A.; Dardiotis, E.; Drakoulis, N. VDR Gene Polymorphisms and Cluster Headache Susceptibility: Case–Control Study in a Southeastern European Caucasian Population. *J. Mol. Neurosci.* **2022**, *72*, 382–392. [CrossRef] [PubMed]
59. Schürks, M.; Kurth, T.; Buring, J.E.; Zee, R.Y.L. A Candidate Gene Association Study of 77 Polymorphisms in Migraine. *J. Pain* **2009**, *10*, 759–766. [CrossRef] [PubMed]

Disclaimer/Publisher's Note: The statements, opinions and data contained in all publications are solely those of the individual author(s) and contributor(s) and not of MDPI and/or the editor(s). MDPI and/or the editor(s) disclaim responsibility for any injury to people or property resulting from any ideas, methods, instructions or products referred to in the content.

Headache and *NOTCH3* Gene Variants in Patients with CADASIL

Oliwia Szymanowicz [1], Izabela Korczowska-Łącka [1], Bartosz Słowikowski [2], Małgorzata Wiszniewska [3,4], Ada Piotrowska [5], Ulyana Goutor [1], Paweł P. Jagodziński [2], Wojciech Kozubski [5] and Jolanta Dorszewska [1,*]

1. Laboratory of Neurobiology, Department of Neurology, Poznan University of Medical Sciences, 61-701 Poznan, Poland
2. Department of Biochemistry and Molecular Biology, Poznan University of Medical Sciences, 61-701 Poznan, Poland
3. Faculty of Health Care, Stanislaw Staszic University of Applied Sciences in Pila, 64-920 Pila, Poland
4. Department of Neurology, Specialistic Hospital in Pila, 64-920 Pila, Poland
5. Chair and Department of Neurology, Poznan University of Medical Sciences, 61-701 Poznan, Poland
* Correspondence: jolanta.dorszewska@ump.edu.pl or dorszewskaj@yahoo.com

Abstract: Autosomal dominant cerebral arteriopathy with subcortical infarcts and leukoencephalopathy (CADASIL) is an inherited vascular disease characterized by recurrent strokes, cognitive impairment, psychiatric symptoms, apathy, and migraine. Approximately 40% of patients with CADASIL experience migraine with aura (MA). In addition to MA, CADASIL patients are described in the literature as having migraine without aura (MO) and other types of headaches. Mutations in the *NOTCH3* gene cause CADASIL. This study investigated *NOTCH3* genetic variants in CADASIL patients and their potential association with headache types. Genetic tests were performed on 30 patients with CADASIL (20 women aged 43.6 ± 11.5 and 10 men aged 39.6 ± 15.8). PCR-HRM and sequencing methods were used in the genetic study. We described three variants as pathogenic/likely pathogenic (p.Tyr189Cys, p.Arg153Cys, p.Cys144Arg) and two benign variants (p.Ala202=, p.Thr101=) in the *NOTCH3* gene and also presented the *NOTCH3* gene variant (chr19:15192257 T>G). Clinical features including headache associated with NOTCH3 (chr19:15192257 T>G) are described for the first time. Patients with pathogenic/likely pathogenic variants had similar headache courses. People with benign variants showed a more diverse clinical picture. It seems that different *NOTCH3* variants may contribute to the differential presentation of a CADASIL headache, highlighting the diagnostic and prognostic value of headache characteristics in this disease.

Keywords: headache; variants of *NOTCH3* gene; CADASIL

1. Introduction

Cerebral autosomal dominant arteriopathy with subcortical infarcts and leukoencephalopathy (CADASIL) is one of the most common hereditary, progressive diseases of small cerebral vessels. CADASIL has an estimated prevalence of two and five cases per 100,000 individuals [1]. CADASIL is characterized by common clinical manifestations, including migraine with aura (MA), young to mid-age recurrent onset of ischemic stroke, psychiatric symptoms, apathy, and cognitive disorder progressing to dementia. In addition, patients with CADASIL have an increased risk of ischemic stroke and cognitive dysfunction [2,3]. A study has reported that 60–85% of CADASIL patients experience their first and subsequent recurrent ischemic stroke with lacunar syndromes between 45 and 50 years old [4]. MA, commonly an atypical aura, affects 20–40% of patients and is the first symptom of the disease, which begins in the second or third decade of life [4,5]. Moreover, MA can occur decades before a stroke. It has also been proven that a small number of CADASIL patients experience other types of headaches [6–9].

A headache refers to pain in any region of the head. Headaches may occur on one or both sides of the head, may be isolated to a certain location, radiate across the head from a distinct point, or have a viselike quality. A headache can be experienced as a sharp pain, a throbbing sensation, or a dull ache. Headaches can develop gradually or suddenly and can last from anywhere between less than an hour and several days [10–12]. According to the 2018 International Classification of Headache Disorders Third Edition (ICHD-3) [13], more than 200 types of headaches have been identified. Headaches can be divided into three main categories: primary headaches, secondary headaches and neuralgia. Primary headaches are those that are not caused by another disease, i.e., the headache itself is the disease. Primary headaches cause episodic and chronic head pain without an underlying pathologic process, disease, or traumatic injury. The most common are migraine and tension-type headaches (TTH) [14,15]. Secondary headaches are symptoms of other diseases (for example, brain infections such as encephalitis or brain tumors) [16].

As we highlighted above, a few CADASIL patients experience other types of headache, e.g., tension-type headache (TTH) [9,17]. A TTH is generally characterized by patients having mild to moderate pain, often described as feeling like a tight band around the head. Symptoms of a TTH include dull, aching head pain, tightness or pressure across the forehead or on the sides and back of the head, and tenderness in the scalp, neck, and shoulder muscles [18].

However, most CADASIL patients experience headache pain from a migraine. As described above, migraines belong to the primary headache category and can occur even before the onset of the first stroke in CADASIL patients [6]. Migraine headaches can last from a few minutes to many hours or days and may occur daily. According to ICHD-3, the disease has two main clinical subtypes: migraine without aura (MO), commonly known as migraine, and migraine with aura (MA) [13]. MO is the more frequent form of migraine, affecting around 70% of migraineurs [19]. Symptoms include headache pain that occurs without warning and is usually felt on one side of the head, along with nausea, confusion, mood changes, fatigue, and increased sensitivity to light or sound and noise. The second clinical subtype is migraine with aura (MA), affecting about 30% of patients with CADASIL. Patients may temporarily lose part or all of their vision. Classic symptoms include speaking trouble, an abnormal sensation, numbness, muscle weakness on one side of the body, a tingling sensation in the hands or face, and confusion [13,20–23]. The aura may occur without headache pain, which can strike anytime [13]. Also, the nature of migraine headaches can change over a patient's lifetime (for example, during menopause) [24,25].

Despite the high incidence of migraines, its pathogenesis is still unknown. As with other neurological diseases, attention is now being paid to the roles of genes that may be involved in migraine pain [26]. The first genetic migraine studies focused on a rare monogeneous subtype of MA, namely familial hemiplegic migraine (FHM). In the pathogenesis of FHM type 1, 2, and 3, mutations in *CACNA1A*, *ATP1A2*, and *SCN1A* genes were identified, respectively [27–29].

As pointed out by de Vries in 2014, insights into the genetic basis of migraines may also come from other monogenic syndromes, such as CADASIL, which is caused by mutations in the *NOTCH3* gene [30]. In one particular study, patients with a mutation in the *NOTCH3* gene showed an increase in white matter hyperintensities on brain MRI, compared to controls, and MA was more common in these subjects than in their controls [31].

An analysis of several large CADASIL families has demonstrated a genetic linkage to a single disease locus on chromosome 19q12 [32]. This disease locus points to a monogenic autosomal-dominant disorder caused by a mutation in the *NOTCH3* gene, localized to chromosome 19, and consisting of 33 exons encoding the 2321 amino acid transmembrane receptor NOTCH3 [33]. The Notch family was discovered one century ago [34]. We know that mammals have four Notch receptors (Notch1, Notch2, Notch3, and Notch4) [35]. The Notch pathway leads to the expression of its target genes via translocation, post-translational modifications, and activation by its ligands. The Notch pathway leads to the expression of its target genes via translocation, post-translational modifications, and activation by its ligands. The Notch receptor, after translation, is modified in the Golgi via proteolytic cleavage at site 1 (S1) by Furin-like convertase; then, it is transported to the cell surface as a heterodimer held together by noncovalent interactions. The receptor on the signal-receiving cell is activated by ligand binding on the cell surface of a neighboring signal-sending cell. Ultimately, this induces a conformational change in the receptor to expose site 2 (S2) for cleavage by a disintegrin and metalloprotease [36,37]. Initially described in proliferating neuroepithelium, the *NOTCH3* gene and over 70% of mutations in CADASIL have been reported to occur in EGF-like repeats 3 and 4 of the Notch3 extracellular domain [38]. These are commonly missense mutations involving a cysteine residue, in which cysteine is replaced with another amino acid, but small in-frame deletions and splice-site mutations can also be found [39–41]. These mutations may involve some mechanisms associated with the mutant Notch3. The first mechanism is the local accumulation of the Notch3 extracellular domain in vascular smooth muscle due to local aggregation and impaired endocytosis. This prevents protein ubiquitination and degradation and leads to the formation of granular osmiophilic material [42,43]. The second mechanism involves reducing the transport of mutant Notch3 to the cell surface, subsequently resulting in intracellular aggregation. Another possibility includes mutations in EGF repeats 10 and 11 that may alter CBF1/RBP-jκ interaction. Mutant Notch3 receptors show no change in affinity for ligand binding, and some mutations may increase signaling [44]. The most common mutations in the *NOTCH3* gene and their protein products are presented in Table 1.

Table 1. Mutations in the *NOTCH3* gene.

Domain of NOTCH3 Protein	Mutations in the *NOTCH3* Gene
Signal peptide	L33 del, A34V
EGF-like 1	C43G, C43F, C49G, C49F, C49Y, R54C, S60C, C65S, C65Y, C67Y, W71C, R75W, R75P, C76R, C76W
EGF-like 2	77–83 del, 80–84 del, C87R, C87Y, R90C, C93F, C93Y, C93 dup, C106W, C108W, C108Y, C108R, R110C, R113Q, 114–120 del, C117F, S118C
EGF-like 3	C123F, C123Y, C128Y, C128G, C128F, G131C, R133C, C134W, D139V, R141C, F142C, C144F, C144S, C144Y, S145C, C146F, C146F, C146Y, G149C, Y150C, 153–155 del, R153C, C155S, C155Y
EGF-like 4, calcium-binding	C162S, C162W, R169C, H170R, G171C, C174F, C174R, C174Y, S180C, R182C, C183F, C183R, C183S, C185G, C185R, Y189C, C194F, C194R, C194S, C194Y
EGF-like 5	C201Y, C201R, A202E, C206Y, C206R, R207C, C209R, C212S, R213K, Y220C, C222G, C222Y, C224Y, C233S, C233Y, C233W
EGF-like 6, calcium-binding	239–253 del, V237M, C240S, C245R, C251R, C251S, C251G, Y258C, C260Y, C271F
EGF-like 7	S299C
EGF-like 8, calcium-binding	A319C, R332C, S335C, Y337C, C338R
EGF-like 9	C366W, CC379S, C379R, G382C, C388Y
EGF-like 10, calcium-binding	C395R, G420R, R421C, P426L, C428Y, C428S
EGF-like 11, calcium-binding	C435R, C440G, C440S, C446S, C446F, R449C, C455R, Y465C
EGF-like 12, calcium-binding	C484F, C484Y, C4884G, C495Y, P496L, S497L
EGF-like 13, calcium-binding	C511R, C516Y, G528C, R532C, C533Y, C542Y
Interdomain	R544C
EGF-like 14, calcium-binding	C549Y, C549R, H556R, R558C, C568Y, R578C, R578H
EGF-like 15, calcium-binding	A587C, C591R, C597W, R607C, R607H
EGF-like 16, calcium-binding	R640C, V644D

Table 1. *Cont.*

Domain of NOTCH3 Protein	Mutations in the *NOTCH3* Gene
EGF-like 17, calcium-binding	G667C, R680H
EGF-like 18	Y710C, R728C
EGF-like 19	R767H, C775S
EGF-like 20 -> EGF-like 23, calcium-binding	-
EGF-like 24	G953C
EGF-like 25	C977S, S978R, F984C, R985C, C988Y, C997G
EGF-like 26	R1006C, C1015R, A1020P, Y1021C, W1028C, R1031C
EGF-like 27	G1058C, C1061Y, D1063C, R1076C
EGF-like 28	C1099Y, Y1106C, N1118Y
EGF-like 29, calcium-binding	H1133Q, C1157W
EGF-like 30, calcium-binding	V1183M
EGF-like 31	R1231C, H1235L, R1242H
EGF-like 32	C1250W, C1261R, C1261Y
EGF-like 33	Q1297L
EGF-like 34	P1357L
LNR 1 -> LNR 3	-
HD?	L1518M, L1547V, I1586V
RAM?	L1691E, G1710D, R1748H, V1762M, R1837H
ANK 1 -> ANK 5	A1850S, A1850D, V1952M, F1995C, P2033T, P2074L, R2109Q, A2223V

Source: https://www.uniprot.org/ (accessed on 10 August 2023), https://www.omim.org/entry/600276 (accessed on 10 August 2023)

Genetic testing is the most sensitive and specific method for diagnosing CADASIL. Furthermore, it can provide a diagnosis at an early stage of life in asymptomatic persons and does not require an MRI [45]. Still, it is difficult to determine the patient's clinical course because they can progress differently, even if they have the same mutation, belong to the same family, or are twins [46].

This study aimed to observe the presence or absence of a correlation between selected genetic variants of the *NOTCH3* gene and the clinical characteristics of patients with CADASIL. This can help determine whether there are differences in the clinical picture between people with pathogenic/likely pathogenic changes and people with benign changes in the *NOTCH3* gene. For this purpose, exons 3, 4, 5, 11, and 12 of the *NOTCH3* gene were subjected to genetic testing. The typical *NOTCH3* gene mutations are localized to exons 2–24 encoding EGF-like domains. Since most mutations are present in exon 4 of *NOTCH3*, genetic analysis should begin with screening this exon and then expand to include the rest [47]. Here, we report pathogenic, likely pathogenic, and benign changes in the selected exons of the *NOTCH3* gene in patients with CADASIL and suspected or diagnosed CADASIL syndrome.

2. Patients and Methods

2.1. Patients

Throughout the period from 2017 to 2023, 53 people (34 women, 19 men) with suspected CADASIL were selected. Participants were hospitalized in the Clinical Hospital of Heliodor Święcicki in Poznań and the Specialist Hospital Stanisław Staszic in Piła. The neurobiologist referred these participants to the Neurobiology Laboratory Department of Neurology at Poznan University of Medical Sciences (PUMS) for genetic testing to detect genetic variants in the *NOTCH3* gene. Genetic changes in this gene were confirmed in

30 subjects (20 females, 10 males; 43.6 ± 11.5, 39.6 ± 15.8, respectively). Of the 30 subjects, 14 were diagnosed with MA, 3 were diagnosed with MO, 12 were diagnosed with another type of headache (e.g., TTH or other headache), and 1 subject was asymptomatic, according to the 2018 International Classification of Headache Disorders Third Edition (ICHD-3) [13]. The patients underwent neuroimaging studies. Table 2 shows the demographic data regarding the study participants with a confirmed variant in the *NOTCH3* gene. This study was approved by the PUMS Local Bioethics Committee (No. 931/17 of 4 December 2017, with extension No. 971/22 of 8 December 2022, valid until 2025).

Table 2. Demographic data of subjects with CADASIL.

Number of People (N = 30)		Female	N = 20	Male	N = 10
Age		43.6 ± 11.5		39.6 ± 15.8	
Age of CADASIL diagnosis		≤45 years old	11	≤45 years old	5
		>45 years old	9	>45 years old	5
Headache		Yes	20	Yes	9
MA		Yes	10	Yes	4
MO		Yes	3	Yes	0
Other types of headaches (N = 12)	TTH (N = 2)	Yes	1	Yes	1
	Headache (N = 10)	Yes	6	Yes	4
Family history of headache		Yes	11	Yes	4
Genetic tests of *NOTCH3*		Yes	20	Yes	10
Stroke in family history		Yes	2	Yes	1
Neuroimaging changes (MRI/CT)		Vascular changes/ischemic stroke	8	Vascular changes/ischemic stroke	2

N—number of people, F—female, M—male, MA—migraine with aura, MO—migraine without aura, TTH—tension-type headache, MRI—magnetic resonance imaging, CT—computed tomography.

2.2. Genetic Analysis

The material for genetic testing was venous blood collected for the presence of disodium edetate (EDTA). The blood samples were stored at −80 °C.

The first step involved isolating genomic DNA from venous blood using the Blood Mini Plus column isolation kit (A&A Biotechnology, Gdansk, Poland). The genetic variants of the *NOTCH3* gene were analyzed via high-resolution melt analysis (HRMA) using the CFX Connect™ Real-Time system (Bio-Rad, Hercules, CA, USA). Primers for HRMA were designed using databases available on the Internet based on the published genome sequence of the *NOTCH3* gene. Variants in exons 3, 4, 5, 11, and 12 of this gene were analyzed. The primer sequences are presented in Table 3.

To improve the conditions of the HRMA process, temperature gradient PCR (MJ Mini™ Gradient Thermal Cycler, Bio-Rad, Hercules, CA, USA) was initially performed for selected pairs of primers, optimizing annealing to the DNA template. The temperature gradient involved PCR at 55 °C–65 °C, followed by 2% agarose gel electrophoresis.

Genomic DNA was used as an intercalating dye for real-time PCR with EvaGreen (SsoFast™ EvaGreen® Supermix, Bio-Rad, USA). Melting analysis was performed, and the data were analyzed using Melting Analysis software (Bio-Rad, Hercules, CA, USA). DNA extraction from agarose using Gel-Out Kit (A&A Biotechnology, Gdansk, Poland) was performed to obtain the best quality material for sequencing. HRMA results were confirmed at an independent facility via Sanger sequencing using a 3130xl genetic analyzer (Applied Biosystems HITACHI, Beverly, MA, USA). The sequence reads were analyzed using the FinchTV application (Geospiza, Inc., Seattle, WA, USA) and confirmed using the

ClinVar (NIH, Bethesda, MD, USA), Ensembl.org (The Ensembl Genomes Project, UK), and Varsome (Saphetor SA, Lausanne, Switzerland) databases.

Table 3. Primer sequences for *NOTCH3* genetic variant analysis.

Genetic Variants of NOTCH3 Gene	Primer Sequences	Exon	Temperature of Annealing	Product Size [Base Pair, bp]
rs3815188 p.Thr101= rs28937321 p.Trp71Cys	Forward: 5′GGCCTCAGARAGAGCTGAACC3′ Reverse: 5′ACCCTCGATCTAAGGACCCC3′	3	65 °C	303 bp
rs1043994 p.Ala202=	Forward: 5′GATGGACGCTTCCTCTGCT3′ Reverse: 5′CACCCCTCTGACTCTCCTGA3′	4	62 °C	300 bp
rs371491165 p.Gln151Glu rs797045014 p.Arg153Cys rs2893369 rs28933697 p.Arg182Cys	Forward: 5′ GATGGACGCTTCCTCTGCT 3′ Reverse: 5′ CATGGTGAGGGTGCACAG 3′	4	63 °C	203 bp
rs797045015 p.Asp105Gly rs137852642 p.Arg133Cys rs371491165 p.Gln151Glu	Forward: 5′AGTCTGGAGGGGAGGTAGTC3′ Reverse: 5′ CACCCGGCACTCATCCAC 3′	4	65 °C	217 bp
rs864621965 p.Asp239_Asp253del	Forward: 5′GACCATCCTTGCCCCCTTC3′ Reverse: 5′CACCTGGCGCATGTCCAC3′	5	65 °C	209 bp
rs35793356 p.Gly594=	Forward: 5′GGCCTCAGARAGAGCTGAACC3′ Reverse: 5′ACCCTCGATCTAAGGACCCC3′	11 12	65 °C	600 bp

2.3. Statistical Analyses

GraphPad (Instant) was used to evaluate the genetic results of the study, which are presented in percentage relationships. Fisher's exact test was also used.

3. Results

In the presence of 30 individuals, our studies showed six different *NOTCH3* genetic variants, with three being described as pathogenic/likely pathogenic (p.Tyr189Cys, p.Arg153Cys, p.Cys144Arg) and two being described as benign variants (p.Ala202=, p.Thr101=). These variants have been previously described in the literature but were examined for the first time in the Polish population in our study. Moreover, we identified the *NOTCH3* gene mutation (chr19:15192257/c.382T>G p.Cys128Gly), displayed in Figure 1, which has only been mentioned once as a "de novo mutation" in CADASIL patients in the literature to date, but this is the first time we have described the clinical features including headache associated with this variant.

According to the Varsome database (accessed on 13 December 2023), the variant chr19:15192257 T>G of the *NOTCH3* gene, identified in exon 4, is located in codon 128 and encodes a cysteine [48].

The chr19:15192257 T>G variant was found in one patient (female, 45 years old) who reported episodes of MO from the age of 34 (>10 years of MO). The MO attacks lasted for at least a few hours and occurred 1–2 times a month. In addition, numerous cases of migraines and strokes have been reported among the family members of this patient. The patient was reported to the neurological ward with symptoms of paresis of the upper limbs and increasing pain in the left eye socket, with an earlier diagnosis of strabismus. Imaging studies (MRI, CT) showed no changes in vascular origin.

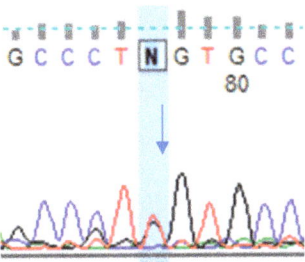

Figure 1. Heterozygous variant in the *NOTCH3* gene, chr19:15192257 T>G. A clinical characteristics of this variant not yet been described in the literature (analyzed according to the following database: https://varsome.com/) (accessed on 13 December 2023).

The pathogenic variant p.Tyr189Cys (c.566A>G) of the *NOTCH3* gene was identified in exon 4, representing a classic pathogenic CADASIL mutation involving a change in the number of cysteine residues from six to seven [49]. This variant was detected in three women belonging to one family. All three subjects (100%) had a common clinical characterization: MA, the onset of migraine around 20 years of age, migraines triggered following highly stressful situations (severe stress in life, partum, pregnancy), attacks lasting approximately two days, 1–2 times or 3–4 times per month with changes of vascular origin in the MRI/CT image.

In one person, out of 30 subjects, the presence of the p.Arg153Cys variant (c.457C>T, rs797045014) of the *NOTCH3* gene was found. In this variant, the A allele was observed instead of the standard G allele, resulting in the addition of an arginine instead of a cysteine in the protein's amino acid sequence [50]. This variant was identified in a 63-year-old woman with headaches lasting less than 24 h and occurring 1–2 times a month. The CT scan showed numerous ischemic changes in the periventricular white matter. In this patient, along with the pathogenic variant, the benign p.Thr101= variant was also detected.

In exon 4, a likely pathogenic variant, p.Cys144Arg (c.1630C>T, rs2046934287), was also identified. According to the ClinVar database, this variant breaks a cysteine residue in the EGF-like repeat domain, which is important for the structure of the protein [51]. The p.Cys144Arg variant was identified in a 53-year-old female. This patient was diagnosed with headaches >4 times per month. In addition, neuroimaging studies showed extensive hypodense changes in the brain's white matter. The patient's medical history contained information regarding numerous strokes occurring in her family members. Two benign variants, p.Ala202= and p.Thr101=, were also detected in this patient.

The first benign variant of the *NOTCH3* gene, p.Ala202= (c.606A>G, rs1043994), was identified in sixteen patients. According to the ClinVar database (NIH, USA), this variant is a synonymous variant in exon 4 that ensures that the replacement of a single nucleotide does not result in a change in the amino acid encoded by the nucleotide sequence [52]. Of the sixteen patients with this variant, nine (57%) had MA, one had MO (6%), one had TTH (6%), four had other headaches (25%), and one was asymptomatic (6%). The headaches lasted for <24 h, 24–48 h, or >48 h in fourteen (88%), one (6%), and one (6%) subjects, respectively. Ten people (63%) had headaches 1–2 times a month, two people (12%) had headaches 3–4 times a month, and four people (25%) had headaches >4 times a month. Only three subjects (19%) reported vascular changes in neuroimaging studies (MRI/CT). Thirteen people (81%) showed no changes regarding vascular origin.

The benign variant p.Ala202= was detected in a family of three whose members presented a different clinical picture. The mother (I-1, 46 years old) has been suffering from MA for ten years (onset at the age of 36), and her 18-year-old son (II-1) has suffered from tension-related disorders for ten years (onset at the age of 8). Both the mother and son had similar headaches, which occurred two to three times a month and lasted several minutes. However, numerous bilateral periventricular ischemic changes were found only in the mother's computed tomography. The second son (II-2, 21 years old), who did not have headaches, was also examined (Figure 2).

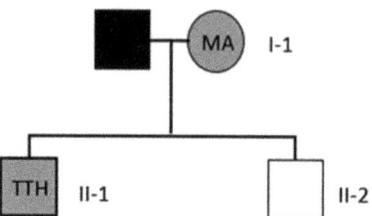

Figure 2. The pedigree of the Polish family with the p.Ala202= NOTCH3 variant. Black—no data; grey—symptomatic patients; white—patients without headache.

The second benign variant of the *NOTCH3* gene, p.Thr101= (c.303C>T, rs3815188), was detected in exon 3. p.Thr101= is a synonymous variant, where the replacement of a single nucleotide does not result in a change in the amino acid [53]. This variant was present in eight individuals with the benign variant p.Ala202=. Of the eight patients, five (61%) had MA, one had MO (13%), one had TTH (13%), and one had other type of headache (13%). Headaches lasted for <24 h, 24–48 h, or >48 h in four subjects (50%), three subjects (37%), and one subject (13%), respectively. Three people (37%) had a headache 1–2 times a month, one person (13%) had a headache 3–4 times a month, and four people (50%) had a headache >4 times a month. Only two (25%) showed vascular changes in the neuroimaging studies (MRI/CT).

The results suggest that the pathogenic/likely pathogenic variants (p.Tyr189Cys, p.Arg153Cys, p.Cys144Arg) of *NOTCH3* were more correlated with MA, while the benign variants (p.Ala202=, p.Thr101= and p.Ala202=) appeared to be more associated with different types of headaches, including MO, tension-type headaches, and other types of headaches (Fisher's exact test, $p = 0.0233$).

Table 4 shows the identified genetic variants of the *NOTCH3* gene and the clinical characteristics of the CADASIL patients in whom these changes were detected.

Table 4. Genetic variants of the *NOTCH3* gene and the clinical characteristics of patients with CADASIL.

NOTCH3 Genetic Variant	Clinical Significance	Number of Patients	Age of Patient [Mean Age ± SD or Single Results]	Type of Headache					Headache Attack Duration [Hours]				Number of Headache Attacks [Per Month]				Changes in the MRI/CT Image		References
				MA	MO	Other Types of Headaches		No Headache	<24	24–48	>48		1–2	3–4	>4		Vascular Changes/Ischemic Stroke	No Changes	
						TTH	Other												
p.Tyr189Cys	Pathogenic	3	34.0 ± 1.0	3	0	0	0	0	0	0	3		2	1	0		2	1	[49]
p.Arg153Cys	Pathogenic	1	63	0	0	0	1	0	1	0	0		1	0	0		1	0	[50]
p.Thr101=	Benign																		
p.Cys144Arg	Likely pathogenic	1	53	0	0	0	1	0	1	0	0		0	0	1		1	0	[51]
p.Ala202= p.Thr101=	Benign																		
p.Ala202=	Benign	16	39.9 ± 13.0	9	1	1	4	1	14	1	1		10	2	4		3	13	[52]
p.Thr101= and p.Ala202=	Benign	8	45.9 ± 13.5	5	1	1	1	0	4	3	1		3	1	4		2	6	[53]
chr19:15192257 T>G, exon 4, codon: 128, Cysteine	Not confirmed in the literature	1	45	0	1	0	0	0	1	0	0		1	0	0		0	1	Varsome page [48]

SD—standard deviation, MA—migraine with aura, MO—migraine without aura, TTH—tension-type headache, MRI—magnetic resonance imaging, CT—computed tomography. Fisher's exact test was used, statistically significant differences between MA and other headaches ($p < 0.05$).

4. Discussion

In this study, we aimed to assess the clinical features of headaches in CADASIL patients whose marked genetic variant determined pathogenicity. Our research contributes to investigating whether MA is the first symptom of CADASIL, appearing several years before the onset of ischemic events. Singhal et al. [54] in 2004 and Narayan et al. in 2012 [55], during their CADASIL studies, focused on MA symptoms and found no relationship between the mutation site and clinical phenotype.

Three pathogenic/likely pathogenic variants, two benign variants, and one variant of the *NOTCH3* gene (chr19:15192257 T>G) have been reported in the literature [48], but the detailed clinical significance last variant and clinical picture of a patient with this variant has not been presented.

Among the three people with the pathogenic p.Tyr189Cys variant of the *NOTCH3* gene, we observed a common phenotype: MA (100%), onset at a young age (around 20 years old), onset of headaches after severe experiences (high stress, pregnancy, childbirth), attacks lasting about 2 days, 1–2 times or 3–4 times a month with changes of vascular origin in the MRI/CT image. A detailed clinical picture of this family was presented by Dorszewska et al. [49]. However, it should be noted that knowledge about the role of the pathogenic p.Tyr189Cys variant of the *NOTCH3* gene in MA and CADASIL remains limited, and further research on this variant is needed.

The second pathogenic variant reported in our study, p.Arg153Cys, is already known, primarily in the context of CADASIL [1,56–60]. In 2016, He et al. [57] confirmed phenotypic changes in a patient with the p.Arg153Cys genetic variant. They performed a skin biopsy, which confirmed the accumulation of GOM in the basal layer of vascular smooth muscle cells, and neuroimaging tests showed diffuse white matter hyperintensities. In 2000, Ceroni et al. [61] described an Italian family with eight affected members who exhibited autosomal dominant migraine with prolonged visual, sensory, motor, and aphasic auras. These symptoms were associated with white matter abnormalities following brain MRI. All living affected members carry the *NOTCH3* (p.Arg153Cys) mutation previously reported with CADASIL. The same situation was described by Guey et al. [62] in 2016. The patient identified with the p.Arg153Cys variant suffered from MA, specifically an atypical aura that included a motor aura. In our study, a woman with the p.Arg153Cys reported headaches without aura or motor and visual abnormalities. Her headaches lasted for <24/h and occurred 1–2 times a month. However, similarly to what was described by Zhu et al. [63], she had ischemic changes in the periventricular white matter, which were made apparent upon MRI imaging. However, it is worth emphasizing that the benign variant p.Thr101= was also present in our patient.

The likely pathogenic variant p.Cys144Arg was detected in only one CADASIL patient, a 53-year-old female who had been reporting headaches for only a year (late-onset at 52). However, she experienced headaches frequently (>4 times a month). In addition, extensive vascular changes in the white matter were detected in the patient. No visual aura, motor abnormalities, or other symptoms related to MA or MO were described in this patient. However, research on this variant is very limited. As described in the ClinVar database, the p.Cys144Arg variant disrupts a cysteine residue in an EGF-like repeat domain, which is important for the structure of the protein. Therefore, it is expected to severely affect the protein's function [51]. Due to the lack of literature data, we assume that this variant may be another genetic variant of probable importance in the diagnosis of CADASIL, but so far, no efforts have been devoted to understanding the influence of this variant in relation to headaches in a patient with CADASIL. Moreover, two benign variants of the *NOTCH3* gene were also identified in this patient: p.Ala202= and p.Thr101=.

A benign variant, p.Thr101=, of the *NOTCH3* gene has been previously studied in the context of CADASIL [64–68]. The results of these types of studies are varied. Keat Wei et al. [69] and González-Giraldo et al. [70] concluded that this mild variant probably does not play a major role in the pathogenesis of CADASIL. He concluded that due to the high prevalence of this variant in the general population, it does not affect the further development of CADASIL in patients suffering from headaches. According to the Ensemble.org database [71], the frequency of the wild-type T allele in the European population is 85%, and the frequency of the alternative C allele in the European population is 15%. The results of our study confirmed its frequent occurrence in the Polish population. We found its presence in 8 of the 30 people tested. In addition, we confirmed the correlation between headaches and CADASIL in approximately 25% of those tested who have been diagnosed with ischemic events. We showed that its presence may be associated with MO (13% of patients). In the Polish population, most subjects with this genetic variant had symptoms of MA (61% of patients). We also showed that the clinical picture pertaining to headaches is not homogenous and can include TTH and other headaches in addition to MA and MO.

The second benign variant, p.Ala202=, was described as probably not a risk factor for migraine in CADASIL because the polymorphic A allele was more common in healthy individuals than in those with migraine [31]. However, in our study, we identified this variant in three people of the same family who had different headache courses in CADASIL. The 46-year-old mother in this family has been suffering from MA for 10 years (onset 36), while her 18-year-old son has suffered from tension-type headaches for 10 years (onset at the age of 8). Both the mother and son have similar headaches that occur 2–3 times a month and last for several minutes. Menon et al. mentioned that CADASIL patients had episodes of headache among their symptoms [72]. Numerous bilateral periventricular ischemic changes were present only in the mother's computed tomography results. The second, older son (21 years old) was shown to have the same genetic variant but has not had any headaches or other symptoms of CADASIL. Moreover, the mother's illness began at the age of 36; thus, it could be associated with pregnancy and childbirth [24,25]. In turn, the younger son's TTH appeared as early as 8 years of age due to the onset of puberty [73,74]. Both cases in the family appear to be hormonal.

The chr19:15192257 T>G variant was first reported by Coto et al. in 2006 [75]. The authors describe a 44-year-old patient with CADASIL symptoms, in whom this genetic variant was confirmed. Interestingly, the authors emphasize that the parents of this patient were neurologically healthy and did not carry this mutation. They also emphasize the need for further analyses of *NOTCH3* gene variants in people with CADASIL symptoms but with a family history. Despite reporting a new mutation in exon 4 of the *NOTCH3* gene, Coto et al. [75] did not provide a detailed clinical picture of the patient with this change. In our study, we described the patient's CADASIL picture depending on the type of headache that was one of the symptoms.

A patient with a chr19:15192257 T>G genetic variant of the *NOTCH3* was diagnosed with MO. The onset of MO occurred at the age of 34. This patient's MO attacks lasted several hours and appeared 1–2 times a month. The patient was reported to the neurological ward with symptoms of paresis of the upper limbs and increasing pain in the left eye socket, with an earlier diagnosis of strabismus. However, neuroimaging studies did not show ischemic changes. Moreover, numerous cases of migraines and strokes have been reported among family members of this patient.

It should be remembered that research on identifying genes involved in the pathogenesis of headaches is still ongoing [76–78]. However, understanding the genes directly involved in headaches may help to diagnose diseases in which headaches are an important symptom that often indicate the onset of an disease. Moreover, it should be remembered that various headaches may occur with CADASIL [79].

5. Conclusions

The present research study has shown that genetic variants of the *NOTCH3* gene may be associated with the presence or absence of headaches during CADASIL or several years before their onset as a harbinger of the disease. Moreover, if the same pathogenic or benign genetic change is present, even in the same family, headache symptoms may vary and present as MA and MO, TTH, and others. Studies with *NOTCH3* genetic variants as a diagnostic and therapeutic factor, especially in the context of headaches, should conduct further research on larger groups of people, including relatives and those without a family history of the condition.

Author Contributions: Conceptualization, J.D.; design and composition, J.D., O.S., I.K.-Ł., B.S., M.W., W.K., A.P. and P.P.J.; writing—original draft preparation, J.D., O.S. and I.K.-Ł.; and writing—review and editing, U.G. and J.D. All authors have read and agreed to the published version of the manuscript.

Funding: This research article received no external funding.

Institutional Review Board Statement: This study was approved by the PUMS Local Bioethics Committee (No. 931/17 of 4 December 2017, with extension No. 971/22 of 8 December 2022, valid until 2025).

Informed Consent Statement: Informed consent was obtained from all subjects involved in the study.

Data Availability Statement: Data is contained within the article.

Conflicts of Interest: The authors declare no conflict of interest.

References

1. Mizuno, T.; Mizuta, I.; Watanabe-Hosomi, A.; Mukai, M.; Koizumi, T. Clinical and genetic aspects of CADASIL. *Front. Aging Neurosci.* **2020**, *12*, 91. [CrossRef] [PubMed]
2. Granild-Jensen, J.A.; Jensen, U.B.; Schwartz, M.; Hansen, U.S. Cerebral autosomal dominant arteriopathy with subcortical infarcts and leukoencephalopathy resulting in stroke in an 11-year-old male. *Dev. Med. Child Neurol.* **2009**, *51*, 754–757. [CrossRef] [PubMed]
3. Pescini, F.; Nannucci, S.; Bertaccini, B.; Salvadori, E.; Bianchi, S.; Ragno, M.; Sarti, C.; Valenti, R.; Zicari, E.; Moretti, M.; et al. The cerebral autosomal-dominant arteriopathy with subcortical infarcts and leukoencephalopathy (CADASIL) scale: A screening tool to select patients for *NOTCH3* gene analysis. *Stroke* **2012**, *43*, 2871–2876. [CrossRef] [PubMed]
4. Chabriat, H.; Joutel, A.; Dichgans, M.; Tournier-Lasserve, E.; Bousser, M.G. Cadasil. *Lancet Neurol.* **2009**, *8*, 643–653. [CrossRef]
5. Di Donato, I.; Bianchi, S.; De Stefano, N.; Dichgans, M.; Dotti, M.T.; Duering, M.; Jouvent, E.; Korczyn, A.D.; Lesnik-Oberstein, S.A.; Malandrini, A.; et al. Cerebral autosomal dominant arteriopathy with subcortical infarcts and leukoencephalopathy (CADASIL) as a model of small vessel disease: Update on clinical, diagnostic, and management aspects. *BMC Med.* **2017**, *15*, 41. [CrossRef]
6. Dichgans, M.; Mayer, M.; Uttner, I.; Brüning, R.; Müller-Höcker, J.; Rungger, G.; Ebke, M.; Klockgether, T.; Gasser, T. The phenotypic spectrum of CADASIL: Clinical findings in 102 cases. *Ann. Neurol.* **1998**, *44*, 731–739. [CrossRef]
7. Chabriat, H.; Vahedi, K.; Iba-Zizen, M.T.; Joutel, A.; Nibbio, A.; Nagy, T.G.; Krebs, M.O.; Julien, J.; Dubois, B.; Ducrocq, X.; et al. Clinical spectrum of CADASIL: A study of 7 families. Cerebral autosomal dominant arteriopathy with subcortical infarcts and leukoencephalopathy. *Lancet* **1995**, *346*, 934–939. [CrossRef]
8. Desmond, D.W.; Moroney, J.T.; Lynch, T.; Chan, S.; Chin, S.S.; Mohr, J.P. The natural history of CADASIL: A pooled analysis of previously published cases. *Stroke* **1999**, *30*, 1230–1233. [CrossRef]
9. Russell, M.B.; Rasmussen, B.K.; Fenger, K.; Olesen, J. Migraine without aura and migraine with aura are distinct clinical entities: A study of four hundred and eighty-four male and female migraineurs from the general population. *Cephalalgia* **1996**, *16*, 239–245. [CrossRef]
10. Digre, K.B. Headaches and other head pain. In *Goldman-Cecil Medicine*, 25th ed.; Saunders Elsevier: Amsterdam, The Netherlands, 2016.
11. Friedman, B.W.; Lipton, R.B. Headache emergencies: Diagnosis and management. *Neurol. Clin.* **2012**, *30*, 43–59. [CrossRef]
12. Green, M.W. Secondary headaches. *Contin. Lifelong Learn. Neurol.* **2012**, *18*, 783–795. [CrossRef] [PubMed]
13. Headache Classification Committee of the International Headache Society (IHS). The International Classification of Headache Disorders, 3rd edition (beta version). *Cephalalgia* **2013**, *33*, 629–808. [CrossRef] [PubMed]
14. Mier, R.W.; Dhadwal, S. Primary Headaches. *Dent. Clin. N. Am.* **2018**, *62*, 611–628. [CrossRef] [PubMed]
15. Stovner, L.; Hagen, K.; Jensen, R.; Katsarava, Z.; Lipton, R.; Scher, A.; Steiner, T.; Zwart, J.A. The global burden of headache: A documentation of headache prevalence and disability worldwide. *Cephalalgia* **2007**, *27*, 193–210. [CrossRef] [PubMed]
16. May, A. Hints on Diagnosing and Treating Headache. *Dtsch. Arztebl. Int.* **2018**, *115*, 299–308. [CrossRef] [PubMed]
17. Lee, Y.C.; Liu, C.S.; Chang, M.H.; Lin, K.P.; Fuh, J.L.; Lu, Y.C.; Liu, Y.F.; Soong, B.W. Population-specific spectrum of NOTCH3 mutations, MRI features and founder effect of CADASIL in Chinese. *J. Neurol.* **2009**, *256*, 249–255. [CrossRef] [PubMed]
18. Hassan, M.; Asaad, T. Tension-type headache, its relation to stress, and how to relieve it by cryotherapy among academic students. *Middle East Curr. Psychiatry* **2020**, *27*, 20. [CrossRef]
19. Mattsson, P.; Lundberg, P.O. Characteristics and prevalence of transient visual disturbances indicative of migraine visual aura. *Cephalalgia* **1999**, *19*, 479–484. [CrossRef]

20. Safiri, S.; Pourfathi, H.; Eagan, A.; Mansournia, M.A.; Khodayari, M.T.; Sullman, M.J.M.; Kaufman, J.; Collins, G.; Dai, H.; Bragazzi, N.L.; et al. Global, regional, and national burden of migraine in 204 countries and territories, 1990 to 2019. *Pain* **2022**, *163*, 293–309. [CrossRef]
21. Woldeamanuel, Y.W.; Cowan, R.P. Migraine affects 1 in 10 people worldwide featuring recent rise: A systematic review and meta-analysis of community-based studies involving 6 million participants. *J. Neurol. Sci.* **2017**, *372*, 307–315. [CrossRef]
22. Polk, A.N.; Smitherman, T.A. A meta-analytic review of acceptance-based interventions for migraine. *Headache* **2023**. *online ahead of print*. [CrossRef] [PubMed]
23. Queiroz, L.P.; Friedman, D.I.; Rapoport, A.M.; Purdy, R.A. Characteristics of migraine visual aura in Southern Brazil and Northern USA. *Cephalalgia* **2011**, *31*, 1652–1658. [CrossRef] [PubMed]
24. Pavlović, J.M. The impact of midlife on migraine in women: Summary of current views. *Womens Midlife Health* **2020**, *6*, 11. [CrossRef] [PubMed]
25. Ripa, P.; Ornello, R.; Degan, D.; Tiseo, C.; Stewart, J.; Pistoia, F.; Carolei, A.; Sacco, S. Migraine in menopausal women: A systematic review. *Int. J. Womens Health* **2015**, *7*, 773–782.
26. Burstein, R.; Noseda, R.; Borsook, D. Migraine: Multiple processes, complex pathophysiology. *J. Neurosci.* **2015**, *35*, 6619–6629. [CrossRef]
27. Ophoff, R.A.; Terwindt, G.M.; Vergouwe, M.N.; Oefner, R.; van Eijk, P.J.; Hoffman, S.M.; Lamerdin, J.E.; Mohrenweiser, H.W.; Bulman, D.E.; Ferrari, M.; et al. Familial hemiplegic migraine and episodic ataxia type-2 are caused by mutations in the Ca^{2+} channel gene CACNL1A4. *Cell* **1996**, *87*, 543–552. [CrossRef]
28. De Fusco, M.; Marconi, R.; Silvestri, L.; Atorino, L.; Rampoldi, L.; Morgante, L.; Ballabio, A.; Aridon, P.; Casari, G. Haploinsufficiency of ATP1A2 encoding the Na^+/K^+ pump alpha2 subunit associated with familial hemiplegic migraine type 2. *Nat. Genet.* **2003**, *33*, 192–196. [CrossRef]
29. Dichgans, M.; Freilinger, T.; Eckstein, G.; Babini, E.; Lorenz-Depiereux, B.; Biskup, S.; Ferrari, M.D.; Herzog, J.; van den Maagdenberg, A.M.; Pusch, M.; et al. Mutation in the neuronal voltage-gated sodium channel SCN1A in familial hemiplegic migraine. *Lancet* **2005**, *366*, 371–377. [CrossRef]
30. de Vries, B.; Haan, J.; van den Maagdenberg, A.M.J.M.; Ferrari, M.D. Migraine. Genetics; In *Encyclopedia of the Neurological Sciences*, 2nd ed.; Aminoff, M.J., Daroff, R.B., Eds.; Academic Press: Oxford, UK, 2014; pp. 42–46.
31. Schwaag, S.; Evers, S.; Schirmacher, A.; Stögbauer, F.; Ringelstein, E.B.; Kuhlenbäumer, G. Genetic variants of the NOTCH3 gene in migraine-a mutation analysis and association study. *Cephalalgia* **2006**, *26*, 158–161. [CrossRef]
32. Tournier-Lasserve, E.; Joutel, A.; Melki, J.; Weissenbach, J.; Mark Lathrop, G.; Chabriat, H.; Mas, J.-L.; Cabanis, E.-A.; Baudrimont, M.; Maciazek, J.; et al. Cerebral autosomal dominant arteriopathy with subcortical infarcts and leukoencephalopathy maps to chromosome 19q12. *Nat. Genet.* **1993**, *3*, 256–259. [CrossRef]
33. Ungaro, C.; Mazzei, R.; Conforti, F.L.; Sprovieri, T.; Servillo, P.; Liguori, M.; Citrigno, L.; Gabriele, A.L.; Magariello, A.; Patitucci, A.; et al. Cadasil: Extended polymorphisms and mutational analysis of the NOTCH3 gene. *J. Neurosci. Res.* **2009**, *87*, 1162–1167. [CrossRef] [PubMed]
34. Wang, M.M. Notch signaling and Notch signaling modifiers. *Int. J. Biochem. Cell Biol.* **2011**, *43*, 1550–1562. [CrossRef] [PubMed]
35. Kopan, R.; Ilagan, M.X. The canonical Notch signaling pathway: Unfolding the activation mechanism. *Cell* **2009**, *137*, 216–233. [CrossRef]
36. Aburjania, Z.; Jang, S.; Whitt, J.; Jaskula-Stzul, R.; Chen, H.; Rose, J.B. The Role of Notch3 in Cancer. *Oncologist* **2018**, *23*, 900–911. [CrossRef] [PubMed]
37. Stephenson, N.L.; Avis, J.M. Direct observation of proteolytic cleavage at the S2 site upon forced unfolding of the Notch negative regulatory region. *Proc. Natl. Acad. Sci. USA* **2012**, *109*, E2757–E2765. [CrossRef] [PubMed]
38. Joutel, A.; Vahedi, K.; Corpechot, C.; Troesch, A.; Chabriat, H.; Vayssière, C.; Cruaud, C.; Maciazek, J.; Weissenbach, J.; Bousser, M.G.; et al. Strong clustering and stereotyped nature of Notch3 muations in CADASIL patients. *Lancet* **1997**, *350*, 1511–1515. [CrossRef]
39. Duering, M.; Karpinska, A.; Rosner, S.; Hopfner, F.; Zechmeister, M.; Peters, N.; Kremmer, E.; Haffner, C.; Giese, A.; Dichgans, M.; et al. Co-aggregate formation of CADASIL-mutant NOTCH3: A single-particle analysis. *Hum. Mol. Genet.* **2011**, *20*, 3256–3265. [CrossRef]
40. Meng, H.; Zhang, X.; Yu, G.; Lee, S.J.; Chen, Y.E.; Prudovsky, I.; Wang, M.M. Biochemical characterization and cellular effects of CADASIL mutants of NOTCH3. *PLoS ONE* **2012**, *7*, 44964. [CrossRef]
41. Opherk, C.; Duering, M.; Peters, N.; Karpinska, A.; Rosner, S.; Schneider, E.; Bader, B.; Giese, A.; Dichgans, M. CADASIL mutations enhance spontaneous multimerization of NOTCH3. *Hum. Mol. Genet.* **2009**, *18*, 2761–2767. [CrossRef]
42. Joutel, A.; Andreux, F.; Gaulis, S.; Domenga, V.; Cecillon, M.; Battail, N.; Piga, N.; Chapon, F.; Godfrain, C.; Tournier-Lasserve, E. The ectodomain of the Notch3 receptor accumulates within the cerebrovasculature of CADASIL patients. *J. Clin. Investig.* **2000**, *105*, 597–605. [CrossRef]
43. Yamamoto, Y.; Craggs, L.J.; Watanabe, A.; Booth, T.; Attems, J.; Low, R.W.; Oakley, A.E.; Kalaria, R.N. Brain microvascular accumulation and distribution of the NOTCH3 ectodomain and granular osmiophilic material in CADASIL. *J. Neuropathol. Exp. Neurol.* **2013**, *72*, 416–431. [CrossRef] [PubMed]

44. Haritunians, T.; Chow, T.; De Lange, R.P.; Nichols, J.T.; Ghavimi, D.; Dorrani, N.; St Clair, D.M.; Weinmaster, G.; Schanen, C. Functional analysis of a recurrent missense mutation in Notch3 in CADASIL. *J. Neurol. Neurosurg. Psychiatry* **2005**, *76*, 1242–1248. [CrossRef] [PubMed]
45. Rutten, J.W.; Dauwerse, H.G.; Gravesteijn, G.; van Belzen, M.J.; van der Grond, J.; Polke, J.M.; Bernal-Quiros, M.; Lesnik-Oberstein, S.A. Archetypal NOTCH3 mutations frequent in public exome: Implications for CADASIL. *Ann. Clin. Transl. Neurol.* **2016**, *3*, 844–853. [CrossRef]
46. Mykkänen, K.; Junna, M.; Amberla, K.; Bronge, L.; Kääriäinen, H.; Pöyhönen, M.; Kalimo, H.; Viitanen, M. Different clinical phenotypes in monozygotic CADASIL twins with a novel NOTCH3 mutation. *Stroke* **2009**, *40*, 2215–2218. [CrossRef] [PubMed]
47. Kowalska, M.; Wize, K.; Wieczorek, I.; Kozubski, W.; Dorszewska, J. Migraine and risk factors of vascular diseases. In *Ischemic Stroke of Brain*; Sanchetee, P., Ed.; IntechOpen: London, UK; Rijeka, Croatia, 2018; pp. 1–20.
48. Varsome.com. Available online: https://varsome.com/position/hg38/19:15192257 (accessed on 13 December 2023).
49. Dorszewska, J.; Kowalska, M.; Grzegorski, T.; Dziewulska, D.; Karmelita-Katulska, K.; Barciszewska, A.; Prendecki, M.; Gorczyński, W.; Kozubski, W. Clinical presentation of Y189C mutation of the *NOTCH3* gene in the Polish family with CADASIL. *Folia Neuropathol.* **2020**, *58*, 83–92. [CrossRef]
50. Varsome.com. Available online: https://varsome.com/variant/hg38/chr19:15192073:T:C? (accessed on 10 August 2023).
51. NCBI.NLM.NIH.GOV Internet Site. Available online: https://www.ncbi.nlm.nih.gov/clinvar/variation/995327/ (accessed on 10 August 2023).
52. NCBI.NLM.NIH.GOV Internet Site. Available online: https://www.ncbi.nlm.nih.gov/clinvar/variation/256148/?oq=rs1043994&m=NM_000435.3(NOTCH3):c.606A%3EG%20(p.Ala202=) (accessed on 10 August 2023).
53. NCBI.NLM.NIH.GOV Internet site. Available online: https://www.ncbi.nlm.nih.gov/clinvar/variation/256131/?oq=rs3815188&m=NM_000435.3(NOTCH3):c.303C%3ET%20(p.Thr101=) (accessed on 10 August 2023).
54. Singhal, S.; Bevan, S.; Barrick, T.; Rich, P.; Markus, H.S. The influence of genetic and cardiovascular risk factors on the CADASIL phenotype. *Brain* **2004**, *127*, 2031–2038. [CrossRef]
55. Narayan, S.K.; Gorman, G.; Kalaria, R.N.; Ford, G.A.; Chinnery, P.F. The minimum prevalence of CADASIL in northeast England. *Neurology* **2012**, *78*, 1025–1027. [CrossRef]
56. Ni, W.; Zhang, Y.; Zhang, L.; Xie, J.-J.; Li, H.-F.; Wu, Z.-Y. Genetic spectrum of NOTCH3 and clinical phenotype of CADASIL patients in different populations. *CNS Neurosci. Ther.* **2022**, *28*, 1779–1789. [CrossRef]
57. He, D.; Chen, D.; Li, X.; Hu, Z.; Yu, Z.; Wang, W.; Luo, X. The comparisons of phenotype and genotype between CADASIL and CADASIL-like patients and population-specific evaluation of CADASIL scale in China. *J. Headache Pain* **2016**, *17*, 55. [CrossRef]
58. Chen, S.; Ni, W.; Yin, X.Z.; Liu, H.Q.; Lu, C.; Zheng, Q.J.; Zhao, G.X.; Xu, Y.F.; Wu, L.; Zhang, L.; et al. Clinical features and mutation spectrum in Chinese patients with CADASIL: A multicenter retrospective study. *CNS Neurosci. Ther.* **2017**, *23*, 707–716. [CrossRef]
59. Dunn, P.J.; Maksemous, N.; Smith, R.A.; Sutherland, H.G.; Haupt, L.M.; Griffiths, L.R. Investigating diagnostic sequencing techniques for CADASIL diagnosis. *Hum. Genom.* **2020**, *14*, 2. [CrossRef]
60. Matsushima, T.; Conedera, S.; Tanaka, R.; Li, Y.; Yoshino, H.; Funayama, M.; Ikeda, A.; Hosaka, Y.; Okuzumi, A.; Shimada, Y.; et al. Genotype-phenotype correlations of cysteine replacement in CADASIL. *Neurobiol. Aging* **2017**, *50*, 1697–16914. [CrossRef] [PubMed]
61. Ceroni, M.; Poloni, T.E.; Tonietti, S.; Fabozzi, D.; Uggetti, C.; Frediani, F.; Simonetti, F.; Malaspina, A.; Alimonti, D.; Celano, M.; et al. Migraine with aura and white matter abnormalities: Notch3 mutation. *Neurology* **2000**, *54*, 1869–1871. [CrossRef] [PubMed]
62. Guey, S.; Mawet, J.; Hervé, D.; Duering, M.; Godin, O.; Jouvent, E.; Opherk, C.; Alili, N.; Dichgans, M.; Chabriat, H. Prevalence and characteristics of migraine in CADASIL. *Cephalalgia* **2016**, *36*, 1038–1047. [CrossRef]
63. Zhu, Y.; Wang, J.; Wu, Y.; Wang, G.; Hu, B. Two novel mutations in *NOTCH3* gene causes cerebral autosomal dominant arteriopathy with subcritical infarct and leucoencephalopathy in two Chinese families. *Int. J. Clin. Exp. Pathol.* **2015**, *8*, 1321–1327. [PubMed]
64. Cappelli, A.; Ragno, M.; Cacchiò, G.; Scarcella, M.; Staffolani, P.; Pianese, L. High recurrence of the R1006C NOTCH3 mutation in central Italian patients with cerebral autosomal dominant arteriopathy with subcortical infarcts and leukoencephalopathy (CADASIL). *Neurosci. Lett.* **2009**, *462*, 176–178. [CrossRef] [PubMed]
65. Guerreiro, R.J.; Lohmann, E.; Kinsella, E.; Brás, J.M.; Luu, N.; Gurunlian, N.; Dursun, B.; Bilgic, B.; Santana, I.; Hanagasi, H.; et al. Exome sequencing reveals an unexpected genetic cause of disease: NOTCH3 mutation in a Turkish family with Alzheimer's disease. *Neurobiol. Aging* **2012**, *33*, 17–23. [CrossRef] [PubMed]
66. Testi, S.; Malerba, G.; Ferrarini, M.; Ragno, M.; Pradotto, L.; Mauro, A.; Fabrizi, G.M. Mutational and haplotype map of NOTCH3 in a cohort of Italian patients with cerebral autosomal dominant arteriopathy with subcortical infarcts and leukoencephalopathy (CADASIL). *J. Neurol. Sci.* **2012**, *319*, 37–41. [CrossRef]
67. Roy, B.; Maksemous, N.; Smith, R.A.; Menon, S.; Davies, G.; Griffiths, L.R. Two novel mutations and a previously unreported intronic polymorphism in the *NOTCH3* gene. *Mutat. Res.* **2012**, *732*, 3–8. [CrossRef]
68. Rutten-Jacobs, L.C.; Traylor, M.; Adib-Samii, P.; Thijs, V.; Sudlow, C.; Rothwell, P.M.; Boncoraglio, G.; Dichgans, M.; Bevan, S.; Meschia, J.; et al. Common NOTCH3 variants and cerebral small-vessel disease. *Stroke* **2015**, *46*, 1482–1487. [CrossRef]
69. Keat Wei, L.; Griffiths, L.R.; Irene, L.; Kooi, C.W. Association of *NOTCH3* gene polymorphisms with ischemic stroke and its subtypes: A Meta-Analysis. *Medicina* **2019**, *55*, 351. [CrossRef]

70. González-Giraldo, Y.; Barreto, G.E.; Fava, C.; Forero, D.A. Ischemic stroke and six genetic variants in *CRP*, *EPHX2*, *FGA*, and *NOTCH3* genes: A meta-analysis. *J. Stroke Cerebrovasc. Dis.* **2016**, *25*, 2284–2289. [CrossRef]
71. Ensembl.org. Available online: https://www.ensembl.org/Homo_sapiens/Variation/Population?r=19:15191914-15192914;v=rs3815188;vdb=variation;vf=202725780 (accessed on 10 August 2023).
72. Menon, S.; Cox, H.C.; Kuwahata, M.; Quinlan, S.; MacMillan, J.C.; Haupt, L.M.; Lea, R.A.; Griffiths, L.R. Association of a Notch 3 gene polymorphism with migraine susceptibility. *Cephalalgia* **2011**, *31*, 264–270. [CrossRef]
73. Monteith, T.S.; Sprenger, T. Tension type headache in adolescence and childhood: Where are we now? *Curr. Pain Headache Rep.* **2010**, *14*, 424–430. [CrossRef]
74. Fonseca, E.; Torres-Ferrús, M.; Gallardo, V.J.; Macaya, A.; Pozo-Rosich, P. Impact of puberty in pediatric migraine: A pilot prospective study. *J. Clin. Neurol.* **2020**, *16*, 416–422. [CrossRef]
75. Coto, E.; Menéndez, M.; Navarro, R.; García-Castro, M.; Alvarez, V. A new de novo Notch3 mutation causing CADASIL. *Eur. J. Neurol.* **2006**, *13*, 628–631. [CrossRef]
76. Grangeon, L.; Lange, K.S.; Waliszewska-Prosół, M.; Onan, D.; Marschollek, K.; Wiels, W.; Mikulenka, P.; Farham, F.; Gollion, C.; Ducros, A. European Headache Federation School of Advanced Studies (EHF-SAS). Genetics of migraine: Where are we now? *J. Headache Pain* **2023**, *24*, 12. [CrossRef]
77. Li, S.J.; Shi, J.J.; Mao, C.Y.; Zhang, C.; Xu, Y.F.; Fan, Y.; Hu, Z.W.; Yu, W.K.; Hao, X.Y.; Li, M.J.; et al. Identifying causal genes for migraine by integrating the proteome and transcriptome. *J. Headache Pain* **2023**, *24*, 111. [CrossRef]
78. de Boer, I.; Terwindt, G.M.; van den Maagdenberg, A.M.J.M. Genetics of migraine aura: An update. *J. Headache Pain* **2020**, *21*, 64. [CrossRef]
79. Katsuki, M.; Matsumori, Y.; Kawahara, J.; Yamagishi, C.; Koh, A.; Kawamura, S.; Kashiwagi, K.; Kito, T.; Oguri, M.; Mizuno, S.; et al. Headache education by leaflet distribution during COVID-19 vaccination and school-based on-demand e-learning: Itoigawa Geopark Headache Awareness Campaign. *Headache* **2023**, *63*, 429–440. [CrossRef]

Disclaimer/Publisher's Note: The statements, opinions and data contained in all publications are solely those of the individual author(s) and contributor(s) and not of MDPI and/or the editor(s). MDPI and/or the editor(s) disclaim responsibility for any injury to people or property resulting from any ideas, methods, instructions or products referred to in the content.

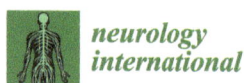

Article

Semi-Automated Recording of Facial Sensitivity in Rat Demonstrates Antinociceptive Effects of the Anti-CGRP Antibody Fremanezumab

Nicola Benedicter [1], Karl Messlinger [1,*], Birgit Vogler [1], Kimberly D. Mackenzie [2], Jennifer Stratton [2], Nadine Friedrich [3] and Mária Dux [3]

[1] Institute of Physiology and Pathophysiology, Friedrich-Alexander-University, D-91054 Erlangen, Germany
[2] Teva Pharmaceuticals, Redwood City, CA 94063, USA
[3] Department of Physiology, University of Szeged, H-6720 Szeged, Hungary; dux.maria@med.u-szeged.hu (M.D.)
* Correspondence: karl.messlinger@fau.de

Abstract: Migraine pain is frequently accompanied by cranial hyperalgesia and allodynia. Calcitonin gene-related peptide (CGRP) is implicated in migraine pathophysiology but its role in facial hypersensitivity is not entirely clear. In this study, we investigated if the anti-CGRP monoclonal antibody fremanezumab, which is therapeutically used in chronic and episodic migraines, can modify facial sensitivity recorded by a semi-automatic system. Rats of both sexes primed to drink from a sweet source had to pass a noxious mechanical or heat barrier to reach the source. Under these experimental conditions, animals of all groups tended to drink longer and more when they had received a subcutaneous injection of 30 mg/kg fremanezumab compared to control animals injected with an isotype control antibody 12–13 days prior to testing, but this was significant only for females. In conclusion, anti-CGRP antibody, fremanezumab, reduces facial sensitivity to noxious mechanical and thermal stimulation for more than one week, especially in female rats. Anti-CGRP antibodies may reduce not only headache but also cranial sensitivity in migraineurs.

Keywords: fremanezumab; monoclonal antibody; behavioral model; mechanical sensitivity; thermal sensitivity; calcitonin gene-related peptide; migraine symptoms

1. Introduction

Calcitonin gene-related peptide (CGRP) is a vasodilating neuropeptide released upon activation of nociceptive afferents in the trigeminovascular system [1]. CGRP is believed to play an important role in migraine pathophysiology, even if the pathomechanisms involved are not yet fully understood [2]. Infusion of CGRP can cause an immediate headache and it is able to trigger delayed migraine-like states in parts of migraineurs with and without aura [3,4]. Based on accumulated knowledge on CGRP, different classes of therapeutics against migraine targeting the CGRP pathway have been developed [5], among them humanised monoclonal anti-CGRP antibodies, which are effective in preventing frequent and chronic migraines [6]. In preclinical models of migraine, anti-CGRP antibodies such as fremanezumab prevented increased trigeminal activity following cortical spreading depression in rats as a likely correlate of migraine aura [7,8].

Facial mechanosensitivity has been determined in rodent models as a measure of facial hypersensitivity in migraine [9,10]. The involvement of CGRP in the control of facial sensitivity is not entirely clear. In mice, intrathecal application of CGRP can cause facial allodynia with elevated expression of the receptor activity-modifying protein-1 (RAMP1), the functionally rate-limiting subunit of the CGRP receptor [11,12]. Intraperitoneal injection of CGRP induced grimace responses which are indicative of pain [13], but the sensitivity to CGRP seems to depend on the mouse strain [14]. Injection of CGRP into the facial skin has been found to cause dose-dependent periorbital allodynia, which could be prevented

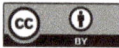

by administration of the CGRP receptor antagonist olcegepant or a monoclonal antibody against CGRP [15]. In rats, injection of CGRP into the facial skin did not induce signs of facial pain unless the rats were sensitized by pre-administration of nitroglycerin [16]. Remarkably, the application of CGRP to the rat dura mater has been shown to cause periorbital hypersensitivity selectively in female animals [17]. Similar responses in different species to CGRP administration through different routes have been reviewed in detail [18]. Assuming that CGRP is involved in facial sensitivity, the hypothesis of the current study was that anti-CGRP antibodies may reduce facial sensitivity in rats.

Using a new orofacial stimulation test device combined with feeding of an attractive solution, we measured facial sensitivity using different parameters such as the number of approaches to the source and the time of consumption before and after treatment with the anti-CGRP antibody fremanezumab or an isotype control antibody that does not target CGRP in rats of both sexes. In addition to a mechanical barrier that allows the approach to the source only under facial noxious mechanical stimulation, the tool also offers the option to apply a thermal barrier, which is a type of stimulation that has limited use so far regarding facial sensitivity. As a main result of the current study, both mechanical and heat barriers reduced the consumption parameters indicating unpleasant facial sensations that lead to avoidance of the barriers. Pre-treatment with fremanezumab partly abolished these changes, suggesting the involvement of CGRP in facial nociceptive sensitivity in rats.

2. Materials and Methods

2.1. Animals

Female and male Wistar rats with a body weight between 200 and 460 g bred and housed in the animal facility of the Institute of Physiology and Pathophysiology were used. Animal housing and all experiments were carried out according to the German guidelines and regulations of the care and treatment of laboratory animals and the European Communities Council Directive of 24 November 1986 (86/609/EEC), amended 22 September 2010 (2010/63/EU). Groups of 3–4 animals were kept in cages in a 12 h day–night-cycle and received pellet food and water ad libitum. Equal numbers of animals were matched according to their sex and weight and allocated to the treatments. The estrus state of females was not checked. The experiments were performed in the same room where the animals were housed, thus their transport to the test cage was not confounded by changes of the surroundings. The animals were weighed weekly on the day at which no barrier tests were performed. The starting weight for females was 180–260 g and for males maximally 230 g to keep the size of their head in a range best suited to the test devices during growth (see below). After completion of the experiment, the animals were used for further experiments such as meningeal CGRP release studies.

2.2. Preparation of Animals for Behavioral Tests

To get used to the behavioral set-up and create sufficient motivation for the subsequent experiments, the rats were primed for the attractive drink in advance. In this scheme, they were offered a 10% sucrose solution (in water) on seven consecutive days. The solution (40 mL per animal) was offered by a standard drinking bottle in the housing cage during the same time slot, in which the experiments were later performed, i.e., at 08:00 a.m.

2.3. Test Cage and Recording Device

The behavioral experiments were carried out with the Orofacial Stimulation Test by Ugo Basile (Lugano, Italy; https://ugobasile.com (accessed on 29 March 2023)). The construction consisted of an acrylic glass cage covered by a mesh (48.5 × 27.5 cm, total height 30.5 cm) with a variable recording device, which separated the cage into two parts. In the larger part with approximately 34 × 27.5 cm, the animal could move freely. The other part contained a drinking bottle, which could be adjusted in height, depth, and inclination. An opening in the center of the wall separating the two rooms could be changed in size and shape by inserting different barriers (Figure 1). The animals could approach the outlet of the drinking bottle with their mouth once they passed the opening with their forehead (Figure 1A,B). Mechanical or thermal stimulation barriers could be inserted reducing the size of this opening. A photo sensor (light barrier) was installed directly behind the separating wall in order to detect movements of the rat's head through the opening. It was important to set the holder for the drinking bottle (filled with 100 mL 10% sucrose solution) correctly so that the light barrier was only interrupted when the animal approached the opening of the bottle to reach the sugar solution. The system automatically recorded the number of drinking trials (approaches) and the duration of intervals when the light barrier was inactivated (finally calculated as the average drinking time per trial and total drinking time). After the experimental period of 15 min had elapsed, the volume of ingested sucrose solution during the test period was determined by measuring the rest of solution in the drinking bottle.

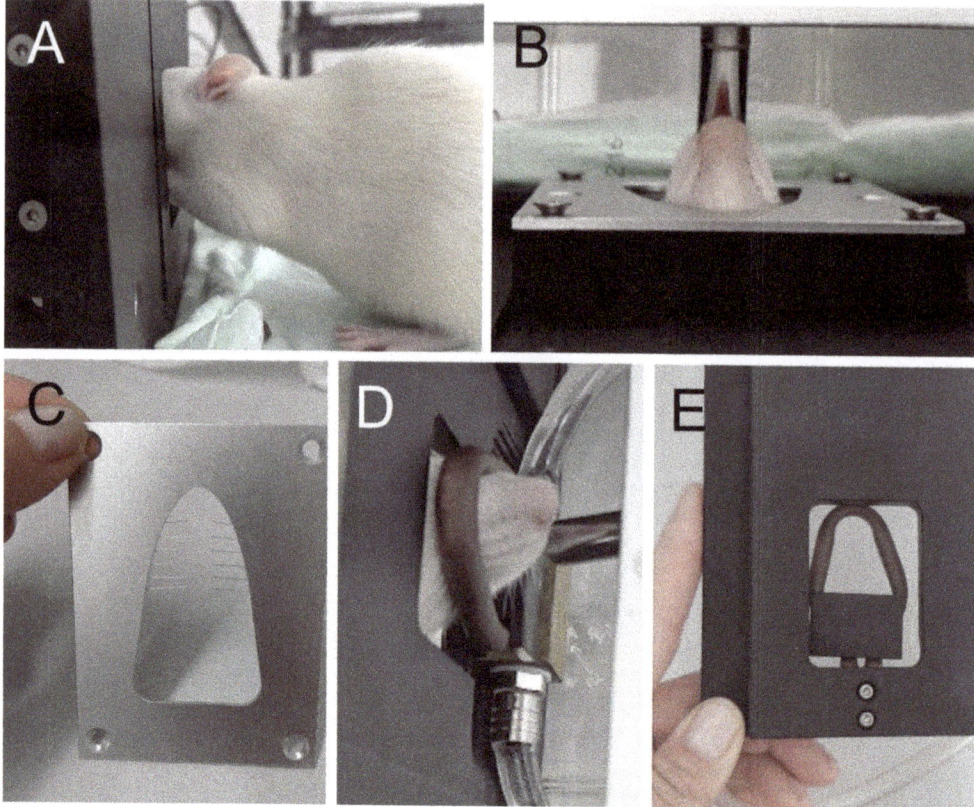

Figure 1. Photographs illustrating details of the experimental setup. The rat sitting in front of the separating wall with the light sensor, has passed the opening with its forehead and is licking the sugar solution from the tube of the drinking bottle (**A**,**B**). A mechanical barrier with 12 bristles (**C**) or a thermal barrier consisting of a U-shaped tube with circulating heated water (**D**,**E**) could be fixed behind the wall.

2.4. Mechanical and Thermal Stimulation Device

The mechanical barrier that was added to the opening consisted of 12 thin bristles made of flexible spring steel wire (0.09 mm in diameter) that reached at a length of 1.6 cm into the opening (Figure 1C). The barrier constricted the opening and left a circular gap of 0.6 cm free of bristles. When the animal approached the drinking bottle, the facial area between the nose and the eyes was touched by the bristles. For thermal stimulation, the barrier consisted of a tube in the form of a rounded triangular loop (adapted to the contours of the rat's head) filled with circulating water at a constant flow, which was heated by a water bath and held at a constant temperature of 50 °C (Figure 1E). The opening of the drinking bottle could be reached by the animal while its cheeks and forehead came into contact with the hot tube (Figure 1D).

2.5. Test Procedures

Behavioral experiments were performed at 8:00 a.m. Each experiment lasted 20 min in total. The rat was first placed in the test chamber without the attractant sugar solution and left there for 5 min to get accustomed to the new cage. After this phase, the drinking bottle with the sucrose solution was fixed and left for 15 min. As soon as the drinking bottle was correctly positioned, the test time was started and the light barrier was activated. The experimenter closed the cage with an air-permeable lid. The recording device measured the activity at the light barrier for 15 min. During this time, the rat could freely access the drinking bottle. Food was not offered during the experiment.

2.6. Test Sequence

All animals in a cage were tested according to the same scheme. The test sequence started after seven days of priming as described above (Figure 2). The tests took place from Tuesday to Thursday for three consecutive weeks. On the first day, each animal was weighed, moved to the test cage, and left there for 5 min to get used to the environment. Then, the drinking bottle filled with 100 mL sugar solution was fixed in place. The program for the test period of 15 min was started. During this period, the cover of the cage remained closed and the animal could move around freely. When this time had elapsed, the cage was opened, the sugar solution removed, and the rat returned to its housing cage. A measuring cylinder was used to read the volume of the sugar solution left and to determine the consumed amount. On the second day of the test sequence, the mechanical barrier was placed into the test cage and the procedure was performed repeating that of the first day. On the third day, the procedure was repeated with the thermal barrier. The entire test sequence in this first week of the experiment was referred to as baseline, while the rats received no antibodies.

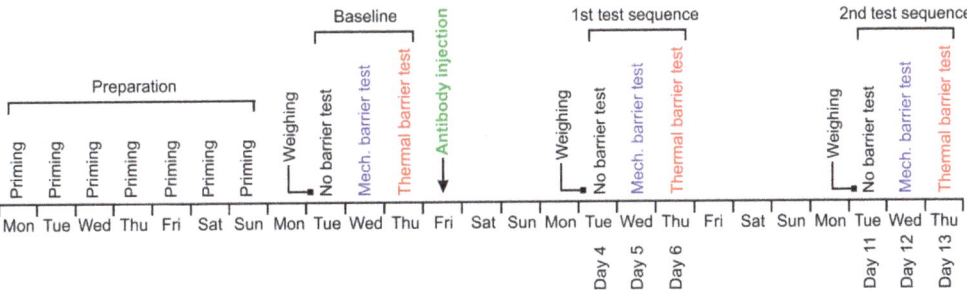

Figure 2. Schematic workflow of the experiments. The first week was used for priming the animals to the attractive source, in the second week baseline measurements without barrier, and with the mechanical and thermal barrier were performed, finished by injection of antibodies (either anti-CGRP antibody fremanezumab or control antibody). In the third and fourth week, the measurements were repeated with the same sequence at days 4–6 and days 11–13 after antibody injection.

On the day after the third (last) baseline measurement, always on a Friday in this sequence, animals received anti-CGRP antibody or isotype control antibody as described below. On the fourth day after the antibody injection, i.e., on the following Tuesday, the same test sequence as described was repeated, starting without the barrier and repeated with the mechanical and the thermal barrier on the following days. The whole test sequence was repeated at day 11 after the antibody injection. The order of the tested animals was always the same. The experimenter was blinded regarding the treatment of the animals during the whole experiment.

2.7. Injection of Antibodies

The animals were divided into two groups, one group that received isotype control antibody and the other anti-CGRP antibody, fremanezumab (Teva Pharmaceuticals, Redwood City, CA, USA). The rats were transferred from their housing cage in a plastic box and anesthetized around 9 a.m. with an increasing concentration up to 4% isoflurane applied by an evaporator (Forane Vapor 19.3, Dräger AG, Lübeck, Germany). The animals were weighed, individually marked at the tail, and shaved in the neck region. After disinfecting the skin with 70% ethanol, 30 mg/kg anti-CGRP antibody or the same dose of isotype control antibody diluted in saline (10 mg/mL) was subcutaneously injected using a syringe with a 27G needle into the shaved area 2 cm left and right from the midline and 5 cm caudal of the occiput. Examiners performing the injections were blinded to the treatment. The animals were placed back into the housing cage where they recovered from anesthesia within 2–3 min. The animals were inspected two times every following day.

2.8. Data Calculation and Statistics

Sequential data (body weight, number of approaches to the drinking source, total drinking time, and drinking volume within 15 min) were calculated for each individual animal. Means were calculated for the whole group and specifically for female and male animals. Statistical analysis was performed with Statistica software (StatSoft, Release 7, Tulsa, OK, USA). Following verification of normal distribution of values, analysis of variance (ANOVA) with repeated measurements was applied, and the factors "antibody" and "sex" were used as independent variables or in combinations. ANOVA was extended by Fisher's least square difference (LSD) test. The level of significance was set at $p < 0.05$. Data are displayed as the means ± SEM (standard error of the mean). Graphical work was produced using Origin 2017 (https://www.originlab.com (accessed on 29 March 2023)) and CorelDraw X7 (https://coreldraw.com (accessed on 29 March 2023)).

3. Results

3.1. Allocation of Animals and Tolerability of Treatments

Female and male animals (each n = 12) were matched according to their age and body weight and, as far as possible, equally allocated into two groups either for control antibody or fremanezumab injection (Figure 2, Baseline). The animals did not take notice of the injection site and did not show any unusual behavior during the following days. During the following two weeks, the animals gained weight, which was more significant in the males than in the females (gain ratio about 4.5:1), but there was no significant difference between the control antibody and fremanezumab groups (Figure 3).

3.2. Baseline Experiments

In the first week after priming of the animals to the attractive source, i.e., before the injection of antibodies (see Figure 2), we aimed to examine the impact of the test apparatus with the barriers. We counted the number of approaches to the drinking source within 15 min of presentation (Figure 4A), the cumulated time in which the animals stayed at the source inactivating the light barrier (Figure 4B), and the consumed drinking volume within this time (Figure 4C). There was no significant difference between the cohorts of animals designated for injection with control antibody or fremanezumab, respectively, regarding the above measurements without, with the mechanical, and with the thermal barrier (Figure 4A–C). However, after insertion of the mechanical barrier, the number of approaches increased in the fremanezumab group (Figure 4A), while both the drinking time and consumed volume decreased dramatically in both groups when the mechanical or the thermal barrier was inserted (Figure 4B,C).

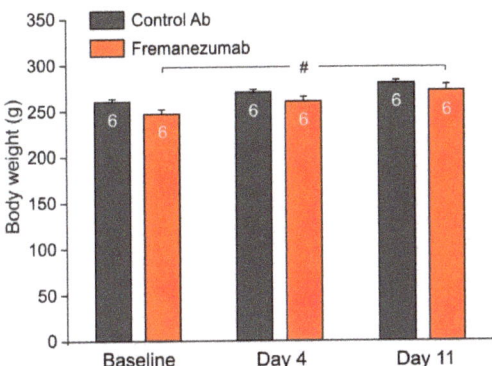

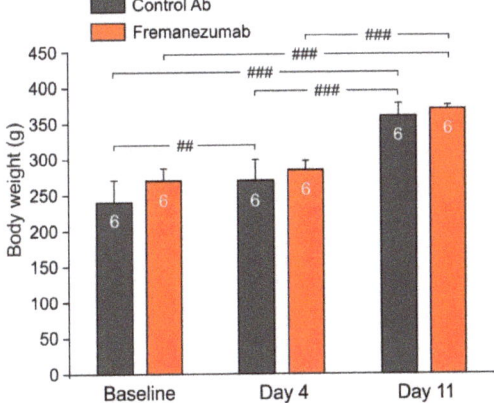

Figure 3. Gain of body weight in animals injected with fremanezumab or control antibody from baseline to the two test sequences at 4 and 11 days. Females (**A**) gained less weight than males (**B**), in which the increase was clearly significant (repeated measures ANOVA with factor antibody, $F_{2,40} = 18.9$, $p < 0.0005$). There was no significant difference between the animals that received fremanezumab or control antibody in any group at any time of measurement. White digits in the bars represent the number of animals tested. Differences between days: # $p < 0.05$, ## $p < 0.005$, ### $p < 0.0005$ (LSD post hoc test).

3.3. Experiments after Antibody Injection

In the second and third week after priming (first and second test sequence), i.e., days 4–6 and days 11–13 after antibody injection, the three parameters, number of approaches, cumulated time at the drinking source and consumed solution, were tested again (Figures 5–7). The aim was to compare these parameters after injection of the tested antibodies at the first and second test sequence with the baseline data.

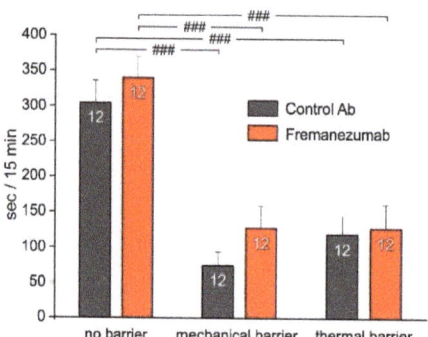

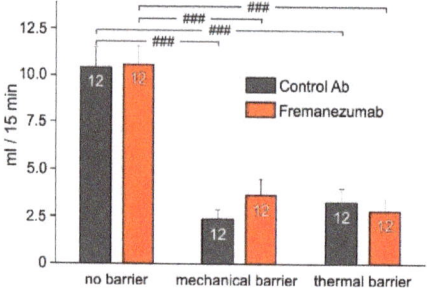

Figure 4. Comparison of baselines for approaches to the source (**A**), drinking time (**B**), and drinking volume (**C**) before the injection of antibodies. Groups designated for the control antibody and fremanezumab, respectively, showed some variance but no significant differences. After inserting the mechanical barrier, the number of trials to approach the source tended to increase (**A**), which was significant in the group designated for fremanezumab (repeated measures ANOVA with factor antibody, $F_{2,44}$ = 3.99, $p < 0.05$ and LSD post hoc test, $p < 0.05$). On the contrary, the mechanical and thermal barriers dramatically reduced both the drinking time (**B**) and drinking volume (**C**) (repeated measures ANOVA, $F_{2,44}$ = 39.17 and 74.03, respectively, $p < 0.0005$). White digits in the bars represent the number of animals tested. Difference between no barrier situation and mechanical and thermal barrier, respectively: # $p < 0.05$, ### $p < 0.0005$ (LSD post hoc test).

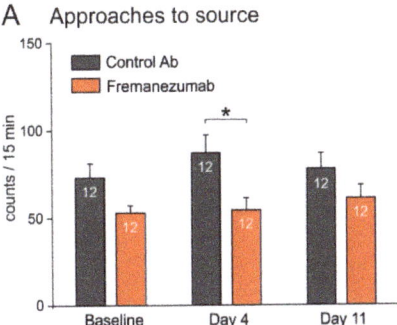
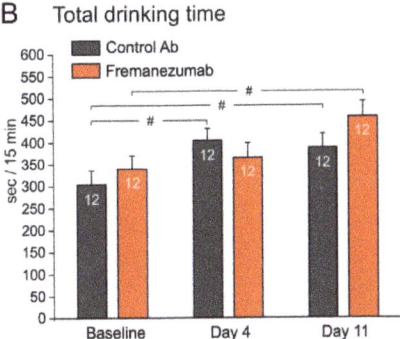
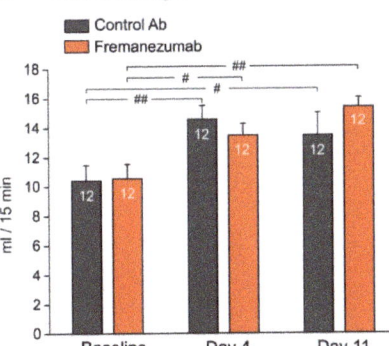

Figure 5. Tests without the barrier before (baseline) and at days 4 and 11 after antibody injection (1st and 2nd test sequence). (**A**) Animals injected with the control antibody tended to approach the drinking source more frequently than animals injected with fremanezumab (repeated measures ANOVA with factor antibody, $F_{2,44} = 6.52$, $p < 0.05$), which was significant at day 4 after antibody injection (LSD post hoc test, $p < 0.05$). (**B**) The cumulated time, during which the animals stayed at the source to drink, increased at days 4 and 11 compared to baseline, independent of the type of antibody injected (repeated measures ANOVA with factor antibody, $F_{2,44} = 8.90$, $p < 0.005$). (**C**) Similarly, the cumulated volume consumed by the animals increased at days 4 and 11 (repeated measures ANOVA, $F_{2,44} = 17.17$, $p < 0.0005$). White digits in bars represent the number of animals tested. Difference between antibodies: * $p < 0.05$; difference in the course of repeated tests: # $p < 0.05$; ## $p < 0.005$ (LSD post hoc tests).

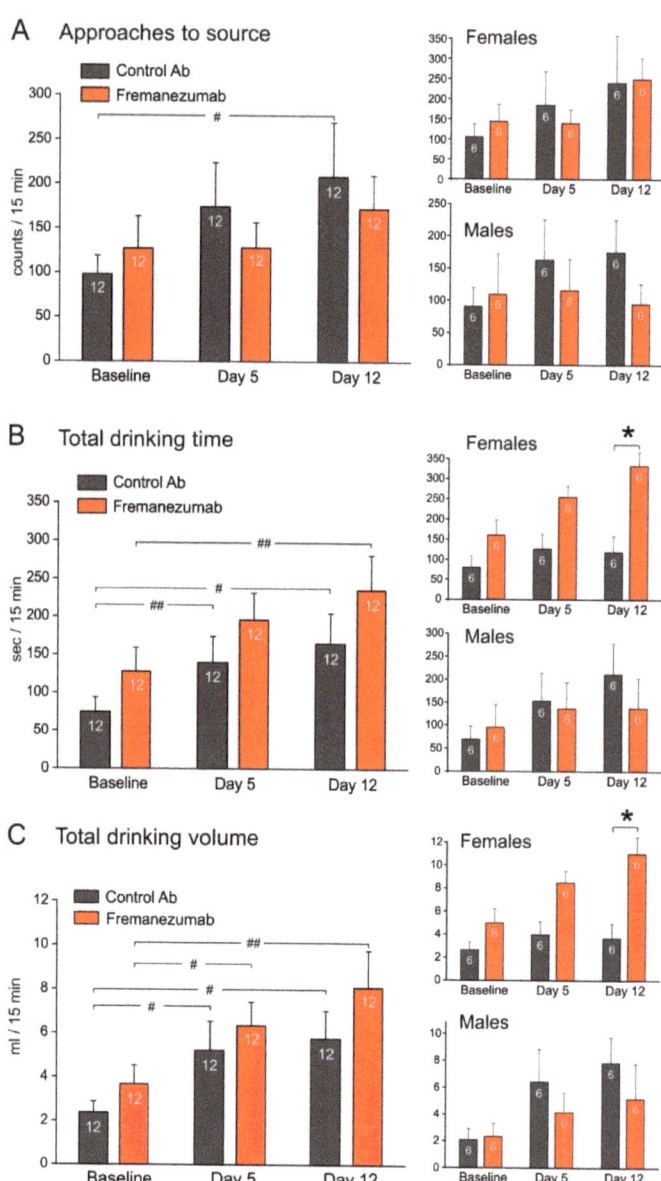

Figure 6. Tests with the mechanical barrier before (baseline) and at days 5 and 12 (1st and 2nd test sequence) after antibody injection. Compared to baseline, the animals tended to approach the drinking source more often (**A**), they stayed longer at the source (**B**), and drank more (**C**), independently of the type of injected antibody (repeated measures ANOVA with factor antibody, $F_{2,44} = 8.90$, $p < 0.005$ for B and $F_{2,44} = 10.44$, $p < 0.0005.81$ for (**C**)). However, ANOVA with the combination of factors antibody and sex indicated significant differences ($F_{1,20} = 7.28$; $p < 0.05$); the LSD post hoc test showed significant differences ($p < 0.05$) in the drinking time and volume exclusively in the female groups at day 12 ((**B**,**C**), right insets). White digits in bars represent the number of animals tested. Difference between antibodies: * $p < 0.05$; difference in the course of repeated tests: # $p < 0.05$; ## $p < 0.005$ (LSD post hoc test).

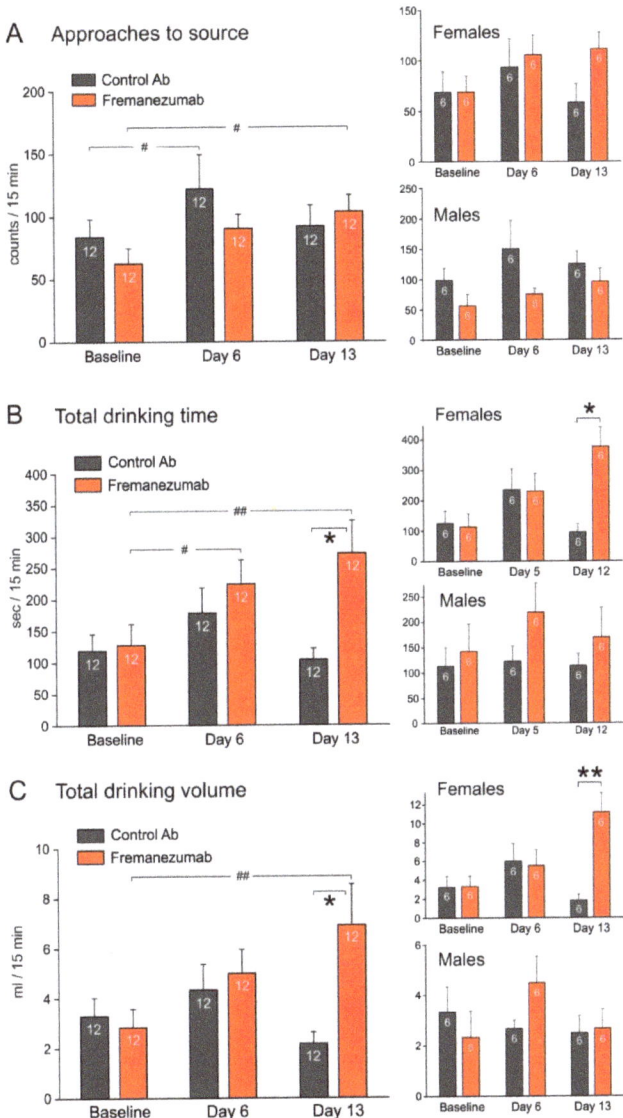

Figure 7. Tests with the thermal barrier before (baseline) and at days 6 and 13 (1st and 2nd test sequence) after antibody injection. At days 6 and 13, the animals partly approached the drinking source more often (**A**) and stayed longer at the source (**B**) compared to baseline, independently of the type of injected antibody (repeated measures ANOVA with factor antibody, $F_{2,44} = 3.92$, $p < 0.05$ for A and $F_{2,44} = 3.60$, $p < 0.05$ for B; $F_{2,44} = 10.44$, $p < 0.0005.81$ for (**C**)). At day 12, the drinking time (**B**) and the consumed volume (**C**) were significantly higher in animals injected with fremanezumab compared to the control antibody (repeated measures ANOVA with combined factors repetition and antibody extended by the LSD post hoc test, $F_{2,44} = 45.10$, $p < 0.05$). The separated analysis of the sexes showed that this was particularly due to the female animals, which drank longer and significantly more when they were injected with fremanezumab ((**B**,**C**), right insets). White digits in bars represent the number of animals tested. Difference between antibodies: * $p < 0.05$, ** $p < 0.005$; difference in the course of repeated tests: # $p < 0.05$; ## $p < 0.005$ (LSD post hoc test).

3.3.1. Experiments without Barrier (Figure 5)

The number of approaches to the drinking source tended to decrease after fremanezumab treatment compared to the control antibody in the baseline experiments; the difference was significant in the first test sequence (day 4 after antibody injection) but there was no significant difference between the first test (baseline) and days 4 and 11 when the same groups of animals were compared (Figure 5A). The drinking time and volume increased in the course from the baseline measurements to the first and second test sequence, which was especially significant regarding the drinking volume, most likely as a compensatory mechanism for the increasing body weight (Figure 5B,C). However, there was no difference between the control antibody and fremanezumab at any of the test sequences. A repeated measures ANOVA with the factors "antibody" and "sex" indicated no significant sex difference.

3.3.2. Experiments with Mechanical Barrier (Figure 6)

The number of approaches to the source tended to increase (Figure 6A), while the drinking time and drinking volume clearly increased in the course from the baseline to the first and second test sequence both in the control antibody and the fremanezumab groups (Figure 6B,C), however, there was no significant difference between the antibodies at same days. At day 12, the drinking time and the consumed volume tended to increase in animals injected with fremanezumab compared to the control antibody. The separated analysis of sexes showed that this was solely due to female animals, which drank longer and significantly more when they were injected with fremanezumab (Figure 6B,C, right insets).

3.3.3. Experiments with Thermal Barrier (Figure 7)

The number of approaches to the source, drinking time, and volume partly increased in the course of the experiments (Figure 7A–C). A repeated measures ANOVA indicated significant differences in the course of the experiments between antibodies and sexes, the post hoc test showed significance in drinking time and volume between the control antibody and fremanezumab at day 13 (Figure 7B,C). Therefore, the analysis was repeated with the factor "sex", where ANOVA extended by the LSD test showed that the differences were specifically based on the female groups (Figure 7B,C, right insets).

4. Discussion

To our knowledge, this is the first study using a semiautomatic test system to determine facial mechanical and thermal sensitivity in rodents after treatment with an anti-CGRP monoclonal antibody. Rats of both sexes were primed to use a pleasant-tasting drinking source, which in the experimental condition they could only approach when they touched an unpleasant mechanical or heat barrier with their face. At days 12 and 13 after treatment with anti-CGRP antibody, female, but not male, animals stayed significantly longer at the source and consumed more volume compared to animals treated with the control antibody. We conclude that animals treated with anti-CGRP antibody, in particular females, show a higher tolerance towards unpleasant facial mechanical and heat stimuli. Our data suggest that facial sensitivity is partly dependent on CGRP levels which are lowered by anti-CGRP antibodies.

4.1. Test Device

The semiautomatic device deployed for this study is new and needed mechanical adjustment for its proper use. In particular, the mechanical barrier with the steel bristles had to be modified and adapted in size for the head of the animals, which required several trials in preliminary experiments. In previous studies, facial sensitivity was most frequently tested by determining the withdrawal threshold with hand-held calibrated von Frey filaments, which requires fixing the animals and repetitive testing at exactly the same site [19–22]. Different to these, in our test device the animals were free to contact the unpleasant barriers and could do this in their individual way, only attracted by the sweet drink. In the course of the test sequence, no differences between the tested antibodies became apparent as long as no barriers were used. This suggests that the animals did not undergo any fundamental change in behavior as a result of antibody application. The mechanical and thermal barriers proved to be effective in terms of nociceptive stimulation of the periorbital area, as was evident from the dramatic drop in drinking time and volume when the barriers were fixed. As a confounding factor, the number of approaches to the source and the duration of drinking was possibly also influenced by psychological factors such as motivation, attendance, and alertness of the animals. The device used in our study is reminiscent of an operant test system previously developed to determine mechanical and thermal orofacial sensitivity [23,24]. Similar to this device, a thermal stimulation paradigm was added in our experiments, which has rarely been used so far regarding facial sensitivity in a behavioral context [25–27]. The observation that heat stimulation yielded very similar results to the mechanical barrier may argue for an involvement of polymodal C-nociceptors in the CGRP-dependent modulation of facial sensitivity [28].

4.2. Proposed Mechanisms of Anti-CGRP Antibody Effects

Fremanezumab is a humanized monoclonal antibody that specifically targets CGRP and antagonizes CGRP-induced cAMP signaling at the canonical human CGRP receptor [29]. This antibody has been shown to also inhibit the vasodilatory effect of rat CGRP in rat cranial arteries [30] and the activity of rat meningeal afferents [7]. In our previous study, fremanezumab reduced CGRP release from rat trigeminal tissues as well as increasing meningeal blood flow evoked by stimulation with the TRPV1 receptor agonist capsaicin [31]. Therefore, although human and rat α- and β-CGRPs differ in four amino acids [32], fremanezumab binds rat CGRP and is suitable for testing CGRP-mediated effects in this species. The results of the present study suggest that the anti-CGRP antibody, fremanezumab, decreased periorbital sensitivity to noxious mechanical and heat stimuli and hence facial sensitivity may be influenced by CGRP. This result was unexpected, since a decrease in the facial mechanical threshold upon inhibition of CGRP signalling has so far only been reported in experiments in which the trigeminal system was sensitized, for example by repetitive electrical stimulation [33] or cortical spreading depolarization [27]. Injection of CGRP into the trigeminal ganglion has also been reported to cause periorbital mechanical allodynia attenuated by sumatriptan [34].

We speculate that the decrease in facial sensitivity following treatment with anti-CGRP antibodies is not merely a function of peripheral CGRP actions but may also include central effects. In a mouse model, CGRP administration produced facial grimace indicative of spontaneous pain, which was blocked by pre-administration of a monoclonal anti-CGRP antibody [13]. Avoidance of unpleasant or painful stimuli is a complex behavior depending on several factors such as motivation and tolerability. The observation that 12–13 days passed until the effect of fremanezumab was apparent may be interpreted with such a behavioral adjustment. In a broader clinical context, these observations are reminiscent of the real life experiences with monoclonal antibodies in the treatment of chronic migraines, which have been found not only to decrease the frequency and duration of migraine attacks but also the severity reported by the patients [35,36].

4.3. Sex Differences

Although the animals seemed to tolerate the mechanical and thermal barrier longer after treatment with fremanezumab in all groups tested, the differences to the control antibody were statistically significant only in female animals. We did not test and correct for the oestrus cycle of the females, which would not have been compatible with the fixed test sequence. Sex differences in facial sensitivity of rodents are known from several reports. In rat models of headache, female animals showed more frequent headache-like behavior [37]. Following meningeal afferent sensitization through application of inflammatory mediators onto the dura mater in rats, females but not males showed increased withdrawal responses to mechanical test stimuli in the periorbital region [38]. Similarly, application of small doses of CGRP onto the dura mater caused periorbital hypersensitivity only in female rats, and particular sex-specific sensitivity to CGRP was caused by the application of interleukin-6 or the NO-donor sodium nitroprusside [17]. In a model of post-traumatic headache, female rats developed pericranial mechanical hyperalgesia that lasted longer than in males and showed elevated CGRP levels in the peripheral blood [39]. Thus, we can conclude that female rats are more sensitive to CGRP, which may be the reason why anti-CGRP antibody treatment may be more efficient in female rats.

The mechanisms underlying the higher sensitivity to CGRP of female rats are not clear. We assume that sex hormones such as estrogen with a higher expression in the female rat body independent of the estrus state contribute to sensitizing the recently proposed CGRP-NO-TRPA1 signalling cascade, inducing facial hypersensitivity [40]. In this cascade CGRP, released mainly from trigeminal C-afferents, is proposed to activate CGRP receptors on adjacent Schwann cells (glial cells of Remak bundles). This induces the expression of nitric oxide (NO) synthase to produce more NO, which in turn acts on TRPA1 receptor channels of adjacent Aδ-afferents causing afferent sensitization. This hypothetical cascade is based on previously published experiments in which this group has demonstrated that subcutaneous injection of CGRP and other migraine-provoking substances cause periorbital mechanical hypersensitivity in mice [15]. Regarding sex differences, it has formerly been shown that inhibition of the vascular NO synthase has different effects in pre- versus post-menopausal women and men in that vasoconstriction was selectively higher in the pre-menopausal state [41], indirectly indicating that sex hormones such as estrogen may contribute to an increase in endogenous NO production. Regarding facial hypersensitivity as an animal model of migraine, it would be interesting to examine whether female migraineurs, particularly in the pre-menopause, may benefit more from a treatment with monoclonal anti-CGRP antibodies than male migraineurs. Overall, these results fit to the generally higher prevalence of migraine in women [42].

4.4. Clinical Relevance and Limitations

Migraine patients frequently show facial allodynia and are also hypersensitive in other body regions [43,44]. To our knowledge, changes in cutaneous sensitivity have not been systematically monitored in patients treated with fremanezumab. Following repetitive treatment with galcanezumab, another anti-CGRP antibody, cutaneous allodynia during migraine attacks has been found to improve, however, without reaching statistical significance after correction for multiple comparison [45]. Similar late responses including the decrease in allodynia to galcanezumab, fremanezumab and the anti-CGRP receptor antibody erenumab have recently been communicated [46]. These data are based on self-reports of patients and did not differentiate between body regions. It would be interesting to test, in addition to facial sensitivity, other regions of the rat's body with the device used in our experiments.

Thermal hypersensitivity is usually not tested in migraine, and patients usually do not report thermal hypersensitivity. Thermal pain thresholds have been shown to be decreased immediately prior to migraine attacks [47]. Derived from the present data, we assume that thermal hypersensitivity in the face of migraineurs may be reduced after treatment with anti-CGRP antibodies. Developing a standard test for the evaluation of mechanical and thermal sensitivity in migraineurs would possibly be very useful for monitoring the effect of treatments targeting CGRP or its receptors.

5. Conclusions

In conclusion, the current experiments together with our previous results about CGRP release [31], and earlier data about reduced trigeminal activity [7] and prevention of periorbital allodynia [48] following pre-treatment with the anti-CGRP antibody fremanezumab strongly argue for a role of CGRP in the development of facial sensitivity and hyperalgesia, at least in female animals. The experiments confirm this rodent model based on semi-automated recording of facial sensitivity is useful for preclinical research on headache therapies targeting CGRP signalling.

Author Contributions: Conceptualization, N.B., K.M., K.D.M., J.S. and M.D.; methodology, N.B., B.V., N.F. and M.D.; software, N.B. and K.M.; validation, N.B., K.M. and M.D.; formal analysis, N.B. and K.M.; investigation, N.B. and B.V.; resources, K.M. and M.D.; data curation, K.M.; writing—original draft preparation, N.B. and K.M.; writing—review and editing, K.M., K.D.M., J.S. and M.D.; visualization, N.B. and K.M.; supervision, K.M. and M.D.; project administration, K.M.; funding acquisition, K.M., K.D.M., J.S. and M.D. All authors have read and agreed to the published version of the manuscript.

Funding: These studies were part of a sponsored research collaboration with Teva, who provided research support and the anti-CGRP antibody, fremanezumab. The project was also partly supported by the research grant K119597 project of the Hungarian National Research, Development and Innovation Office and the Alexander von Humboldt Foundation (Research Group Linkage Program between the Institutes of Physiology of the FAU Erlangen-Nürnberg and the University of Szeged). We acknowledge financial support by the Friedrich-Alexander-Universität Erlangen-Nürnberg within the funding programme "Open Access Publication Funding".

Institutional Review Board Statement: These studies were conducted in accordance with the Declaration of Helsinki. The animal study protocol was approved by the District Government of Mittelfranken (54-2532.1-21/12) after review by the Ethics Committee of the District Government of Unterfranken.

Informed Consent Statement: Not applicable.

Data Availability Statement: Not applicable.

Conflicts of Interest: K.D.M. and J.S. are employees of Teva Pharmaceuticals. The first author (N.B.) performed this work for obtaining the degree "Dr. med." at the Friedrich-Alexander-University Erlangen-Nürnberg (FAU). The other authors declare no conflict of interest.

References

1. Edvinsson, L.; Ekman, R.; Jansen, I.; McCulloch, J.; Uddman, R. Calcitonin Gene-Related Peptide and Cerebral Blood Vessels: Distribution and Vasomotor Effects. *J. Cereb. Blood Flow Metab.* **1987**, *7*, 720–728. [CrossRef] [PubMed]
2. Edvinsson, L.; Goadsby, P.J. Neuropeptides in Migraine and Cluster Headache. *Cephalalgia* **1994**, *14*, 320–327. [CrossRef] [PubMed]
3. Lassen, L.H.; Haderslev, P.A.; Jacobsen, V.B.; Iversen, H.K.; Sperling, B.; Olesen, J. Cgrp May Play A Causative Role in Migraine. *Cephalalgia Int. J. Headache* **2002**, *22*, 54–61. [CrossRef] [PubMed]
4. Hansen, J.M.; Hauge, A.W.; Olesen, J.; Ashina, M. Calcitonin gene-related peptide triggers migraine-like attacks in patients with migraine with aura. *Cephalalgia* **2010**, *30*, 1179–1186. [CrossRef]
5. Benemei, S.; Cortese, F.; Labastida-Ramírez, A.; Marchese, F.; Pellesi, L.; Romoli, M.; Vollesen, A.L.; Lampl, C.; Ashina, M.; School of Advanced Studies of the European Headache Federation (EHF-SAS). Triptans and CGRP blockade—Impact on the cranial vasculature. *J. Headache Pain* **2017**, *18*, 103. [CrossRef]
6. Charles, A.; Pozo-Rosich, P. Targeting calcitonin gene-related peptide: A new era in migraine therapy. *Lancet* **2019**, *394*, 1765–1774. [CrossRef]
7. Melo-Carrillo, A.; Strassman, A.M.; Nir, R.-R.; Schain, A.J.; Noseda, R.; Stratton, J.; Burstein, R. Fremanezumab—A Humanized Monoclonal Anti-CGRP Antibody—Inhibits Thinly Myelinated (Aδ) But Not Unmyelinated (C) Meningeal Nociceptors. *J. Neurosci.* **2017**, *37*, 10587–10596. [CrossRef]
8. Melo-Carrillo, A.; Noseda, R.; Nir, R.-R.; Schain, A.J.; Stratton, J.; Strassman, A.M.; Burstein, R. Selective Inhibition of Trigeminovascular Neurons by Fremanezumab: A Humanized Monoclonal Anti-CGRP Antibody. *J. Neurosci.* **2017**, *37*, 7149–7163. [CrossRef]
9. Burstein, R.; Yamamura, H.; Malick, A.; Strassman, A.M. Chemical Stimulation of the Intracranial Dura Induces Enhanced Responses to Facial Stimulation in Brain Stem Trigeminal Neurons. *J. Neurophysiol.* **1998**, *79*, 964–982. [CrossRef]
10. Edelmayer, R.M.; Ossipov, M.H.; Porreca, F. An Experimental Model of Headache-Related Pain. *Methods Mol. Biol.* **2012**, *851*, 109–120. [CrossRef]
11. Zhang, Z.; Winborn, C.S.; de Prado, B.M.; Russo, A.F. Sensitization of Calcitonin Gene-Related Peptide Receptors by Receptor Activity-Modifying Protein-1 in the Trigeminal Ganglion. *J. Neurosci.* **2007**, *27*, 2693–2703. [CrossRef]
12. De Prado, B.M.; Hammond, D.; Russo, A.F. Genetic Enhancement of Calcitonin Gene-Related Peptide-Induced Central Sensitization to Mechanical Stimuli in Mice. *J. Pain* **2009**, *10*, 992–1000. [CrossRef]
13. Rea, B.J.; Wattiez, A.-S.; Waite, J.S.; Castonguay, W.C.; Schmidt, C.M.; Fairbanks, A.M.; Robertson, B.R.; Brown, C.J.; Mason, B.N.; Moldovan-Loomis, M.-C.; et al. Peripherally administered calcitonin gene–related peptide induces spontaneous pain in mice: Implications for migraine. *Pain* **2018**, *159*, 2306–2317. [CrossRef]

14. Mogil, J.S.; Miermeister, F.; Seifert, F.; Strasburg, K.; Zimmermann, K.; Reinold, H.; Austin, J.-S.; Bernardini, N.; Chesler, E.J.; Hofmann, H.A.; et al. Variable sensitivity to noxious heat is mediated by differential expression of the CGRP gene. *Proc. Natl. Acad. Sci. USA* **2005**, *102*, 12938–12943. [CrossRef]
15. Landini, L.; Janal, M.N.; Simone, L.P.; Pierangelo, G.; Romina, N. Migraine-provoking substances evoke periorbital allodynia in mice. *J. Headache Pain* **2019**, *20*, 18. [CrossRef]
16. Capuano, A.; Greco, M.C.; Navarra, P.; Tringali, G. Correlation between algogenic effects of calcitonin-gene-related peptide (CGRP) and activation of trigeminal vascular system, in an in vivo experimental model of nitroglycerin-induced sensitization. *Eur. J. Pharmacol.* **2014**, *740*, 97–102. [CrossRef]
17. Avona, A.; Burgos-Vega, C.; Burton, M.D.; Akopian, A.N.; Price, T.J.; Dussor, G. Dural Calcitonin Gene-Related Peptide Produces Female-Specific Responses in Rodent Migraine Models. *J. Neurosci.* **2019**, *39*, 4323–4331. [CrossRef]
18. Wattiez, A.-S.; Wang, M.; Russo, A.F. CGRP in Animal Models of Migraine. In *Calcitonin Gene-Related Peptide (CGRP) Mechanisms*; Brain, S.D., Geppetti, P., Eds.; Springer International Publishing: Cham, Switzerland, 2018; pp. 85–107.
19. Gazerani, P.; Dong, X.; Wang, M.; Kumar, U.; Cairns, B.E. Sensitization of rat facial cutaneous mechanoreceptors by activation of peripheral N-methyl-d-aspartate receptors. *Brain Res.* **2010**, *1319*, 70–82. [CrossRef]
20. Wei, X.; Edelmayer, R.M.; Yan, J.; Dussor, G. Activation of TRPV4 on dural afferents produces headache-related behavior in a preclinical rat model. *Cephalalgia* **2011**, *31*, 1595–1600. [CrossRef]
21. Garrett, F.G.; Hawkins, J.L.; Overmyer, A.E.; Hayden, J.B.; Durham, P.L. Validation of a novel rat-holding device for studying heat- and mechanical-evoked trigeminal nocifensive behavioral responses. *J. Orofac. Pain* **2012**, *26*, 337–344.
22. Wang, S.; Wang, J.; Liu, K.; Bai, W.; Cui, X.; Han, S.; Gao, X.; Zhu, B. Signaling Interaction between Facial and Meningeal Inputs of the Trigeminal System Mediates Peripheral Neurostimulation Analgesia in a Rat Model of Migraine. *Neuroscience* **2020**, *433*, 184–199. [CrossRef] [PubMed]
23. Neubert, J.K.; Rossi, H.L.; Malphurs, W.; Vierck, C.J.; Caudle, R.M. Differentiation between capsaicin-induced allodynia and hyperalgesia using a thermal operant assay. *Behav. Brain Res.* **2006**, *170*, 308–315. [CrossRef] [PubMed]
24. Nolan, T.A.; Hester, J.; Bokrand-Donatelli, Y.; Caudle, R.M.; Neubert, J.K. Adaptation of a novel operant orofacial testing system to characterize both mechanical and thermal pain. *Behav. Brain Res.* **2011**, *217*, 477–480. [CrossRef] [PubMed]
25. Kobayashi, A.; Shinoda, M.; Sessle, B.J.; Honda, K.; Imamura, Y.; Hitomi, S.; Tsuboi, Y.; Okada-Ogawa, A.; Iwata, K. Mechanisms Involved in Extraterritorial Facial Pain following Cervical Spinal Nerve Injury in Rats. *Mol. Pain* **2011**, *7*, 12. [CrossRef] [PubMed]
26. Honda, K.; Shinoda, M.; Kondo, M.; Shimizu, K.; Yonemoto, H.; Otsuki, K.; Akasaka, R.; Furukawa, A.; Iwata, K. Sensitization of TRPV1 and TRPA1 via peripheral mGluR5 signaling contributes to thermal and mechanical hypersensitivity. *Pain* **2017**, *158*, 1754–1764. [CrossRef]
27. Kitagawa, S.; Tang, C.; Unekawa, M.; Kayama, Y.; Nakahara, J.; Shibata, M. Sustained Effects of CGRP Blockade on Cortical Spreading Depolarization-Induced Alterations in Facial Heat Pain Threshold, Light Aversiveness, and Locomotive Activity in the Light Environment. *Int. J. Mol. Sci.* **2022**, *23*, 13807. [CrossRef]
28. Strassman, A.M.; Vos, B.P.; Mineta, Y.; Naderi, S.; Borsook, D.; Burstein, R. Fos-like immunoreactivity in the superficial medullary dorsal horn induced by noxious and innocuous thermal stimulation of facial skin in the rat. *J. Neurophysiol.* **1993**, *70*, 1811–1821. [CrossRef]
29. Bhakta, M.; Vuong, T.; Taura, T.; Wilson, D.S.; Stratton, J.R.; Mackenzie, K.D. Migraine therapeutics differentially modulate the CGRP pathway. *Cephalalgia* **2021**, *41*, 499–514. [CrossRef]
30. Grell, A.-S.; Haanes, K.A.; Johansson, S.E.; Edvinsson, L.; Sams, A. Fremanezumab inhibits vasodilatory effects of CGRP and capsaicin in rat cerebral artery—Potential role in conditions of severe vasoconstriction. *Eur. J. Pharmacol.* **2019**, *864*, 172726. [CrossRef]
31. Dux, M.; Vogler, B.; Kuhn, A.; Mackenzie, K.D.; Stratton, J.; Messlinger, K. The Anti-CGRP Antibody Fremanezumab Lowers CGRP Release from Rat Dura Mater and Meningeal Blood Flow. *Cells* **2022**, *11*, 1768. [CrossRef]
32. Hay, D.L.; Garelja, M.L.; Poyner, D.R.; Walker, C.S. Update on the pharmacology of calcitonin/CGRP family of peptides: IUPHAR Review 25. *Br. J. Pharmacol.* **2018**, *175*, 3–17. [CrossRef]
33. Zhang, Q.; Han, X.; Wu, H.; Zhang, M.; Hu, G.; Dong, Z.; Yu, S. Dynamic changes in CGRP, PACAP, and PACAP receptors in the trigeminovascular system of a novel repetitive electrical stimulation rat model: Relevant to migraine. *Mol. Pain* **2019**, *15*, 1744806918820452. [CrossRef]
34. Araya, E.I.; Turnes, J.D.M.; Barroso, A.R.; Chichorro, J.G. Contribution of intraganglionic CGRP to migraine-like responses in male and female rats. *Cephalalgia* **2020**, *40*, 689–700. [CrossRef]
35. Caronna, E.; Gallardo, V.J.; Alpuente, A.; Torres-Ferrus, M.; Pozo-Rosich, P. Anti-CGRP monoclonal antibodies in chronic migraine with medication overuse: Real-life effectiveness and predictors of response at 6 months. *J. Headache Pain* **2021**, *22*, 120. [CrossRef]
36. Blumenfeld, A.; Durham, P.L.; Feoktistov, A.; Hay, D.L.; Russo, A.F.; Turner, I. Hypervigilance, Allostatic Load, and Migraine Prevention: Antibodies to CGRP or Receptor. *Neurol. Ther.* **2021**, *10*, 469–497. [CrossRef]
37. Benbow, T.; Ekbatan, M.R.; Wang, G.H.Y.; Teja, F.; Exposto, F.G.; Svensson, P.; Cairns, B.E. Systemic administration of monosodium glutamate induces sexually dimorphic headache- and nausea-like behaviours in rats. *Pain* **2022**, *163*, 1838–1853. [CrossRef]
38. Stucky, N.L.; Gregory, E.; Winter, M.K.; He, Y.-Y.; Hamilton, E.S.; McCarson, K.; Berman, N.E. Sex Differences in Behavior and Expression of CGRP-Related Genes in a Rodent Model of Chronic Migraine. *Headache* **2011**, *51*, 674–692. [CrossRef]

39. Bree, D.; Mackenzie, K.; Stratton, J.; Levy, D. Enhanced post-traumatic headache-like behaviors and diminished contribution of peripheral CGRP in female rats following a mild closed head injury. *Cephalalgia* **2020**, *40*, 748–760. [CrossRef]
40. De Logu, F.; Nassini, R.; Hegron, A.; Landini, L.; Jensen, D.D.; Latorre, R.; Ding, J.; Marini, M.; de Araujo, D.S.M.; Ramírez-Garcia, P.; et al. Schwann cell endosome CGRP signals elicit periorbital mechanical allodynia in mice. *Nat. Commun.* **2022**, *13*, 646. [CrossRef]
41. Majmudar, N.G.; Robson, S.C.; Ford, G.A. Effects of the Menopause, Gender, and Estrogen Replacement Therapy on Vascular Nitric Oxide Activity. *J. Clin. Endocrinol. Metab.* **2000**, *85*, 1577–1583. [CrossRef]
42. Burch, R.; Rizzoli, P.; Loder, E.; Loder, E. The prevalence and impact of migraine and severe headache in the United States: Updated age, sex, and socioeconomic-specific estimates from government health surveys. *Headache* **2021**, *61*, 60–68. [CrossRef] [PubMed]
43. Burstein, R.; Noseda, R.; Borsook, D. Migraine: Multiple Processes, Complex Pathophysiology. *J. Neurosci.* **2015**, *35*, 6619–6629. [CrossRef] [PubMed]
44. Goadsby, P.J. Migraine, Allodynia, Sensitisation and All of That . . . . *Eur. Neurol.* **2005**, *53* (Suppl. S1), 10–16. [CrossRef] [PubMed]
45. Silvestro, M.; Tessitore, A.; Orologio, I.; De Micco, R.; Tartaglione, L.; Trojsi, F.; Tedeschi, G.; Russo, A. Galcanezumab effect on "whole pain burden" and multidimensional outcomes in migraine patients with previous unsuccessful treatments: A real-world experience. *J. Headache Pain* **2022**, *23*, 69. [CrossRef]
46. Barbanti, P.; Aurilia, C.; Egeo, G.; Torelli, P.; Proietti, S.; Cevoli, S.; Bonassi, S. For the Italian Migraine Registry Study Group. Late Response to Anti-CGRP Monoclonal Antibodies in Migraine: A Multicenter, Prospective, Observational Study. *Neurology* **2023**. [CrossRef]
47. Sand, T.; Zhitniy, N.; Nilsen, K.B.; Helde, G.; Hagen, K.; Stovner, L.J. Thermal pain thresholds are decreased in the migraine preattack phase. *Eur. J. Neurol.* **2008**, *15*, 1199–1205. [CrossRef]
48. Kopruszinski, C.M.; Xie, J.Y.; Eyde, N.M.; Remeniuk, B.; Walter, S.; Stratton, J.; Bigal, M.; Chichorro, J.; Dodick, D.; Porreca, F. Prevention of stress- or nitric oxide donor-induced medication overuse headache by a calcitonin gene-related peptide antibody in rodents. *Cephalalgia* **2017**, *37*, 560–570. [CrossRef]

Disclaimer/Publisher's Note: The statements, opinions and data contained in all publications are solely those of the individual author(s) and contributor(s) and not of MDPI and/or the editor(s). MDPI and/or the editor(s) disclaim responsibility for any injury to people or property resulting from any ideas, methods, instructions or products referred to in the content.

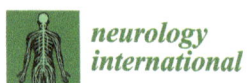 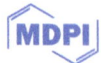

Article
Neurite Damage in Patients with Migraine

Yasushi Shibata [1,*] and Sumire Ishiyama [2]

[1] Department of Neurosurgery, Headache Clinic, Mito Medical Center, University of Tsukuba, Mito Kyodo General Hospital, Mito 3100015, Japan
[2] Center for Medical Sciences, Ibaraki Prefectural University of Health Sciences, Ami 3000394, Japan
* Correspondence: yshibata@md.tsukuba.ac.jp

Abstract: We examined neurite orientation dispersion and density imaging in patients with migraine. We found that patients with medication overuse headache exhibited lower orientation dispersion than those without. Moreover, orientation dispersion in the body of the corpus callosum was statistically negatively correlated with migraine attack frequencies. These findings indicate that neurite dispersion is damaged in patients with chronic migraine. Our study results indicate the orientation preference of neurite damage in migraine.

Keywords: migraine; neurite; MRI

Citation: Shibata, Y.; Ishiyama, S. Neurite Damage in Patients with Migraine. *Neurol. Int.* **2024**, *16*, 299–311. https://doi.org/10.3390/neurolint16020021

Academic Editor: Marcello Moccia

Received: 26 December 2023
Revised: 20 February 2024
Accepted: 26 February 2024
Published: 29 February 2024

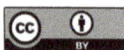

Copyright: © 2024 by the authors. Licensee MDPI, Basel, Switzerland. This article is an open access article distributed under the terms and conditions of the Creative Commons Attribution (CC BY) license (https://creativecommons.org/licenses/by/4.0/).

1. Introduction

Migraine has a high prevalence and causes high levels of disability worldwide and is ranked second among the diseases in terms of the years lived with disability in the Global Burden of Disease Study in 2016 [1]. The International Classification of Headache Disorders, third edition (ICHD-3), is the world's standard classification and diagnostic criteria of headache [2]. This classification and diagnostic criteria for migraine are based only on a patient's history, symptoms, and clinical findings. Calcitonin-gene-related peptide (CGRP) is the molecule responsible for the pathology of migraine [3]. Specific anti-CGRP monoclonal or anti-CGRP receptor antibodies have been developed and are clinically effective in preventing migraine attacks [4–6]. The small molecules of CGRP antagonists have also been used for both the prevention and acute treatment of migraine attacks in some countries [7–10]. The CGRP concentration in saliva is higher in chronic migraine (CM) patients than in episodic migraine (EM) patients [11,12]. However, the diagnostic credibility of CGRP concentration in saliva has not been investigated. Thus, to the best of our knowledge, no biomarker has been identified for diagnosing migraine.

Neuroimaging is a standard clinical examination used to diagnose neurological diseases. Magnetic resonance imaging (MRI) is noninvasive and has high spatial resolution and high contrast; thus, it is used to diagnose various brain diseases, including cerebrovascular diseases, brain tumors, traumatic hematomas, epilepsy, congenital neural diseases, hydrocephalus, intracranial infection, psychiatric diseases, and neurodegenerative diseases [13–18].

Patients with migraine have a higher prevalence of cerebellar and brain stem infarction and white matter T2 hyperintense lesions than healthy controls according to the Cerebral Abnormalities in Migraine, Epidemiological Risk Analysis study [19,20]. The authors of this study discussed the possibility of impaired adaptive cerebral hemodynamic mechanisms in the posterior circulation of migraine patients being the cause of these ischemic lesions [20]. Another study on women with migraine showed a strong trend toward an association with lacunar stroke and no association with atherosclerotic and cardio-embolic strokes [21]. This study indicated no difference in the risk of stroke between the anterior and posterior regions. The association between migraine and cerebral infarction and white matter hyperintense lesions has been reported [22–24]. Most of these studies have a cross-sectional design;

thus, the causal and temporal associations of these regions with migraine are unclear. In one longitudinal study [22], the progression of white matter hyperintense lesions was not observed among migraine patients during the 8–12-year study period. They speculated that brain lesions in migraine patients may occur early in life.

Migraine is predominantly observed in young women [25,26]. Migraine with aura, oral hormonal contraceptives, and tobacco smoking are risk factors for ischemic stroke in young women [21,24,27–29]. Although the incidence of ischemic stroke among young women is low, women with migraine with aura should be advised to stop smoking or stop using oral contraceptives.

Patent foramen ovale causes intracardiac right–left shunt and paradoxical embolus. Cases of cryptogenic stroke accompanied by migraine have a high prevalence (79%) among patients with patent foramen ovale who have right-to-left shunting [30]. A meta-analysis of case–control studies revealed an association between the presence of patent foramen ovale and migraine with aura but not with migraine without aura [31]. Given that cerebral ischemia lesions are related to migraine with aura, microembolization and ischemia are speculated to be the cause of cortical spreading depression [32], which is the primary cause of migraine aura [33,34]. However, a series of studies of regional cerebral blood flow during migraine attacks showed reduced regional cerebral blood flow posteriorly spreading slowly and contiguously anteriorly and crossing borders of the supply of major cerebral arteries [35]. Human studies showed initial hyperemia followed by prolonged hypoperfusion. Therefore, cortical spreading depression is not simply caused by ischemia. Moreover, most migraine attacks are not accompanied by aura, which are then diagnosed as migraines without aura. Therefore, cortical spreading depression could not fully explain the pathology of most migraines [35].

Migraine premonitory symptoms, including general fatigue, irritability, food cravings, and yawning, were observed 2 days before the migraine attacks [36]. The activation of the hypothalamus demonstrated by functional MRI [37] is considered the pathology of these premonitory symptoms. Therefore, the hypothalamus is considered the generator of migraine attacks.

Cerebral microbleeds are indicators of cerebral vascular damage. Migraine patients showed a significantly higher prevalence of infratentorial microbleeds than healthy controls [38]. However, standard anatomical MRI revealed no abnormalities that are specific for patients with migraine.

Volume analysis, i.e., volumetry, is a popular method for analyzing brain morphological changes. Migraine patients showed decreased gray matter volume in the posterior–opercular regions, prefrontal cortex, and anterior cingulate cortex compared with healthy controls [39]. Most volume studies were cross-sectional and compared migraine patients with healthy controls. Liu et al. analyzed the longitudinal MRI volume changes in patients with migraine and reported progressive gray matter volume reductions in the dorsolateral and medical parts of the superior frontal gyrus, orbitofrontal cortex, hippocampus, precuneus, and primary and secondary somatosensory cortices during the 1-year observation period in patients with early migraine without aura [40]. In this study, changes in diffusion tensor imaging (DTI), which is a method used to measure the direction of water diffusion, were not observed during the same period [41].

Cerebral cortical thickness was investigated using MRI. Compared with healthy controls, patients with migraine showed cortical thickening in the caudal somatosensory cortex, which is responsible for the head and face [42]. Another study showed cortical thickening in the left rostral middle frontal and bilateral postcentral gyri [43]. The average thickness of the bilateral postcentral gyri was positively correlated with migraine disease duration and headache frequency. Another study indicated cortical thinning at the somatosensory cortex, right fusiform gyrus, and right temporal pole in patients with migraine, as compared with healthy controls [44]. These cortical thickness changes were investigated in relation to migraine attack frequencies. Somatosensory cortical thickness was thin and thick in low- and high-frequency episodic migraine (EM) patients, respectively, as compared with healthy controls [45]. Another study indicated reduced cortical thickness and cortical surface area in the regions subserving pain processing, and conversely, the cortical thickness and surface area were increased in the migraine in regions involved in executive functions and visual motion processing [46]. These cortical thickness and surface area abnormalities were related to aura and white matter hyperintensities but not to migraine disease duration and attack frequency. In this study, the cortical surface area abnormalities were more pronounced and more widely distributed than the cortical thickness abnormalities. Cortical surface area normally increases during late fetal development as a consequence of cortical folding, whereas cortical thickness changes throughout the life span as a consequence of development and disease. Therefore, these results might indicate a congenital condition rather than consequences of repeated migraine attacks. The discrepancies between several studies may be explained by different patient populations, analytical and statistical methods, applied thresholds, and included covariates. Neural plasticity must have significant effects, especially on cortical thickness, in the long term.

However, some abnormal findings of advanced MRI methods, including DTI and functional MRI (fMRI), have been reported [47–51]. The amount of longitudinal and perpendicular diffusions are expressed as axial diffusivity (AD) and radial diffusivity (RD), respectively, and the mean value of the three mutually perpendicular diffusivities is referred to as the mean diffusivity (MD) [41]. Fractional anisotropy (FA) is defined as the index of the directionality of diffusion. In free water, water molecules freely diffuse in every direction; hence, FA is defined as 0. If diffusion is restricted to only one direction, FA becomes 1. In the central nervous system, homogenously directed neural fibers, including the corpus callosum and internal capsule, have high FA values; hence, these regions are good targets for DTI investigation. We previously reported significantly lower FA in the white matter of patients with migraine with aura and medication overuse headache using 1.5 Tesla MRI [47]. Planchuelo-Gómez et al. reported DTI findings in migraine patients [52]. They found considerably reduced AD in CM patients as compared with EM patients. Nonetheless, these findings are insufficient for diagnosing migraine at present. Therefore, a new biomarker for migraine diagnosis is required.

Neurite orientation dispersion and density imaging (NODDI) is an advanced imaging method that automatically divides tissues into the following three components: free water, extraneurite, and intraneurite [53]. The fraction of isovolume (Fiso), which is the fraction of free water, is a marker of inflammation [54–57]. An extraneurite, such as the cell body, is analyzed using the DTI model. Intraneurites, including axons and dendrites, are analyzed using a stick model. Intracellular volume fraction (Ficvf) is a marker of neurite density, and orientation dispersion index (ODI) is a marker of neurite dispersion. DTI parameters, including FA and AD, depend on both brain neurite density and dispersion. FA reduction may occur due to decreased neurite density or increased neurite ODI, which can only be assessed via NODDI [53,58].

NODDI has been used to analyze various physiological and pathological conditions. In physiological situations, increased neurite ODI is associated with brain development, whereas reduced neurite density is linked with brain aging [53]. Structural alterations in neurites have been linked to numerous neurological disorders [59]. The value of the gray-matter ODI is reportedly significantly lower in the temporal pole, anterior parahippocampal gyrus, and hippocampus of patients with schizophrenia than in healthy controls [60]. Brain tumors with high Ficvf in the tumor parenchyma (icvfTP) and low Ficvf in the peritumoral region (icvfPT) are more likely to be high-grade gliomas, whereas lesions with low icvfTP and high icvfPT are more likely to be low-grade gliomas [61]. Decreased dendritic arborization, dendritic spine loss, and synapse loss have been observed in neuropathological studies of Alzheimer's disease and are associated with cognitive deficits. The ODI values of multiple cortical regions were significantly lower in patients with Alzheimer's disease [62]. The cortical ODI is associated with Mini-mental State Examination performance. In the injured brain in mouse models of closed traumatic brain injury, only the NODDI-derived Ficvf was significantly lower [63]. The ODI values computed using the NODDI model were nearly identical to those obtained via electron microscopy. Ficvf was related to cognitive functioning in patients with moyamoya disease, and all NODDI parameters were significantly correlated with positron emission computed tomographic parameters and clinical severity [64]. Neurite density and network complexity decreased with the increasing severity of the ischemic burden and increased interstitial fluid. ODI was higher in gadolinium-enhancing multiple sclerosis lesions than in nonenhancing lesions [65]. Some other studies have indicated that NODDI may be useful in determining seizure focus in patients with focal cortical dysplasia [66]. Decreased neurite density has been observed in temporal lobe epilepsy, mainly in the ipsilateral temporal areas [67].

However, to the best of our knowledge, no study has evaluated NODDI in patients with migraine. Therefore, we examined the DTI and NODDI in patients with migraine and compared them with those of healthy controls.

2. Materials and Methods

2.1. Study Population

Overall, 29 patients with migraine (mean age: 44.5 years; two men) and 23 healthy controls (mean age: 44.9 years; six men) were recruited (Table 1). All patients were diagnosed and treated at the Mito Medical Center, Mito Kyodo General Hospital, University of Tsukuba, Japan. The patients met the ICHD-3 criteria for the diagnosis of migraine [2]. The ICHD-3 was also used to diagnose EM, CM, and medication overuse headache (MOH). Migraine was episodic in 17 patients and chronic in 12 patients, and MOH was diagnosed in 4 migraine patients (Tables 2 and 3). The mean ages of the EM and CM groups were 46.6 and 41.4 years, respectively, with the difference being not statistically significant. The mean ages of MOH and non-MOH patients were 37.8 and 45.6 years, respectively, with the difference being not statistically significant. The mean disease duration of all migraine patients was 21.4 years. The mean disease durations of EM and CM were 23.9 and 17.6 years, respectively, and this difference was not statistically significant. The mean disease durations of MOH and non-MOH patients were 7.5 and 23.6 years, respectively, with the difference being statistically significant (t-test, $p < 0.01$). There was no history of neurological disease, severe headache, head trauma, psychiatric disorder, or any intracranial abnormalities on anatomical MRI in the healthy controls. None of the migraine patients had any clinical and radiological neurological diseases such as stroke and dementia or any systematic diseases such as hypertension and malignancy. We obtained institutional review board approval prior to conducting this study (No. 20-56) on 2021-March-25 and informed consent from the patients.

Table 1. The characteristics of migraine patients and healthy volunteers.

	Migraine	Healthy Volunteer	p
n	29	23	-
Male/female	2/27	6/17	ns
Mean age ±SD	44.5 ± 13.5	44.9 ± 12.7	ns
Duration ± SD	21.4 ± 15.7	-	-
MOH(Yes/No)	4/25	-	-
EM/CM	17/12	-	-

Table 2. Characteristics of EM and CM patients.

	EM	CM	p
n	17	12	
Male/female	0/17	1/11	
Mean age +SD	46.6 ± 14.6	41.4 ± 11.0	0.3
Duration +SD	23.9 ± 15.4	17.6 ± 15.3	0.32

Table 3. Characteristics of MOH and non-MOH patients.

	MOH	Non-MOH	p
n	4	25	
Male/female	0/4	1/24	
Mean age + SD	37.8 ± 7.1	45.6 ± 13.9	0.155
Duration + SD	7.5 ± 4.6	23.6 ± 15.7	<0.01

2.2. Imaging Protocols

The patients and healthy controls underwent DTI and NODDI using a 3.0-Tesla MR scanner (Siemens, Erlangen, Germany) with a 32-channel head coil. All participants were instructed to close their eyes and not fall asleep. Structural imaging, including T1-weighted volume using magnetization-prepared rapid acquisition with gradient echo and T2 (fluid-attenuated inversion recovery), was performed. For T1-weighted imaging, the following parameters were used: repetition time (TR)/echo time (TE) = 2300/2.32 ms, 192 slices, and slice thickness = 0.9 mm. The following single-shot echo planar imaging parameters were used for diffusion-weighted acquisition: TR/TE = 7500/95 ms; matrix size = 128 × 128; 50 axial slices; slice thickness = 3 mm with no gap; field of view = 230 × 230 mm; 65 axial slices; number of excitations = 1; generalized autocalibrating partially parallel acquisitions (GRAPPA) factor = 2; 30 non-collinear axes; and b values of 0, 1000, and 2000 s/mm^2. The FA, MD, AD, RD, Fiso, ODI, and Ficvf in the whole brain were analyzed using tract-based spatial statistics (TBSS). The region of interest (ROI) was placed on the corpus callosum. All MR images were examined during the interictal phase of the migraine.

2.3. Statistical Analysis

Statistical analyses were performed using SPSS version 28.00 (IBM, Tokyo, Japan). Fisher's exact test and the two-sample unpaired t-test were used for the comparison of the sex and age distributions between the two groups. DTI and NODDI were analyzed using the randomize program of FMRIB, Oxford, UK Software Library (software 6.0v; http://www.fmrib.ox.ac.uk/fsl (accessed on 25 March 2021)). The significance level was set at a p-value of < 0.05. The mean FA, MD, AD, RD, Ficvf, and ODI in the ROIs were calculated and analyzed using the corresponding t-test program, MATLAB (R2017a, MathWorks, Natick, MA, USA).

3. Results

There were no significant differences in the DTI and NODDI parameters between the migraine patients and healthy controls. Additionally, there were no significant differences in the DTI and NODDI parameters between migraine patients with and without MOH. The Fiso was not significantly different between the EM and CM patients and between the MOH and migraine patients.

The Ficvf of the CM patients was slightly lower than that of the EM patients in the right temporal lobe, although this difference was not statistically significant (Figure 1). The Ficvf of the patients with MOH was lower than that of patients with migraine in the bilateral cerebrum, although this difference was not statistically significant (Figure 2). No significant correlation was observed between migraine attack frequency and Ficvf in the genu, body, and splenium of the corpus callosum (Figure 3).

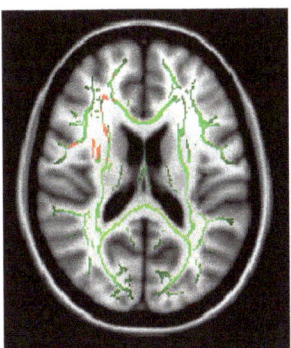

Figure 1. Ficvf (EM > CM): Green skeleton showed no difference, red skeleton showed difference at $p = 0.07$.

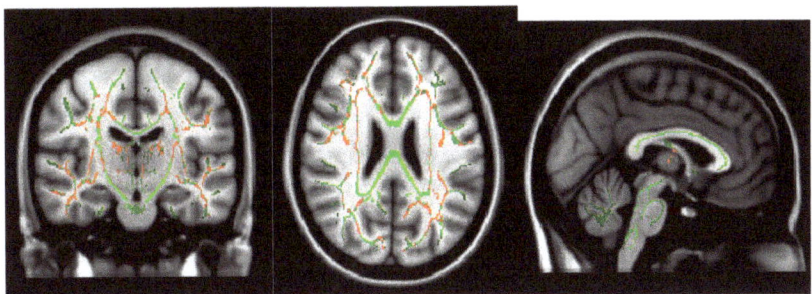

Figure 2. Ficvf (migraine > MOH): Green skeleton showed no difference, red skeleton showed difference at $p < 0.2$.

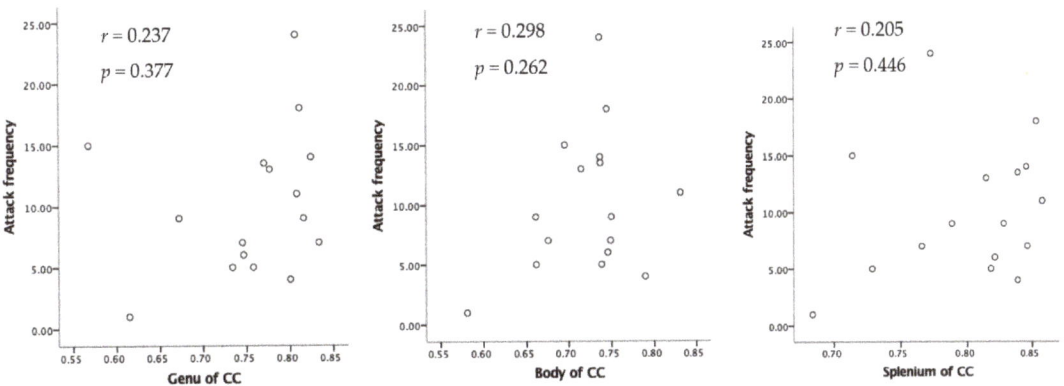

Figure 3. Relation between attack frequency and Ficvf in the corpus callosum.

The ODI in the bilateral cerebellum and brain stem was significantly lower in MOH patients than in patients with migraine (Figure 4). Migraine attack frequency and the ODI in the corpus callosum in the genu, body, and splenium showed negative correlations. In particular, the body in the corpus callosum showed a statistically significant correlation (Figure 5).

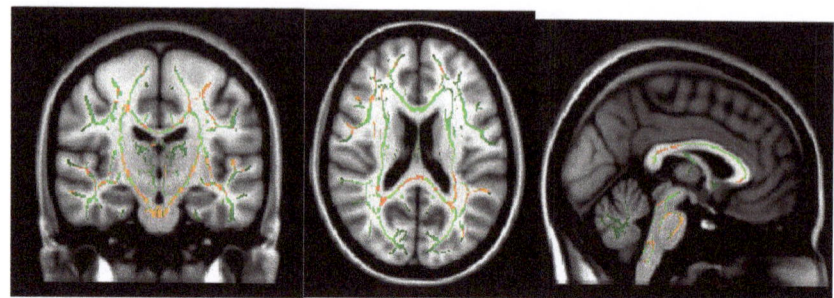

Figure 4. ODI (migraine > MOH) $p < 0.05$.

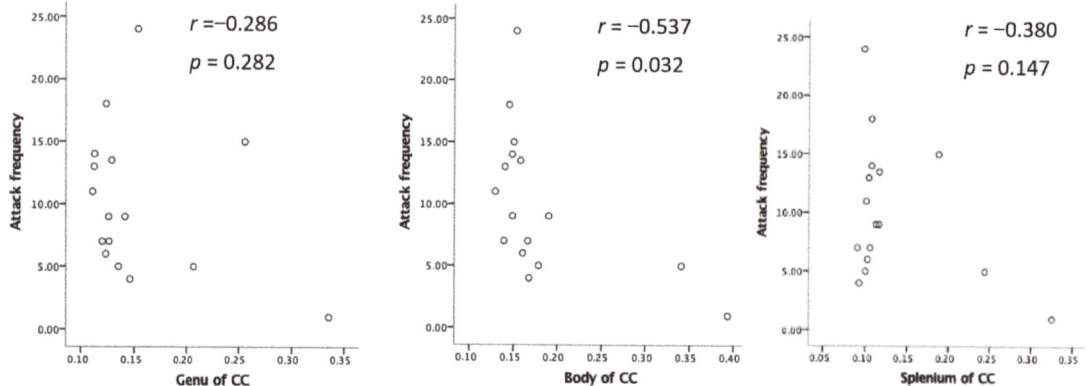

Figure 5. Negative relation between attack frequency and ODI.

4. Discussion

In the present study, we did not find any significant differences in the DTI and NODDI parameters between migraine patients and healthy controls. Fiso has been reported as a marker of neuroinflammation [54–57]. In acute neural inflammatory diseases, including demyelinating diseases such as multiple sclerosis and neurodegenerative diseases such as Parkinson's disease, neural inflammation precedes neural degeneration. Therefore, the fraction of free water volume increases before pathological microstructural changes are detectable with DTI. Given that we could not find any significant differences in Fiso, the neural tissue in patients with migraine does not demonstrate neural inflammation, or at least those that are detectable in NODDI. We did not observe the increase in free water volume in the neural tissue, which may have been caused by the fact that we only examined the migraine patients during the interictal period. During the migraine cycle, some parts of the nervous tissue, including the brainstem, hypothalamus, and trigeminal nerve, may demonstrate an increase in free water content.

We found that patients with MOH exhibited lower ODIs than those without MOH. Moreover, ODI in the corpus callosum was statistically negatively correlated with migraine attack frequency. These findings indicate that neurite dispersion is damaged in patients with MOH and CM.

MOH and CM showed pathological changes in DTI and fMRI using a 3.0-Tesla MRI scanner [52,68]. Schmitz et al. investigated the MRI findings of 28 adult female patients with migraine and compared them with those of age-matched female controls [69] using voxel-based morphometry for whole-brain analysis. Patients with migraine showed significantly reduced FA values in the superior frontal bole, middle frontal lobe, brain stem, and cerebellum as compared with the control patients. Individuals with long disease duration as compared with those with short have reduced frontal anisotropy. The differences between EM and CM groups have been demonstrated in various modalities, including electro- and magneto-physiological brain activity (M/EEG) and neurovascular and metabolic recordings from fMRI and positron emission tomography [70]. We also demonstrated significant differences between EM, CM, and MOH using DTI [47].

There are several methods to analyze the DTI data. The region of interest method is the most simple; the investigator can put the region of interest on the images. Only the selected area is analyzed, and the location and area are intentionally selected, so bias cannot be avoided. In the tract-specific analysis, specific tracts are selected and analyzed. Given that there are individual variations in brain morphology, the comparison between different individuals requires the standardization of brain morphology. Voxel-based analysis is a whole-brain analysis after standardization. Given that whole-brain analysis involves a large amount of data, a longer time for analysis is required. Some image transactions, including smoothing, are required. These image transactions and partial volume effects decrease the sensitivity of the differences. TBSS analysis is a new method for summarizing the whole-brain DTI data into white matter skeletons [71]. Whole-brain standardization was not required because only white matter skeletons were analyzed. In the present method, only limited data were analyzed within an acceptable time window. Moreover, this technique has low noise and high sensitivity. Therefore, the TBSS analysis is the standard method for analyzing DTI [71].

Szabo et al. performed a TBSS analysis of the MRI data of patients with migraine [72] and found reduced FA, increased MD, and increased RD in the right frontal white matter. They did not find any associations between migraine attack frequency or disease duration and the intensity of DTI structural changes.

Yu et al. also compared DTI findings of 20 migraine patients without aura with those of 20 age-, education-, and sex-matched healthy volunteers [73]. Migraine patients without aura showed significantly lower FA, MD, and AD in multiple brain regions, specifically in the genu, body, and splenium of the corpus callosum, than the healthy controls. Some of these white matter changes were significantly correlated with headache duration and frequency. Given that a difference in RD was observed, they speculated that these decreases in FA, AD, and MD may reveal axonal loss in migraine patients without aura.

Li et al. examined the DTI data of 12 migraine patients without a depressive/anxious disorder, 12 patients complicated with depressive/anxious disorder, and 12 age- and sex-matched healthy individuals [74]. The FA values from the migraine groups were significantly lower than those from the control group, and the FA values from the group complicated with a depressive/anxious disorder were significantly lower than those from the group without a depressive/anxious disorder. This study indicated common pathological changes in the neural microstructure among patients with migraine and depressive/anxious disorders.

Rocca et al. also analyzed the DTI data of seven migraine patients with aura and eight migraine patients without aura and healthy controls [75]. No difference was found for any white matter bundles between the healthy controls and migraine patients without aura. However, the migraine patients with aura had reduced FA of both optic radiations as compared with healthy controls and reduced average FA of the right optic radiation as compared with migraine patients without aura. These findings indicate that aura may cause neural damage in optic radiation.

Microstructural changes were observed within the migraine attack cycle. During the interictal phase, migraine patients without aura had shown significantly higher FA and slightly lower MD values in the bilateral thalami than healthy volunteers [76]. These abnormal values normalized during an attack. They speculated that these changes were related to plastic peri-ictal modifications in regional branching and the crossing of neural fibers. Given that FA is affected by various neural tissues, these FA changes could not be explained only by the neural changes, but rather, the glial changes may contribute to these results.

A previous study performed a voxel-based morphometry analysis of structural T1-weighted MRI over the course of the migraine cycle [77]. Interictally, migraine patients without aura had a significantly lower gray matter density within the right inferior parietal lobule, right temporal inferior gyrus, right superior temporal gyrus, and left temporal pole than healthy volunteers. Ictally, gray matter density increased with the left temporal pole, bilateral insula, and right lenticular nuclei. These rapid changes in gray matter density may not be explained by the neural changes in the axon or cell body; however, spinal change could be responsible.

Yuan et al. investigated DTI and resting-state functional connectivity at the same time in migraine patients without aura [78]. Twenty-one migraine patients without aura and 21 age-, sex-, and education-matched healthy controls were examined. The results of the TBSS analysis revealed reduced FA values in the genu and splenium of the corpus callosum in migraine patients. Functional connectivity analysis showed decreased interhemispheric functional connectivity of the anterior cingulate cortex in migraine patients without aura as compared to the healthy controls. The reduced FA values of the genus of the corpus callosum correlated with decreased interhemispheric resting-state functional connectivity of the anterior corpus callosum. They discussed how reduced FA of the corpus callosum modulates interhemispheric connectivity in migraine patients without aura.

Most previous DTI studies were cross-sectional; therefore, these studies could not demonstrate the longitudinal change. Liu et al. examined these structural changes between repeated observations that were 1 year apart in a group of early-stage migraine patients without aura [40]. A gray matter volume reduction was observed in the dorsolateral and medical regions of the superior frontal gyrus, orbitofrontal cortex, hippocampus, precuneus, and primary and secondary somatosensory cortices. No significant differences in the FA, AD, RD, and MD of white matter were observed in the migraine patients without aura within a year. They speculated that the gray matter volume reduction in sensory-discriminative brain regions may occur in migraine patients in its early stage and that the white matter evolves slowly during migraine chronicity. DTI mainly reflects white matter structures; therefore, DTI may not be able to detect the early changes in the sensory cortex in patients with migraine.

Most previous DTI studies used a 3.0-Tesla MRI scanner. We have reported significant DTI changes using 1.5-Tesla MRI for patients with MOH and CM [47]. This study revealed that even 1.5-Tesla MRI could demonstrate significant imaging differences between patients with migraine and healthy controls.

In the present study, DTI revealed no abnormalities between patients with migraine and healthy controls. This discrepancy from the results of a previous study may be due to the different patient populations and the number of patients analyzed. However, NODDI demonstrated significant changes in patients with MOH and CM. Therefore, NODDI may be more sensitive than DTI for investigating neurite changes in patients with migraine.

Some fMRI studies have revealed dynamic changes in functional connectivity during a migraine attack cycle [37]. Various neuroimaging studies including arterial spin labeling, positron emission tomography, and DTI reported significant changes in migraine's pre-ictal or premonitory phase [79]. One DTI study demonstrated interictal diffusivity fluctuation in the midbrain, dorsomedial pons, and spinal trigeminal nucleus over the migraine cycle [80]. These dynamic changes seem not to be caused by neural or axonal anatomical changes. Contrarily, neurite change may occur during a migraine attack cycle, although this speculation should be examined in the future.

If all neurites are equally damaged during a migraine attack, both neurite density and dispersion should decrease. However, the Ficvf in the corpus callosum showed no statistically significant correlation with migraine attack frequency. These results indicate that a high migraine attack frequency caused considerable damage to neurite dispersion as compared with neurite density. This may be caused by neurite damage only in the cross-section with an axon. Therefore, our study results indicate the orientation preference of neurite damage during a migraine attack.

This study has several limitations. The study participants were recruited from a single institution. Consequently, the study population, especially for the patients with MOH, was small and limited to Japanese individuals. Moreover, most patients were adults with a long history of migraine disease and had been medically treated for it. However, our study demonstrated significant findings. In the future, we plan to perform NODDI analyses for various populations of patients with migraine. Furthermore, we did not perform imaging during migraine attacks. Finally, our cross-sectional study compared patients with migraine with healthy controls. Thus, we do not have any longitudinal data regarding therapeutic interventions. Future investigations on the dynamic and longitudinal changes in NODDI findings in patients with migraine are warranted. We did not have any pathological data. In the future, a pathological study to demonstrate neurite damage in patients with migraine is expected.

5. Conclusions

Our study demonstrated that patients with MOH exhibited lower ODIs than those without MOH. Neurite damage in patients with CM and MOH was not observed in the DTI study. Therefore, a high migraine attack frequency and MOH caused considerable damage to neurite dispersion as compared with the neurite density. This may be caused by neurite damage only in the cross-section with an axon. Therefore, our study results indicate the orientation preference of neurite damage in patients with migraine. NODDI may be useful in understanding the pathophysiology of migraine.

Author Contributions: Conceptualization, Y.S.; formal analysis, Y.S., S.I.; investigation, Y.S., S.I.; writing—original draft preparation, Y.S.; writing—review and editing, Y.S.; funding acquisition, Y.S. All authors have read and agreed to the published version of the manuscript.

Funding: This research was funded by grant number JP20K08099 from JSPS KAKENHI.

Institutional Review Board Statement: The study was conducted in accordance with the Declaration of Helsinki and approved by the Institutional Review Board of Mito medical Center, University of Tsukuba, Mito Kyodo general hospital for studies involving humans (No. 20-56) on 25 March 2021.

Informed Consent Statement: Informed consent was obtained from all subjects involved in the study.

Data Availability Statement: The data are not publicly available due to privacy or ethical restrictions.

Conflicts of Interest: The authors declare no conflicts of interest.

References

1. Vos, T.; Abajobir, A.A.; Abate, K.H.; Abbafati, C.; Abbas, K.M.; Abd-Allah, F.; Abdulkader, R.S.; Abdulle, A.M.; Abebo, T.A.; Abera, S.F.; et al. Global, regional, and national incidence, prevalence, and years lived with disability for 328 diseases and injuries for 195 countries, 1990–2016: A systematic analysis for the Global Burden of Disease Study 2016. *Lancet* **2017**, *390*, 1211–1259. [CrossRef] [PubMed]
2. Headache Classification Committee of the International Headache Society (IHS). The International Classification of Headache Disorders, 3rd edition. *Cephalalgia* **2018**, *38*, 1–211. [CrossRef] [PubMed]
3. Lassen, L.H.; Haderslev, P.A.; Jacobsen, V.B.; Iversen, H.K.; Sperling, B.; Olesen, J. Cgrp May Play a Causative Role in Migraine. *Cephalalgia* **2002**, *22*, 54–61. [CrossRef] [PubMed]
4. Tepper, S.; Ashina, M.; Reuter, U.; Brandes, J.L.; Doležil, D.; Silberstein, S.; Winner, P.; Leonardi, D.; Mikol, D.; Lenz, R. Safety and efficacy of erenumab for preventive treatment of chronic migraine: A randomised, double-blind, placebo-controlled phase 2 trial. *Lancet Neurol.* **2017**, *16*, 425–434. [CrossRef]
5. Silberstein, S.; Dodick, D.; Bigal, M.; Yeung, P.; Goadsby, P.; Blankenbiller, T.; Grozinski-Wolff, M.; Yang, R.; Ma, Y.; Aycardi, E. Fremanezumab for the Preventive Treatment of Chronic Migraine. *N. Engl. J. Med.* **2017**, *377*, 2113–2122. [CrossRef]
6. Förderreuther, S.; Zhang, Q.; Stauffer, V.L.; Aurora, S.K.; Láinez, M.J.A. Preventive effects of galcanezumab in adult patients with episodic or chronic migraine are persistent: Data from the phase 3, randomized, double-blind, placebo-controlled EVOLVE-1, EVOLVE-2, and REGAIN studies. *J. Headache Pain* **2018**, *19*, 121. [CrossRef]
7. Croop, R.; Lipton, R.B.; Kudrow, D.; Stock, D.A.; Kamen, L.; Conway, C.M.; Stock, E.G.; Coric, V.; Goadsby, P.J. Oral rimegepant for preventive treatment of migraine: A phase 2/3, randomised, double-blind, placebo-controlled trial. *Lancet* **2021**, *397*, 51–60. [CrossRef]

8. Ailani, J.; Lipton, R.B.; Goadsby, P.J.; Guo, H.; Miceli, R.; Severt, L.; Finnegan, M.; Trugman, J.M. Atogepant for the Preventive Treatment of Migraine. *N. Engl. J. Med.* **2021**, *385*, 695–706. [CrossRef] [PubMed]
9. Dodick, D.W.; Lipton, R.B.; Ailani, J.; Halker Singh, R.B.; Shewale, A.R.; Zhao, S.; Trugman, J.M.; Yu, S.Y.; Viswanathan, H.N. Ubrogepant, an Acute Treatment for Migraine, Improved Patient-Reported Functional Disability and Satisfaction in 2 Single-Attack Phase 3 Randomized Trials, ACHIEVE I and II. *Headache J. Head Face Pain* **2020**, *60*, 686–700. [CrossRef]
10. Ailani, J.; Lipton, R.B.; Hutchinson, S.; Knievel, K.; Lu, K.; Butler, M.; Yu, S.Y.; Finnegan, M.; Severt, L.; Trugman, J.M. Long-Term Safety Evaluation of Ubrogepant for the Acute Treatment of Migraine: Phase 3, Randomized, 52-Week Extension Trial. *Headache J. Head Face Pain* **2020**, *60*, 141–152. [CrossRef] [PubMed]
11. Alpuente, A.; Gallardo, V.J.; Asskour, L.; Caronna, E.; Torres-Ferrus, M.; Pozo-Rosich, P. Salivary CGRP can monitor the different migraine phases: CGRP (in)dependent attacks. *Cephalalgia* **2021**, *42*, 186–196. [CrossRef] [PubMed]
12. Alpuente, A.; Gallardo, V.J.; Asskour, L.; Caronna, E.; Torres-Ferrus, M.; Pozo-Rosich, P. Salivary CGRP and Erenumab Treatment Response: Towards Precision Medicine in Migraine. *Ann. Neurol.* **2022**, *92*, 846–859. [CrossRef] [PubMed]
13. Wechsler, L.R. Imaging Evaluation of Acute Ischemic Stroke. *Stroke* **2011**, *42*, S12–S15. [CrossRef] [PubMed]
14. Robert, J.; Young, E.A.K. Brain MRI: Tumor evaluation. *J. Magn. Reson. Imaging* **2006**, *24*, 709–724.
15. Wintermark, M.; Sanelli, P.C.; Anzai, Y.; Tsiouris, A.J.; Whitlow, C.T. Imaging Evidence and Recommendations for Traumatic Brain Injury: Advanced Neuro- and Neurovascular Imaging Techniques. *Am. J. Neuroradiol.* **2015**, *36*, E1–E11. [CrossRef] [PubMed]
16. Glenn, O.A.; Barkovich, A.J. Magnetic Resonance Imaging of the Fetal Brain and Spine: An Increasingly Important Tool in Prenatal Diagnosis, Part 1. *AJNR Am. J. Neuroradiol.* **2006**, *27*, 1604–1611. [PubMed]
17. Greitz, D.; Hannerz, J.; Rähn, T.; Bolander, H.; Ericsson, A. MR imaging of cerebrospinal fluid dynamics in health and disease. *Acta Radiol.* **1994**, *35*, 204–211. [CrossRef] [PubMed]
18. Kakeda, S.; Korogi, Y. The efficacy of a voxel-based morphometry on the analysis of imaging in schizophrenia, temporal lobe epilepsy, and Alzheimer's disease/mild cognitive impairment: A review. *Neuroradiology* **2010**, *52*, 711–721. [CrossRef]
19. Kruit, M.C.; van Buchem, M.A.; Hofman, P.A.M.; Bakkers, J.T.N.; Terwindt, G.M.; Ferrari, M.D.; Launer, L.J. Migraine as a Risk Factor for Subclinical Brain Lesions. *JAMA* **2004**, *291*, 427–434. [CrossRef]
20. Kruit, M.C.; Launer, L.J.; Ferrari, M.D.; van Buchem, M.A. Brain stem and cerebellar hyperintense lesions in migraine. *Stroke* **2006**, *37*, 1109–1112. [CrossRef]
21. MacClellan, L.R.; Giles, W.; Cole, J.; Wozniak, M.; Stern, B.; Mitchell, B.D.; Kittner, S.J. Probable Migraine with Visual Aura and Risk of Ischemic Stroke: The Stroke Prevention in Young Women Study. *Stroke* **2007**, *38*, 2438–2445. [CrossRef]
22. Hamedani, A.G.; Rose, K.M.; Peterlin, B.L.; Mosley, T.H.; Coker, L.H.; Jack, C.R.; Knopman, D.S.; Alonso, A.; Gottesman, R.F. Migraine and white matter hyperintensities: The ARIC MRI study. *Neurology* **2013**, *81*, 1308–1313. [CrossRef]
23. Monteith, T.; Gardener, H.; Rundek, T.; Dong, C.; Yoshita, M.; Elkind, M.S.V.; DeCarli, C.; Sacco, R.L.; Wright, C.B. Migraine, White Matter Hyperintensities, and Subclinical Brain Infarction in a Diverse Community: The Northern Manhattan Study. *Stroke* **2014**, *45*, 1830–1832. [CrossRef]
24. Øie, L.R.; Kurth, T.; Gulati, S.; Dodick, D.W. Migraine and risk of stroke. *J. Neurol. Neurosurg. Psychiatry* **2020**, *91*, 593–604. [CrossRef] [PubMed]
25. Sakai, F.; Igarashi, H. Prevalence of migraine in Japan: A nationwide survey. *Cephalalgia* **1997**, *17*, 15–22. [CrossRef] [PubMed]
26. Chu, M.; Kim, D.-W.; Kim, B.-K.; Kim, J.-M.; Jang, T.-W.; Park, J.; Lee, K.; Cho, S.-J. Gender-specific influence of socioeconomic status on the prevalence of migraine and tension-type headache: The results from the Korean headache survey. *J. Headache Pain* **2013**, *14*, 82. [CrossRef] [PubMed]
27. Fazekas, F.; Koch, M.; Schmidt, R.; Offenbacher, H.; Payer, F.; Freidl, W.; Lechner, H. The prevalence of cerebral damage varies with migraine type: A MRI study. *Headache* **1992**, *32*, 287–291. [CrossRef] [PubMed]
28. Boudreau, G.; Leroux, E. The complications of migraine classified under the international classification of headache disorders: A review. *Headache Care* **2006**, *3*, 85–90. [CrossRef]
29. Kurth, T.; Winter, A.C.; Eliassen, A.H.; Dushkes, R.; Mukamal, K.J.; Rimm, E.B.; Willett, W.C.; Manson, J.E.; Rexrode, K.M. Migraine and risk of cardiovascular disease in women: Prospective cohort study. *BMJ* **2016**, *353*, i2610. [CrossRef]
30. West, B.H.; Noureddin, N.; Mamzhi, Y.; Low, C.G.; Coluzzi, A.C.; Shih, E.J.; Gevorgyan Fleming, R.; Saver, J.L.; Liebeskind, D.S.; Charles, A.; et al. Frequency of Patent Foramen Ovale and Migraine in Patients with Cryptogenic Stroke. *Stroke* **2018**, *49*, 1123–1128. [CrossRef]
31. Takagi, H.; Umemoto, T. A meta-analysis of case-control studies of the association of migraine and patent foramen ovale. *J. Cardiol.* **2016**, *67*, 493–503. [CrossRef]
32. Pezzini, A.; Grassi, M.; Lodigiani, C.; Patella, R.; Gandolfo, C.; Casoni, F.; Musolino, R.; Calabro, R.S.; Bovi, P.; Adami, A.; et al. Predictors of Migraine Subtypes in Young Adults with Ischemic Stroke: The Italian Project on Stroke in Young Adults. *Stroke* **2011**, *42*, 17–21. [CrossRef]
33. Lance, J.W. The pathophysiology of migraine. *Ann. Acad. Med. Singap.* **1985**, *14*, 4–11. [PubMed]
34. Hadjikhani, N.; Sanchez del Rio, M.; Wu, O.; Schwartz, D.; Bakker, D.; Fischl, B.; Kwong, K.K.; Cutrer, F.M.; Rosen, B.R.; Tootell, R.B.H.; et al. Mechanisms of migraine aura revealed by functional MRI in human visual cortex. *Proc. Natl. Acad. Sci. USA* **2001**, *98*, 4687–4692. [CrossRef] [PubMed]
35. Tfelt-Hansen, P.C. History of migraine with aura and cortical spreading depression from 1941 and onwards. *Cephalalgia* **2009**, *30*, 780–792. [CrossRef]

36. Burstein, R.; Noseda, R.; Borsook, D. Migraine: Multiple Processes, Complex Pathophysiology. *J. Neurosci. Off. J. Soc. Neurosci.* **2015**, *35*, 6619–6629. [CrossRef] [PubMed]
37. Schulte, L.H.; Mehnert, J.; May, A. Longitudinal Neuroimaging over 30 Days: Temporal Characteristics of Migraine. *Ann. Neurol.* **2020**, *87*, 646–651. [CrossRef]
38. Arkink, E.B.; Terwindt, G.M.; de Craen, A.J.M.; Konishi, J.; van der Grond, J.; van Buchem, M.; Ferrari, M.D.; Kruit, M.C. Infratentorial Microbleeds. *Stroke* **2015**, *46*, 1987–1989. [CrossRef]
39. Dai, Z.; Zhong, J.; Xiao, P.; Zhu, Y.; Chen, F.; Pan, P.; Shi, H. Gray matter correlates of migraine and gender effect: A meta-analysis of voxel-based morphometry studies. *Neuroscience* **2015**, *299*, 88–96. [CrossRef]
40. Liu, J.; Lan, L.; Li, G.; Yan, X.; Nan, J.; Xiong, S.; Yin, Q.; von Deneen, K.M.; Gong, Q.; Liang, F.; et al. Migraine-Related Gray Matter and White Matter Changes at a 1-Year Follow-Up Evaluation. *J. Pain* **2013**, *14*, 1703–1708. [CrossRef]
41. Shibata, Y.; Goto, M.; Ishiyama, S. Analysis of Migraine Pathophysiology by Magnetic Resonance Imaging. *OBM Neurobiol.* **2022**, *6*, 115. [CrossRef]
42. DaSilva, A.F.M.; Granziera, C.; Nouchine Hadjikhani, J.S. Thickening in the somatosensory cortex of patients with migraine. *Neurology* **2007**, *69*, 1990–1995. [CrossRef]
43. Kim, J.H.; Kim, J.B.; Suh, S.I.; Seo, W.K.; Oh, K.; Koh, S.B. Thickening of the somatosensory cortex in migraine without aura. *Cephalalgia* **2014**, *34*, 1125–1133. [CrossRef]
44. Chong, C.D.; Dodick, D.W.; Schlaggar, B.L.; Schwedt, T.J. Atypical age-related cortical thinning in episodic migraine. *Cephalalgia* **2014**, *34*, 1115–1124. [CrossRef] [PubMed]
45. Maleki, N.; Becerra, L.; Brawn, J.; Bigal, M.; Burstein, R.; Borsook, D. Concurrent functional and structural cortical alterations in migraine. *Cephalalgia* **2012**, *32*, 607–620. [CrossRef] [PubMed]
46. Messina, R.; Rocca, M.A.; Colombo, B.; Valsasina, P.; Horsfield, M.A.; Copetti, M.; Falini, A.; Comi, G.; Filippi, M. Cortical Abnormalities in Patients with Migraine: A Surface-based Analysis. *Radiology* **2013**, *268*, 170–180. [CrossRef] [PubMed]
47. Shibata, Y.; Ishiyama, S.; Matsushita, A. White matter diffusion abnormalities in migraine and medication overuse headache: A 1.5-Tesla tract-based spatial statistics study. *Clin. Neurol. Neurosurg.* **2018**, *174*, 167–173. [CrossRef]
48. Schwedt, T.J.; Si, B.; Li, J.; Wu, T.; Chong, C.D. Migraine Subclassification via a Data-Driven Automated Approach Using Multimodality Factor Mixture Modeling of Brain Structure Measurements. *Headache J. Head Face Pain* **2017**, *57*, 1051–1064. [CrossRef] [PubMed]
49. Planchuelo-Gómez, Á.; García-Azorín, D.; Guerrero, Á.L.; de Luis-García, R.; Rodríguez, M.; Aja-Fernández, S. Alternative Microstructural Measures to Complement Diffusion Tensor Imaging in Migraine Studies with Standard MRI Acquisition. *Brain Sci.* **2020**, *10*, 711. [CrossRef]
50. Schramm, S.; Börner, C.; Reichert, M.; Baum, T.; Zimmer, C.; Heinen, F.; Bonfert, M.V.; Sollmann, N. Functional magnetic resonance imaging in migraine: A systematic review. *Cephalalgia* **2023**, *43*, 03331024221128278. [CrossRef]
51. Ishiyama, S.; Shibata, Y.; Ayuzawa, S.; Matsushita, A.; Matsumura, A.; Ishikawa, E. The Modifying of Functional Connectivity Induced by Peripheral Nerve Field Stimulation using Electroacupuncture for Migraine: A Prospective Clinical Study. *Pain Med.* **2022**, *23*, 1560–1569. [CrossRef] [PubMed]
52. Planchuelo-Gómez, Á.; García-Azorín, D.; Guerrero, Á.L.; Aja-Fernández, S.; Rodríguez, M.; de Luis-García, R. White matter changes in chronic and episodic migraine: A diffusion tensor imaging study. *J. Headache Pain* **2020**, *21*, 1. [CrossRef]
53. Zhang, H.; Schneider, T.; Wheeler-Kingshott, C.A.; Alexander, D.C. NODDI: Practical in vivo neurite orientation dispersion and density imaging of the human brain. *NeuroImage* **2012**, *61*, 1000–1016. [CrossRef] [PubMed]
54. Seyedmirzaei, H.; Nabizadeh, F.; Aarabi, M.H.; Pini, L. Neurite Orientation Dispersion and Density Imaging in Multiple Sclerosis: A Systematic Review. *J. Magn. Reson. Imaging* **2023**, *58*, 1011–1029. [CrossRef]
55. Andica, C.; Kamagata, K.; Hatano, T.; Saito, A.; Uchida, W.; Ogawa, T.; Takeshige-Amano, H.; Zalesky, A.; Wada, A.; Suzuki, M.; et al. Free-Water Imaging in White and Gray Matter in Parkinson's Disease. *Cells* **2019**, *8*, 839. [CrossRef] [PubMed]
56. Nakaya, M.; Sato, N.; Matsuda, H.; Maikusa, N.; Shigemoto, Y.; Sone, D.; Yamao, T.; Ogawa, M.; Kimura, Y.; Chiba, E.; et al. Free water derived by multi-shell diffusion MRI reflects tau/neuroinflammatory pathology in Alzheimer's disease. *Alzheimer Dement.* **2022**, *8*, e12356. [CrossRef]
57. Kraguljac, N.V.; Guerreri, M.; Strickland, M.J.; Zhang, H. Neurite Orientation Dispersion and Density Imaging in Psychiatric Disorders: A Systematic Literature Review and a Technical Note. *Biol. Psychiatry Glob. Open Sci.* **2023**, *3*, 10–21. [CrossRef]
58. Timmers, I.; Roebroeck, A.; Bastiani, M.; Jansma, B.; Rubio-Gozalbo, E.; Zhang, H. Assessing Microstructural Substrates of White Matter Abnormalities: A Comparative Study Using DTI and NODDI. *PLoS ONE* **2016**, *11*, e0167884. [CrossRef]
59. Penzes, P.; Cahill, M.E.; Jones, K.A.; VanLeeuwen, J.-E.; Woolfrey, K.M. Dendritic spine pathology in neuropsychiatric disorders. *Nat. Neurosci.* **2011**, *14*, 285–293. [CrossRef]
60. Nazeri, A.; Mulsant, B.H.; Rajji, T.K.; Levesque, M.L.; Pipitone, J.; Stefanik, L.; Shahab, S.; Roostaei, T.; Wheeler, A.L.; Chavez, S.; et al. Gray Matter Neuritic Microstructure Deficits in Schizophrenia and Bipolar Disorder. *Biol. Psychiatry* **2017**, *82*, 726–736. [CrossRef]
61. Zhao, J.; Li, J.-B.; Wang, J.-Y.; Wang, Y.-L.; Liu, D.-W.; Li, X.-B.; Song, Y.-K.; Tian, Y.-S.; Yan, X.; Li, Z.-H.; et al. Quantitative analysis of neurite orientation dispersion and density imaging in grading gliomas and detecting IDH-1 gene mutation status. *NeuroImage Clin.* **2018**, *19*, 174–181. [CrossRef]

62. Parker, T.D.; Slattery, C.F.; Zhang, J.; Nicholas, J.M.; Paterson, R.W.; Foulkes, A.J.M.; Malone, I.B.; Thomas, D.L.; Modat, M.; Cash, D.M.; et al. Cortical microstructure in young onset Alzheimer's disease using neurite orientation dispersion and density imaging. *Hum. Brain Mapp.* **2018**, *39*, 3005–3017. [CrossRef]
63. Wu, Y.-C.; Mustafi, S.M.; Harezlak, J.; Kodiweera, C.; Flashman, L.A.; McAllister, T.W. Hybrid Diffusion Imaging in Mild Traumatic Brain Injury. *J. Neurotrauma* **2018**, *35*, 2377–2390. [CrossRef] [PubMed]
64. Hara, S.; Hori, M.; Ueda, R.; Hayashi, S.; Inaji, M.; Tanaka, Y.; Maehara, T.; Ishii, K.; Aoki, S.; Nariai, T. Unraveling Specific Brain Microstructural Damage in Moyamoya Disease Using Diffusion Magnetic Resonance Imaging and Positron Emission Tomography. *J. Stroke Cerebrovasc. Dis.* **2019**, *28*, 1113–1125. [CrossRef]
65. Sacco, S.; Caverzasi, E.; Papinutto, N.; Cordano, C.; Bischof, A.; Gundel, T.; Cheng, S.; Asteggiano, C.; Kirkish, G.; Mallott, J.; et al. Neurite Orientation Dispersion and Density Imaging for Assessing Acute Inflammation and Lesion Evolution in MS. *Am. J. Neuroradiol.* **2020**, *41*, 2219–2226. [CrossRef] [PubMed]
66. Winston, G.P. The potential role of novel diffusion imaging techniques in the understanding and treatment of epilepsy. *Quant. Imaging Med. Surg.* **2015**, *5*, 279–287.
67. Sone, D.; Sato, N.; Ota, M.; Maikusa, N.; Kimura, Y.; Matsuda, H. Abnormal neurite density and orientation dispersion in unilateral temporal lobe epilepsy detected by advanced diffusion imaging. *NeuroImage Clin.* **2018**, *20*, 772–782. [CrossRef]
68. Schwedt, T.J.; Chong, C.D. Medication Overuse Headache: Pathophysiological Insights from Structural and Functional Brain MRI Research. *Headache J. Head Face Pain* **2017**, *57*, 1173–1178. [CrossRef] [PubMed]
69. Schmitz, N.; Admiraal-Behloul, F.; Arkink, E.B.; Kruit, M.C.; Schoonman, G.G.; Ferrari, M.D.; Van Buchem, M.A. Attack Frequency and Disease Duration as Indicators for Brain Damage in Migraine. *Headache J. Head Face Pain* **2008**, *48*, 1044–1055. [CrossRef]
70. Gomez-Pilar, J.; Martínez-Cagigal, V.; García-Azorín, D.; Gómez, C.; Guerrero, Á.; Hornero, R. Headache-related circuits and high frequencies evaluated by EEG, MRI, PET as potential biomarkers to differentiate chronic and episodic migraine: Evidence from a systematic review. *J. Headache Pain* **2022**, *23*, 95. [CrossRef]
71. Smith, S.M. Tract-based spatial statistics. *NeuroImage* **2006**, *31*, 1487–1505. [CrossRef]
72. Szabó, N.; Kincses, Z.T.; Párdutz, Á.; Tajti, J.; Szok, D.; Tuka, B.; Király, A.; Babos, M.; Vörös, E.; Bomboi, G.; et al. White matter microstructural alterations in migraine: A diffusion-weighted MRI study. *Pain* **2012**, *153*, 651–656. [CrossRef] [PubMed]
73. Yu, D.; Yuan, K.; Qin, W.; Zhao, L.; Dong, M.; Liu, P.; Yang, X.; Liu, J.; Sun, J.; Zhou, G.; et al. Axonal loss of white matter in migraine without aura: A tract-based spatial statistics study. *Cephalalgia* **2013**, *33*, 34–42. [CrossRef] [PubMed]
74. Li, X.L.; Fang, Y.N.; Gao, Q.C.; Lin, E.J.; Hu, S.H.; Ren, L.; Ding, M.H.; Luo, B.N. A Diffusion Tensor Magnetic Resonance Imaging Study of Corpus Callosum from Adult Patients with Migraine Complicated with Depressive/Anxious Disorder. *Headache J. Head Face Pain* **2011**, *51*, 237–245. [CrossRef]
75. Rocca, M.A.; Pagani, E.; Colombo, B.; Tortorella, P.; Falini, A.; Comi, G.; Filippi, M. Selective diffusion changes of the visual pathways in patients with migraine: A 3-T tractography study. *Cephalalgia* **2008**, *28*, 1061–1068. [CrossRef]
76. Coppola, G.; Tinelli, E.; Lepre, C.; Iacovelli, E.; Di Lorenzo, C.; Di Lorenzo, G.; Serrao, M.; Pauri, F.; Fiermonte, G.; Bianco, F.; et al. Dynamic changes in thalamic microstructure of migraine without aura patients: A diffusion tensor magnetic resonance imaging study. *Eur. J. Neurol.* **2014**, *21*, 287-e13. [CrossRef]
77. Coppola, G.; Di Renzo, A.; Tinelli, E.; Iacovelli, E.; Lepre, C.; Di Lorenzo, C.; Di Lorenzo, G.; Di Lenola, D.; Parisi, V.; Serrao, M.; et al. Evidence for brain morphometric changes during the migraine cycle: A magnetic resonance-based morphometry study. *Cephalalgia* **2015**, *35*, 783–791. [CrossRef] [PubMed]
78. Yuan, K.; Qin, W.; Liu, P.; Zhao, L.; Yu, D.; Dong, M.; Liu, J.; Yang, X.; von Deneen, K.M.; Liang, F.; et al. Reduced fractional anisotropy of corpus callosum modulates inter-hemispheric resting state functional connectivity in migraine patients without aura. *PLoS ONE* **2012**, *7*, e45476. [CrossRef]
79. Karsan, N.; Goadsby, P.J. Neuroimaging in the pre-ictal or premonitory phase of migraine: A narrative review. *J. Headache Pain* **2023**, *24*, 106. [CrossRef]
80. Kasia, K.M.; Noemi, M.; Flavia Di, P.; Vaughan, G.M.; Paul, M.M.; Luke, A.H. Fluctuating Regional Brainstem Diffusion Imaging Measures of Microstructure across the Migraine Cycle. *Eneuro* **2019**, *6*, 5–19.

Disclaimer/Publisher's Note: The statements, opinions and data contained in all publications are solely those of the individual author(s) and contributor(s) and not of MDPI and/or the editor(s). MDPI and/or the editor(s) disclaim responsibility for any injury to people or property resulting from any ideas, methods, instructions or products referred to in the content.

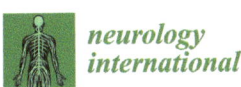

Article

Depression and Anxiety Symptoms in Headache Disorders: An Observational, Cross-Sectional Study

Leonidas Mantonakis [1], Ioanna Belesioti [2], Christina I. Deligianni [2,3], Vasilis Natsis [1], Euthimia Mitropoulou [2], Elina Kasioti [2], Maria Lypiridou [2] and Dimos D. Mitsikostas [2,*]

1. First Psychiatry Department, Aeginition Hospital, Medical School, National & Kapodistrian University of Athens, V. Sofia's Avenue 74, 11528 Athens, Greece; lmantonakis@gmail.com (L.M.); bill.natsis@hotmail.com (V.N.)
2. First Neurology Department, Aeginition Hospital, Medical School, National & Kapodistrian University of Athens, V. Sofia's Avenue 74, 11528 Athens, Greece; belesioti.ioanna@gmail.com (I.B.); cdchristina@gmail.com (C.I.D.); goranbeauty@yahoo.gr (E.M.); elkasioti@hotmail.com (E.K.); marialypiridou@gmail.com (M.L.)
3. Neurology Department, Athens Naval Hospital, Deinokratous 70, 11521 Athens, Greece
* Correspondence: dmitsikostas@uoa.gr; Tel./Fax: +30-2107289282

Citation: Mantonakis, L.; Belesioti, I.; Deligianni, C.I.; Natsis, V.; Mitropoulou, E.; Kasioti, E.; Lypiridou, M.; Mitsikostas, D.D. Depression and Anxiety Symptoms in Headache Disorders: An Observational, Cross-Sectional Study. *Neurol. Int.* 2024, *16*, 356–369. https://doi.org/10.3390/neurolint16020026

Academic Editor: Yasushi Shibata

Received: 11 January 2024
Revised: 13 March 2024
Accepted: 14 March 2024
Published: 18 March 2024

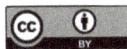

Copyright: © 2024 by the authors. Licensee MDPI, Basel, Switzerland. This article is an open access article distributed under the terms and conditions of the Creative Commons Attribution (CC BY) license (https:// creativecommons.org/licenses/by/ 4.0/).

Abstract: Background: Headache disorders have been associated with anxiety and depressive disorders. The aim of this study was to assess symptoms of anxiety and depression in a large sample of individuals with different headache disorders (HDs) in order to determine whether their frequency differs by headache type. Methods: Consecutive individuals with headache attending a headache outpatient clinic were interviewed with the HAM-D and HAM-A, along with age, sex, and education matched non-headache individuals. Results: Individuals numbering 2673 with headache (females 71.2%) and 464 non-headache individuals (females 70.9%) were interviewed (with participation rates of 98.3% and 91.0%, respectively). Migraine was diagnosed in 49.7%, tension-type headache in 38%, cluster headache 5.2%, and medication overuse (MO) in 21.8%. Participants with HD scored more in HAM-A (OR = 4.741, CI95%: 3.855–5.831, $p < 0.001$) and HAM-D scales (OR = 2.319, CI95%: 1.892–2.842, $p < 0.001$) than non-headache individuals. Participants with chronic HDs ($\geq$15 days with headache for $\geq$3 consecutive months; 52.5%) scored higher for both HAM-A (OR = 1.944, CI95%: 1.640–2.303, $p < 0.001$) and HAM-D (OR = 1.625, CI95%: 1.359–1.944, $p < 0.001$) than those with episodic HDs (33.1%), as did participants with MO vs. participants without MO (OR = 3.418, CI95%: 2.655–4.399, $p < 0.001$ for HAM-A, OR = 3.043, CI95%: 2.322–3.986, $p < 0.001$ for HAM-D). Female and low-educated participants scored higher on both scales. Conclusion: Because symptoms of anxiety and depression are substantial in people with HD, the treating physicians should look out for such symptoms and manage them appropriately.

Keywords: depression; anxiety; migraine; tension-type headache; medication overuse headache; cluster headache

1. Introduction

Headache and depressive disorders stood among the most prevalent health concerns, ranking within the top 15 causes of disability across 369 diseases and injuries globally in the year 2019 [1]. Notably, the burden of disorders has increased markedly over the last 20 years, within the young and productive age group of people, where both disorders are leading causes [1]; this underscores the pressing need for comprehensive understanding and effective management. Compounding this issue is the observation that headache and depressive disorders often coexist within the same individuals [2,3], multiplying the burden of both conditions and limiting the therapeutical outcome [4].

The undeniable association between headache and depressive disorders has prompted extensive research into the intricate mechanisms underlying this relationship. Genetic studies have shed light on a bidirectional influence [5], introducing complexity to our understanding of this comorbidity. This intricate interplay raises crucial questions about the mutual influence of these conditions and the underlying factors that contribute to their coexistence. Additionally, anxiety and depression have been identified as potential co-factors in the chronification of headaches, leading to suggestions of including anxiety and/or depression treatment as part of migraine management strategies [6].

This cross-sectional study seeks to contribute to the existing knowledge by estimating the prevalence of anxiety and depression-like symptoms in individuals with headache disorders (HDs). Thus, our aim was to explore potential associations with specific headache disorders, such as migraine, tension-type headache (TTH), and medication overuse (MO). To our knowledge there has been no controlled study investigating mood and anxiety symptoms in a sample of people with different HDs, although there are several studies that have focused on individual HDs, e.g., people with migraine, cluster headache, or TTH. Moreover, no study has so far investigated whether specific symptoms of anxiety or depression are more common in certain headache types, so we also aimed to compare the prevalence of gastrointestinal, sleep, and cardiovascular-related symptoms in different HDs. These symptoms are reported commonly by people with HD, people with additional anxiety and or depression in particular [6], and if present, require special management.

By elucidating these intricate connections, we aimed to provide valuable insights that can inform more targeted and effective interventions for individuals presenting with the dual challenges of headache and depressive disorders.

2. Materials and Methods

Consecutive individuals with HDs seeking medical treatment at the Aeginition Headache outpatient clinic, formed the participant pool for this cross-sectional study. Recruitment, interviewing, and clinical examination of participants were performed prospectively. The study encompassed a thorough examination of the main demographic features, clinical headache characteristics, and associated factors potentially contributing to the complexity of these disorders.

For each participant, detailed information on demographic features including age, sex, and educational background was systematically collected. Clinical headache features such as disease duration, frequency, and concurrent autonomic symptoms were carefully recorded during a comprehensive history-taking session. Provoking factors, including habits such as alcohol consumption, smoking, and coffee intake, were scrutinized to identify potential triggers.

Furthermore, a comprehensive assessment of coexisting somatic and mental disorders was integral to our investigation. This multifaceted exploration was facilitated through a structured questionnaire administered during the history-taking process. The questionnaire was designed to capture a spectrum of relevant details, ensuring a nuanced understanding of the participants' health profiles. A crucial aspect of our methodology involved a meticulous physical and neurological examination for all participants.

Additionally, a specialized interview was conducted using the Hamilton Anxiety Rating Scale (HAM-A) and Hamilton Depression Rating Scale (HAM-D). The HAM-A was one of the first rating scales developed to measure the severity of anxiety symptoms and is still widely used today in both clinical and research settings. The administration time takes 10–15 min. The scale consists of 14 items, each defined by a series of symptoms measuring mental and somatic symptoms and scored on a scale of 0 (not present) to 4 (severe), with a total score range of 0–56, where <17 indicates mild severity, 18–24 mild to moderate severity, and 25–30 moderate to severe [7]. Similarly, the HAM-D, consisting of 17 items assessing both mental and somatic depressive symptoms, was utilized to gauge the severity of depression. The scale, ranges from 0 to 68, where 10–13 indicates mild depression; 14–17 mild to moderate; >17 moderate to severe depression [8,9]. The Cronbach's alpha coefficient for the HAM-A and HAM-D varies depending on the specific version of the questionnaire and the population it is administered to. However, studies have reported

Cronbach's alpha values for the HAM-A and HAM-D ranging from around 0.70 to 0.90, indicating good to excellent internal consistency reliability.

Headache disorder diagnoses were conducted in accordance with the International Classification of Headache Disorders, 3rd edition (ICHD-3beta) [10]. Individuals with more than one HD were classified according to the most severe and disabling headache type. People with concomitant changes in cerebrospinal fluid pressure were excluded from the study population. All participants were stratified based on their education levels, categorized into three tiers (primary, secondary, and tertiary education). Outpatients who did not consent to participate in the study or did not agree to be interviewed for the HAM-A and HAM-D were excluded from the study.

We conducted a meticulous screening process using data from our hospital's headache specialty clinic database to establish a diverse control group, encompassing both healthy individuals and patients without headache concerns. Control group participants underwent thorough evaluation procedures consistent with clinic standards, ensuring precise classification and eligibility for the study's comparative analysis. Our paramount objective was to uphold data integrity and maintain exact participant selection throughout the study.

Signed informed consent was given by all participants and the study protocol was approved by the Ethical Committee of the Aeginition Hospital (ADA: ΩNKO46Ψ8N2-2BΨ).

Statistics

Descriptive statistics served as the cornerstone for comparing the main demographic and clinical characteristics, providing a comprehensive snapshot of our diverse study cohort. Analysis of variance (ANOVA) was harnessed to scrutinize mean values of continuous variables, enhancing our understanding of the dataset's variability.

Data analysis was conducted using SPSS 22. An independent t-test was performed to compare the mean scores on the Hamilton Anxiety Scale and between the episodic headaches group and the chronic headaches group. The t-test assumes normality and equal variances between groups. An independent samples t-test was conducted to compare depression symptom severity, as measured by the Hamilton Depression Scale, between patients with episodic and chronic headache types. The assumption of equal variances was met ($p > 0.05$).

A One-Way Between Subjects ANOVA test was conducted to examine the differences in anxiety symptom severity and depression symptom severity among patients with different headache types, e.g., episodic migraine, chronic migraine, episodic TTH, chronic TTH, episodic cluster headache (CH), new daily persistent headache (NDPH), and other types of headaches. Levene's test confirmed the equality of variances across groups. Post hoc comparisons using the Bonferroni correction were performed to further elucidate these differences.

The statistical analysis aimed to explore the relationship between severe anxiety and depression scores and various headache characteristics, including episodic versus chronic headaches and the presence of medication overuse (MO). Binary logistic regression analysis was conducted to examine the relationship between severe anxiety scores (HAM-A $\geq$ 25) and the presence or absence of headaches, episodic or chronic headaches, and presence or absence of medication overuse. The logistic regression model allowed for the estimation of odds ratios (OR) and corresponding 95% confidence intervals (CI) to assess the strength and direction of the associations. In this study, we investigated the relationship between severe depression scores, categorized based on the Hamilton Depression Rating Scale (HAM-D) (cutoff > 17 indicating severe depression), and different patient groups, including those with headaches, episodic versus chronic headaches, and those with medication overuse. Logistic regression analysis was performed to examine the relationship between severe depression scores (binary outcome variable: yes/no severe depression) and patient groups (predictor variables: presence of headaches, type of headaches, medication overuse). Adjustments were made for potential confounders such as age and gender.

Logistic regression analyses were conducted to assess the associations between various symptoms (sleep disturbances, gastrointestinal symptoms, and cardiovascular symptoms) and headache disorder subtype, as well as medication overuse.

3. Results

The study unfolded across a substantial time frame, spanning from January 2018 to January 2021, involving a robust participant pool of 2673 individuals grappling with various forms of headache disorders (HD). Regarding the gender distribution within this cohort, the headache group consisted of 1902 women (71.2%) and 771 men (28.8%). On the other hand, 464 headache-free participants willingly accepted the opportunity to contribute to the study, resulting in participation rates of 98.3% and 91.0% for those with HD and those without, respectively. The analysis revealed migraine diagnoses in 1328 participants (49.7%), TTH in 1015 individuals (38%), CH in 139 cases (5.2%), and MO in 583 participants (21.8%). The demographic characteristics of the participants, stratified by headache disorder, are presented in Table 1, offering a clear snapshot of the diverse composition of the study cohort.

Table 1. Descriptive statistics.

Headache Disorder	No of Participants	Mean Age Years (SD)	Male N, (%)	Female N (%)	Primary Education	Secondary Education	Tertiary Education	Disease Duration Years (SD)
All	2.673	40.9 (12.1)	771 (28.8)	1902 (71.2)	417 (15.6%)	947 (35.4%)	1307 (48.9%)	24.2 (15.5)
Migraine	1328 (49.7%)	41.0 (12.0)	253 (19.1)	1075 (80.9)	173 (13)	495 (37.3)	659 (49.7)	24.0 (15.4)
Episodic Migraine	886 (33.2%)	41.5 (12.4)	174 (19.6)	712 (80.4)	98 (11.1)	320 (36.2)	467 (52.8)	24.5 (14.9)
Chronic Migraine	442 (16.5%)	40.0 (11.1)	79 (17.9)	363 (82.1)	75 (17)	174 (39.4)	193 (43.7)	22.9 (16.4)
TTH	1015 (38%)	41.3 (12.5)	337 (33.2)	678 (66.8)	196 (19.3)	337 (33.2)	482 (47.5)	24.8 (15.5)
Episodic TTH	437 (16.3%)	41.5 (11.9)	141 (32.3)	296 (67.7)	67 (15.3)	139 (31.8)	231 (52.9)	25.1 (15.2)
Chronic TTH	578 (21.6%)	41.2 (12.9)	196 (33.9)	382 (66.1)	129 (22.3)	198 (34.3)	251 (43.4)	24.5 (15.7)
Cluster Headache	139 (5.2%)	40.5 (11.4)	104 (74.8)	35 (25.2)	15 (10.8)	55 (39.6)	69 (49.6)	24.5 (15.5)
Episodic CH	89 (3.3%)	39.5 (11.3)	71 (79.8)	18 (20.2)	10 (11.2)	36 (40.4)	43 (48.3)	22.9 (14.9)
Chronic CH	50 (1.9%)	42.1 (11.6)	33 (66)	17 (34)	5 (10)	19 (38)	26 (52)	27.4 (16.4)
MO	583 (21.8%)	43.8 (13.1)	110 (18.9)	473 (81.1)	144 (24.7)	204 (35.0)	234 (40.1)	27.0 (14.7)
NDPH	35 (1.3%)	37.4 (8.9)	14 (40.0)	21 (60.0)	3 (8.6)	12 (34.3)	20 (57.1)	18.85 (16.2)
Other HD	156 (5.8%)	39.3 (11.7)	63 (40.4)	93 (59.6)	31 (19.9)	48 (30.8)	77 (49.4)	23.43 (15.2)
Headache Free participants	464	41.6 (14.6)	135 (29.1%)	329 (70.9%)	71 (15.3%)	165 (35.5%)	228 (49.1%)	

Legend. TTH: Tension-Type Headache; CH: Cluster Headache; MO: Medication Overuse; NDPH: New Daily Persistent Headache; HD: Headache Disorders; SD: Standard Deviation.

3.1. Scores by Headache Type

For participants with migraine, the mean scores for HAM-A and HAM-D stood at 19.61 ± 7.69 and 14.12 ± 6.66, respectively, in contrast to participants without headaches who recorded scores of 13.09 ± 8.14 and 12.03 ± 6.96 on the corresponding scales (Table 2, Figures 1 and 2). Participants with TTH reported mean HAM-A and HAM-D scores of 20.81 ± 7.54 and 15.43 ± 6.59, respectively. The mean HAM-A and HAM-D scores for participants with CH were 13.35 ± 6.69 and 10.61 ± 6.31, respectively. Participants with MO had higher scores for both HAM-A and HAM-D scales vs. participants without MO (Table 2). Furthermore, more participants with MO than participants without MO were scored ≥ 18 or ≥ 25 in HAM-A and ≥ 10 or ≥ 17 in HAM-D, indicating that more participants with MO were suffering from mild or mild to moderate or moderate to severe anxiety or mild, mild to moderate or moderate to severe depression-like condition than those without MO, respectively (Table 2).

Table 2. Participants with anxiety or depression like conditions by headache type.

	Participants without HDs		Participants with HDs		OR	CI
	N	(%)	N	(%)		
HAM-A $\geq$ 18	173	37.3	1973	73.8	4.741	3.855–5.831
HAM-A $\geq$ 25	57	12.3	736	27.5	2.713	2.030–3.625
HAM-D $\geq$ 10	262	56.5	2006	75.0	2.319	1.892–2.842
HAM-D $\geq$ 17	115	24.8	987	36.9	1.777	1.419–2.225
	Participants with episodic HD		Participants with chronic HD			
HAM-A $\geq$ 18	889	63.0	968	76.8	1.944	1.640–2.303
HAM-A $\geq$ 25	250	17.7	486	38.5	2.915	2.441–3.481
HAM-D $\geq$ 10	1000	70.8	1006	79.8	1.625	1.359–1.944
HAM-D $\geq$ 17	431	30.5	556	44.1	1.795	1.532–2.104
	Participants without MO		Participants with MO			
HAM-A $\geq$ 18	1354	64.8	503	86.3	3.418	2.655–4.399
HAM-A $\geq$ 25	500	23.9	236	40.5	2.163	1.782–2.625
HAM-D $\geq$ 10	1491	71.3	515	88.3	3.043	2.322–3.986
HAM-D $\geq$ 17	660	31.6	327	56.1	2.768	2.294–3.339

Legend. MO: Medication Overuse; HD: Headache Disorder (s); HAM-A: Hamilton Rating Scale for Anxiety; HAM-D: Hamilton Rating Scale for Depression; OR: Odds Ratio; CI: Confidential Interval.

Participants with HDs exhibited mean scores of 19.62 ± 7.79 and 14.39 ± 6.71 on the HAM-A and HAM-D, respectively. On the contrary, participants without headaches recorded lower scores of 13.09 ± 8.15 and 12.03 ± 6.96 on the respective scales.

The ANOVA revealed a significant difference in anxiety symptom severity among the various headache groups ($F(7, 2665) = 47.97$, $p < 0.001$). Post hoc comparisons using the Bonferroni correction were performed to further elucidate these differences. Significant differences in HAM-A severity were found between the headache groups:

- Chronic migraine patients reported significantly higher anxiety symptom severity compared to episodic migraine, episodic TTH, episodic cluster, chronic cluster, NDPH, and other types of headaches (all $p < 0.05$).
- Episodic migraine patients did not significantly differ in anxiety symptom severity from episodic TTH, NDPH, and other types of headaches (all $p > 0.05$).
- Chronic TTH patients reported significantly higher anxiety symptom severity compared to all other headache types except chronic migraine (all $p < 0.05$).
- The control group reported significantly lower anxiety symptom severity compared to patients with episodic migraine ($p < 0.001$), chronic migraine ($p < 0.001$), episodic TTH

($p < 0.001$), chronic TTH ($p < 0.001$), NDPH ($p < 0.001$), and other types of headaches ($p < 0.001$).
- There was no significant difference in anxiety symptom severity between the control group and patients with episodic or chronic CH.

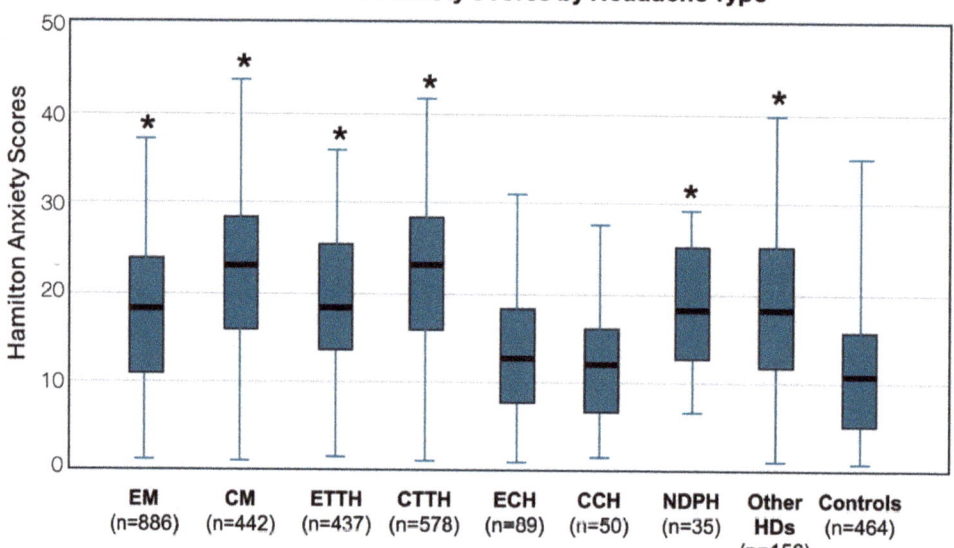

Figure 1. Whisker Plots of scores of Hamilton rating scales for anxiety by headache disorder. EM: Episodic Migraine; CM: Chronic Migraine; ETTH: Episodic Tension-Type Headache; CTTH: Chronic Tension-Type Headache; ECH: Episodic Cluster Headache; CCH: Chronic Cluster Headache; NDPH: New Daily Persistent Headache; HDs: Headache Disorders; Controls: Non-headache participants; * $p < 0.001$ vs. control.

A One-Way Between Subjects ANOVA test was conducted, revealing a significant difference in depression symptoms across headache types (F(7, 2665) = 23.67, $p < 0.001$). Variances were found to be equal across the groups, as confirmed by Levene's test. Bonferroni-corrected post hoc comparisons were performed to elucidate specific differences in depression symptoms between different headache types.

- Episodic migraine participants had significantly lower depression symptom scores compared to chronic migraine patients ($p < 0.001$) and chronic TTH patients ($p < 0.001$).
- Chronic migraine participants exhibited significantly higher depression symptom scores compared to episodic migraine patients ($p < 0.001$) and episodic CH patients ($p < 0.001$). NDPH participants showed significantly higher depression symptom scores compared to chronic migraine patients ($p = 0.011$), chronic TTH patients ($p = 0.026$), and chronic CH participants ($p = 0.023$).
- Participants with other headache types demonstrated significant differences in depression symptom scores compared to chronic TTH patients ($p < 0.001$) and chronic CH participants ($p < 0.001$).
- Participants with chronic HDs (e.g., chronic migraine, chronic TTH) tend to report higher levels of depression symptoms compared to those with episodic HDs.
- Significant differences in depression symptom severity were found between various headache types, with chronic migraine and chronic TTH showing particularly elevated levels.

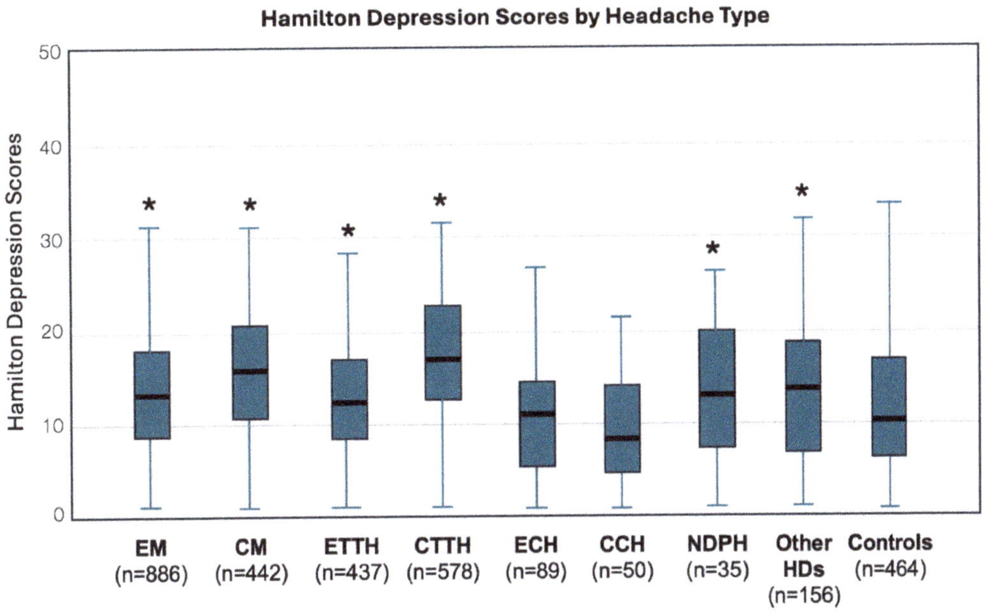

Figure 2. Whisker Plots of scores of Hamilton rating scales for depression by headache disorder. EM: Episodic Migraine; CM: Chronic Migraine; ETTH: Episodic Tension-Type Headache; CTTH: Chronic Tension-Type Headache; ECH: Episodic Cluster Headache; CCH: Chronic Cluster Headache; NDPH: New Daily Persistent Headache; HDs: Headache Disorders; Controls: Non-headache participants; * $p < 0.001$ vs. control.

3.2. Gender, Education, Age, and Use of Anti-Depressants

Gender, education, and age were studied as confounders of the coexistence of elevated assessment for anxiety and depression in participants with headache and in the control group. Specific association for MO was additionally made.

- Gender influence: Females, both within headache and non-headache groups, consistently exhibited higher scores for anxiety (HAM-A) and depression (HAM-D). This trend persisted across various headache disorders, with episodic cluster headache being an exception (Figure 3).
- Education as a co-factor: The level of education was an important co-factor as well. Except for CH and NDPH, low education level was related with high scores in HAM-A and HAM-D in all HD (Figure 3).
- Impact of age: Age did not significantly contribute to the configuration of HAM-A and HAM-D scores, when analysed by headache types.
- Medication Overuse: For the case of MO, gender and education were significant co-factors. Females with MO had higher scores for both HAM-A and HAM-D than males, while low educated participants with MO also had higher scores for HAM-A and HAM-D than participants with MO and high education level. Age did not significantly affect the scoring in the context of MO.
- At the time of examination, only a small percentage of participants were under treatment with antidepressants (4.6%), while 15.5% of participants had a history of previous antidepressant treatment. Individuals with this history were more likely to score higher on both scales, but we did not find an association of prior or concurrent antidepressant use with a specific headache type among the different HD types.
- To investigate the possible impact of the COVID-19 pandemic on our study data, we performed a retrospective analysis of data collected during 2018–2019, i.e., before

COVID-19, against data collected in 2020–2021. We found no significant difference, so we did not proceed with individual analyses for each headache condition.

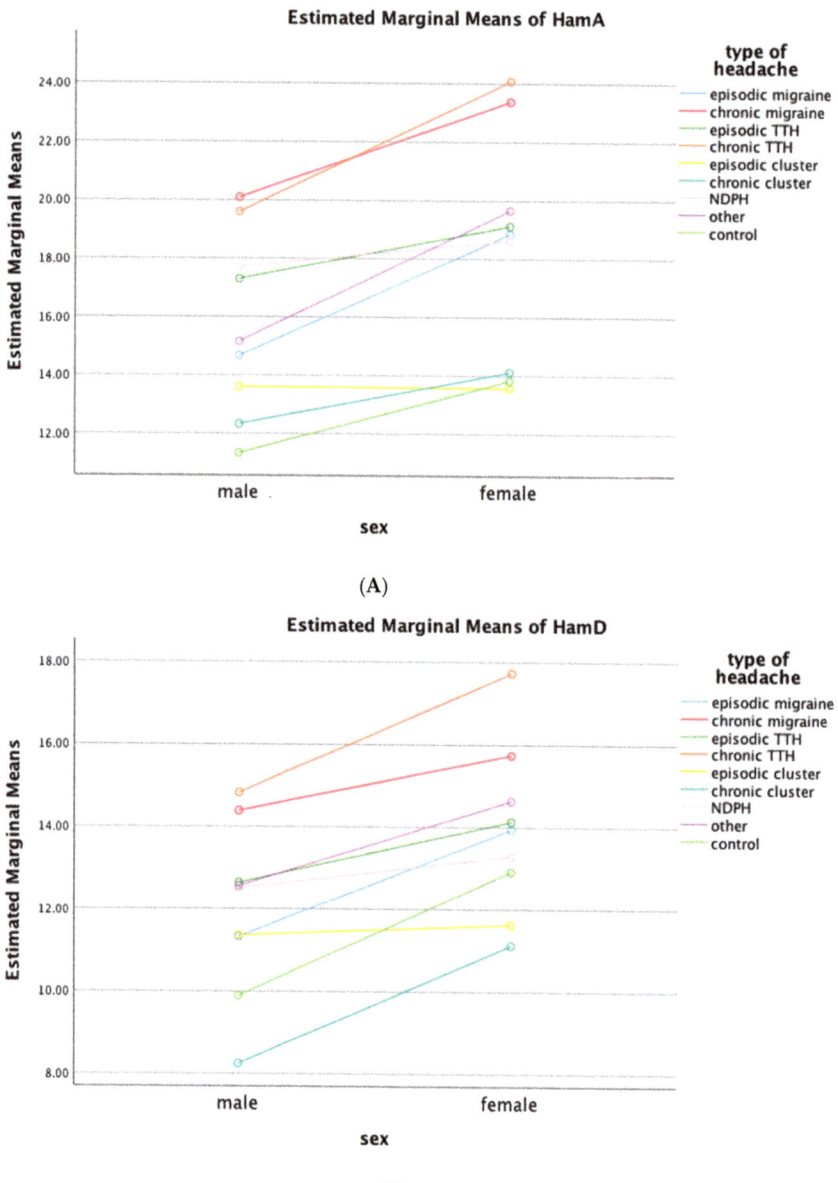

Figure 3. *Cont.*

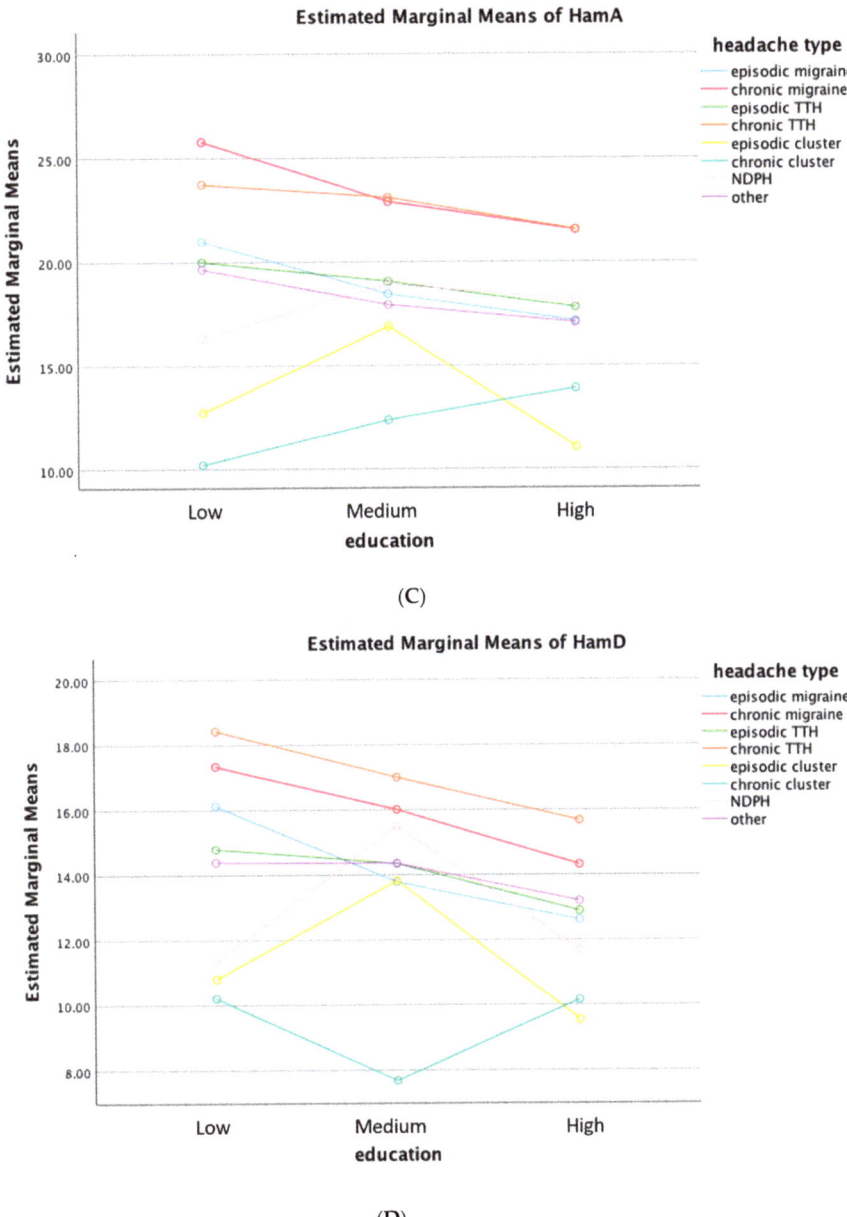

(C)

(D)

Figure 3. Estimated marginal means of Hamilton rating scales for Anxiety (**A**) and Depression (**B**) by headache disorder and gender or education. (**A**,**B**) Female participants had higher scores for both Hamilton rating scales in headache and non-headache participants and in all headache disorders, except for episodic cluster headache. (**C**,**D**) Except for CH and NDPH, low education level was related with high scores in both Hamilton rating scales in all HDs. HamA: Hamilton rating scales for Anxiety; HamD: Hamilton rating scales for Depression; TTH: Tension-Type Headache; NDPH: New Daily Persistent Headache; HDs: Headache Disorders; Other: participants with other Headache Disorders; Control: Non-headache participants.

3.3. Anxiety and Depression Symptoms

Symptoms of interest from the anxiety and depression scales were further examined, to explore potential associations with specific headache types. The logistic regression analyses revealed significant associations between headache types and various symptoms including sleep disturbances, gastrointestinal symptoms, and cardiovascular symptoms.

- Sleep symptoms: Sleep disturbances emerged as a very frequent feature among participants with HD, intensifying notably within the domain of chronic HD (OR = 1.252, 95% CI: 1.075–1459, p = 0.004) and MO (OR = 1.917, 95% CI: 1.592–2.309, p < 0.001) vs. participants with episodic HD and no MO, respectively.
- GI symptoms: The same pattern was observed for gastrointestinal (GI) symptoms with logistic regression analyses indicating a significant association between chronic HD and GI symptoms (OR = 1.394, 95% CI: 1.193–1.629, p < 0.001), as well as between MO and GI symptoms (OR = 1.510, 95% CI: 1.255–1817, p < 0.001).
- Cardiovascular Symptoms: While cardiovascular symptoms were notably common among participants with chronic HD, as evidenced by an odds ratio of 1.394 compared to episodic HD (95% CI: 1.193–1.629, p = 0.04), the influence of MO did not significantly affect the reporting of cardiovascular symptoms vs. participants without MO.

4. Discussion

In this cross-sectional survey encompassing 2673 individuals attending the Aeginition outpatient headache clinic, we uncovered a significant burden of severe anxiety and depressive symptoms within the headache population. Approximately 27.5% of participants with headache exhibited severe anxiety symptoms (HAM-A score $\geq$ 25), and 26.9% displayed severe depressive symptoms (HAM-D score $\geq$ 17). Notably, those grappling with chronic headache disorders (HDs) or medication overuse (MO) showcased markedly higher scores for both HAM-A (38.5% and 40.5%) and HAM-D (44.1% and 56.1%) than those with episodic HDs or no MO, respectively. Participants with migraine exhibited higher HAM-A and HAM-D scores than those with TTH or CH. Gender and education were important co-factors, but age was not. Female participants had higher scores for both HAM-A and HAM-D in headache and non-headache participants and in all HD types, except for episodic CH. Low education level was related with high scores in HAM-A and HAM-D in all HD, but not for CH and NDPH. Sleep, GI and cardiovascular symptoms were commonly reported, most often in participants with chronic than in participants with episodic HDs.

The insights garnered from a recent meta-analysis encompassing 4.19 million individuals with HDs parallel the findings of our present study. The meta-analysis identified the most prevalent comorbidities as depressive disorders (23%; 95%CI: 20–26%), hypertension (24%; 95%CI: 22–26%), and anxiety disorders (25%; 95%CI: 22–28%). These estimates closely align with the prevalence observed in our study, reinforcing the robustness of our findings. Like our study, females exhibited higher comorbidity rates, but our findings did not align with the meta-analysis regarding the association between young age and increased risk for anxiety and depression [11]. Education was not reported as a potential covariable. Why our study did not show that age is an important factor in the comorbidity of HDs with affective disorders, although the sample count was large, is not clear. It seems that other factors overshadow this relationship, possibly genetic, environmental, or even cultural. It is also highly likely that there is no such association between age and comorbidities of migraine with depression and anxiety [5,12,13]. It is noteworthy that the meta-analysis authors themselves acknowledged that their finding regarding age and comorbidity might not signify a genuine relationship. Instead, differences in the average age of subjects enrolled in the studies, particularly those above or below the age of 40, could have influenced their observations [11].

In consonance with the meta-analysis, our study underscores the significance of gender and education as co-factors in the comorbidity of anxiety and/or depression-like symptoms with HDs. Unraveling the mechanistic underpinnings of this association remains elusive, prompting the formulation of several hypothetical etiopathogenetic theories. A prevailing hypothesis, supported by a majority, suggests an interdependent relationship between anxiety, depression, and HDs. However, even within this model, discerning causation becomes intricate—whether anxiety or depression caused the headache or vice versa remains ambiguous. Instead, it appears more plausible that the coexistence of these conditions exacerbates both, demanding heightened therapeutic efforts from physicians [5,6,12,13]. Twin and family studies indicate that this bidirectional relationship can be explained, at least partly, by shared underlying genetically determined disease mechanisms. Although no genes have been robustly associated with the aetiology of both migraine and depression, genes from serotonergic, dopaminergic, and GABAergic systems together with variants in the MTHFR and BDNF genes remain strong candidates [5]. This potential genetic interplay emphasizes the intricate nature of the relationship, offering a glimpse into the complex interweaving of biological factors contributing to the co-occurrence of headache disorders and affective symptoms.

To treat these interrelated conditions, there are specific medicinal agents that have proven efficacy in the treatment of both anxiety/depressive disorders and HDs, such as the antidepressants amitriptyline and venlafaxine in the treatment of migraine [14], and amitriptyline, venlafaxine, and mirtazapine in the treatment of TTH [15]. These treatments should be the first treatment option for the specific comorbidities. Additionally, non-pharmacological therapeutic approaches, such as cognitive-behavioral treatment, physical therapy, and neurostimulation should also be considered [14–16], adding a multifaceted dimension to the comprehensive management of individuals navigating the intricate interplay of headache disorders and affective symptoms.

As was shown previously [3], the coexistence of depressive and anxiety like symptoms in people with HD and MO is higher compared to those without drug overuse. In other recent surveys confirming the findings of our study, individuals with MO showed a subtle psychopathological pattern characterized by impaired social adaptation [17] and depression, anxiety, and stress [18]. This nuanced understanding emphasizes the need for a thorough assessment in individuals with HDs engaged in symptomatic drug overuse. Therefore, a person with an HD who overuses symptomatic drugs for headaches should be thoroughly checked for possible coexistence of anxiety or affective disorder. Such a person, who, in addition to very frequent headaches, also has symptoms of anxiety or depression, suffers a greater deterioration in his daily quality of life and needs special care.

In our study, a special post hoc analysis was made for specific symptoms that we believe may be contributing to the chronification of primary episodic into chronic HDs. Sleep symptoms, for example, were found to be very common in participants with chronic HDs and MO, underscoring our initial hypothesis, while the same was recorded with the GI symptoms. Cardiovascular symptoms were more common in participants with chronic HD but not in participants with MO. Therefore, it appears that sleep and digestive function are disrupted much more frequently in people with chronic HD or MO, or, when an HD and anxiety or depression coexist, sleep and GI are disturbed.

Another finding that is difficult to explain is the absence of an association of cluster headache with symptoms of anxiety and depression. Cluster headache ranks as one among the most intensely painful conditions faced by man today [19], so it is reasonable to expect an increase in symptoms of anxiety and depression in those people with CH, as other studies have shown [20]. It should be noted that only a percentage of participants with CH were in an active cluster period when assessed and this may partly explain the absence of association. However, it seems that even in the case of chronic CH there is no correlation, which is troubling, because in these people the symptoms of anxiety and depression are very often intense. People with CH may often develop personality disorders, e.g., psychological dysregulation and low social engagement [20], but this cannot negate our concern regarding the absence of symptoms of anxiety and depression in this sample of people we studied. One could consider that the number of participants with CH is relatively small compared to other CH groups, and for this no significant difference was obtained, but the prevalence of CH in the general population is about 100 times lower than the prevalence of migraine and TTH, making the number of participants in the CH group in our study comparable to the number of participants in the other headache groups. In other words, the sample sizes in each HD group represent reality, so a statistically significant difference should be found, if it exists in that sample. In addition, we found only one controlled study conducted to investigate anxiety and depression symptoms in different headache types in the early 1980s. Although the classification of headaches was quite different at the time and the sample size in this survey was limited, the researchers found minimal distress in people with CH compared to people with migraine or TTH [21].

Female and low-educated participants were more likely to achieve high scores in both HAM-A and HAM-D across most, but not all, of the different headache types we investigated. In the case of CH, females did not score higher than males. One could hypothesize that most participants with CH were males in our study (104 males vs. 35 females) and this difference obscured the effect of gender, or, simply, that gender does not affect the prevalence of anxiety or depressive symptoms in people with CH, which remains low anyway. Low education was a risk factor for higher HAM-A and HMA-D scores in participants with migraine and TTH, but not in those with CH and NDPH. For the case of migraine and TTH, several studies showed an association of low education with increased burden of the conditions [15,22].

There are several methodological limitations that should be acknowledged. The survey was cross-sectional; therefore, it carries several disadvantages, e.g., it cannot be used to analyze behavior over a period of time and it does not help determine cause and effect. In addition, the timing of the snapshot is not guaranteed to be representative. Data from individuals with MO headache (MOH) are not reported, only individuals with MO, because the latter consist of individuals who although overusing medications, their headache frequency is not fulfilling the "chronic criterion" (defined as having headache for more than 15 days per month for more than three consecutive months). These individuals are at high risk of headache chronification and for MOH. Migraine with aura was not one of the conditions studied in the present study. Among the several co-factors we investigated, income is missing. Finally, the variability in headache types and the potential limitations of clustering them together for analysis should be taken under consideration.

On the other hand, the study design used in this survey offers the opportunity to compare many different variables at the same time. This inclusive approach allows for a comprehensive exploration of factors such as gender, age, and headache type in relation to the coexistence of depression and/or anxiety-like symptoms with HDs. The multifaceted analysis enriches our understanding of the complex interplay between these variables. Another advantage of this study is the relatively large sample of participants, given the fact that all they underwent was a face-to-face interview along with full neurological and physical examination to establish the diagnosis of headache. Finally, this research assessed distress in a range of different HDs and provided comparative data. There has been no other similar report over the last 40 years and none using the current headache classification.

5. Conclusions

In conclusion, this survey illuminates the pervasive presence of anxiety and depression-like symptoms among individuals with HDs, especially within the chronic subtypes or those grappling with MO. It is speculated that these symptoms might trigger headache attacks, acting as potential amplifiers of HD. This insight underscores the crucial role of treating physicians, emphasizing the need for comprehensive screening of individuals with headaches. Identifying and addressing anxiety and mood symptoms promptly becomes paramount, as their management holds the potential not only to alleviate these psychopathological burdens but also to mitigate the risk of headache recurrence or chronification. This proactive approach ensures a holistic and effective strategy in enhancing the overall well-being of individuals grappling with the complex interplay of headache disorders and associated mood symptoms.

Author Contributions: Conceptualization, D.D.M. and L.M.; Methodology, D.D.M. and L.M.; Software, E.M., C.I.D., E.K. and M.L.; Validation, E.M., E.K. and M.L.; Formal Analysis, I.B., C.I.D., E.M., E.K. and M.L.; Investigation, I.B., M.L., V.N., E.M., E.K. and M.L.; Resources, I.B.; Data Curation, I.B., E.M., E.K., V.N. and M.L.; Writing—Original Draft Preparation, L.M., C.I.D., I.B. and V.N.; Writing—Review and Editing, L.M. and D.D.M.; Visualization, C.I.D. and V.N.; Supervision, D.D.M.; Project Administration, D.D.M.; Funding Acquisition, none. All authors have read and agreed to the published version of the manuscript.

Funding: This research received no external funding.

Institutional Review Board Statement: The study was conducted according to the guidelines of the Declaration of Helsinki, and the study protocol was approved by the Ethical Committee of the Aeginition Hospital (ADA: ΩNKO46Ψ8N2-2BΨ).

Informed Consent Statement: All participants signed special informed consent.

Data Availability Statement: Data available upon request due to restrictions. The data presented in the study are available on request from the corresponding author due to personal data protection.

Acknowledgments: We are extremely grateful to the participants of this survey.

Conflicts of Interest: Leonidas Mantonakis, Euthimia Mitropoulou, Elina Kasioti, and Maria Lypiridou, have nothing to declare. Christina I. Deligianni received the International Headache Society 2021 research grant, and she is a member of the Executive Board of the European Headache Federation. Vasilis Natsis received honoraria for lecturing from Janssen-Cilag. D.D. Mitsikostas received honoraria, consultation and research or travel grants from Abbvie/Allergan, Bristol Mayer Squibb, Eli Lilly, Genesis Pharma, Lundbeck, Merck-Serono, Merz, Novartis, Sanofi, Roche, Teva. He participated as principal investigator in clinical trials for Amgen, Abbvie/Allergan, Eli Lilly, ElectroCore, Genesis Pharma, Lundbeck, Merz, Mylan, Merck-Serono, Novartis, Sanofi-Genzyme, and Teva. He is currently co-chair of the Headache Panel at the European Academy of Neurology and President of the Hellenic Headache Society.

References

1. GBD 2019 Diseases and Injuries Collaborators. Global burden of 369 diseases and injuries in 204 countries and territories, 1990–2019: A systematic analysis for the Global Burden of Disease Study 2019. *Lancet* **2020**, *396*, 1204–1222. [CrossRef]
2. Merikangas, K.R.; Angst, J.; Isler, H. Migraine and psychopathology: Results of the Zurich cohort study of young adults. *Arch. Gen. Psychiatry* **1990**, *47*, 849–853. [CrossRef]
3. Mitsikostas, D.; Thomas, A. Comorbidity of headache and depressive disorders. *Cephalalgia* **1999**, *19*, 211–217. [CrossRef]
4. Guidetti, V.; Galli, F.; Fabrizi, P.; Giannantoni, A.S.; Napoli, L.; Bruni, O.; Trillo, S. Headache and psychiatric comorbidity: Clinical aspects and outcome in an 8-year follow-up study. *Cephalalgia* **1998**, *18*, 455–462. [CrossRef] [PubMed]
5. Yang, Y.; Ligthart, L.; Terwindt, G.M.; Boomsma, D.I.; Rodriguez-Acevedo, A.J.; Nyholt, D.R. Genetic epidemiology of migraine and depression. *Cephalalgia* **2016**, *36*, 679–691. [CrossRef] [PubMed]
6. Deligianni, C.I.; Vikelis, M.; Mitsikostas, D.D. Depression in headaches: Chronification. *Curr. Opin. Neurol.* **2012**, *25*, 277–283. [CrossRef] [PubMed]
7. Hamilton, M. The assessment of anxiety states by rating. *Br. J. Med. Psychol.* **1959**, *32*, 50–55. [CrossRef] [PubMed]
8. Hamilton, M. Development of a rating scale for primary depressive illness. *Br. J. Soc. Clin. Psychol.* **1967**, *6*, 278–296. [CrossRef]
9. Zimmerman, M.; Martinez, J.H.; Young, D.; Chelminski, I.; Dalrymple, K. Severity classification on the Hamilton Depression Rating Scale. *J. Affect. Disord.* **2013**, *150*, 384–388. [CrossRef] [PubMed]
10. Headache Classification Committee of the International Headache Society (IHS). The International Classification of Headache Disorders, 3rd edition (beta version). *Cephalalgia* **2013**, *33*, 629–808. [CrossRef] [PubMed]
11. Caponnetto, V.; Deodato, M.; Robotti, M.; Koutsokera, M.; Pozzilli, V.; Galati, C.; Nocera, G.; De Matteis, E.; De Vanna, G.; Fellini, E.; et al. Comorbidities of primary headache disorders: A literature review with meta-analysis. *J. Headache Pain* **2021**, *22*, 71. [CrossRef]
12. Zhang, Q.; Shao, A.; Jiang, Z.; Tsai, H.; Liu, W. The exploration of mechanisms of comorbidity between migraine and depression. *J. Cell. Mol. Med.* **2019**, *23*, 4505–4513. [CrossRef]
13. Baksa, D.; Gonda, X.; Juhasz, G. Why are migraineurs more depressed? A review of the factors contributing to the comorbidity of migraine and depression. *Neuropsychopharmacol. Hung.* **2017**, *19*, 37–44.
14. Ashina, M.; Buse, D.C.; Ashina, H.; Pozo-Rosich, P.; Peres, M.F.P.; Lee, M.J.; Terwindt, G.M.; Halker Singh, R.; Tassorelli, C.; Do, T.P.; et al. Migraine: Integrated approaches to clinical management and emerging treatments. *Lancet* **2021**, *397*, 1505–1518. [CrossRef]

15. Ashina, S.; Mitsikostas, D.D.; Lee, M.J.; Yamani, N.; Wang, S.J.; Messina, R.; Ashina, H.; Buse, D.C.; Pozo-Rosich, P.; Jensen, R.H.; et al. Tension-type headache. *Nat. Rev. Dis. Primers* **2021**, *7*, 24. [CrossRef]
16. Fernández-de-Las-Peñas, C.; Florencio, L.L.; Plaza-Manzano, G.; Arias-Buría, J.L. Clinical reasoning behind non-pharmacological interventions for the management of headaches: A narrative literature review. *Int. J. Environ. Res. Public Health* **2020**, *17*, 4126. [CrossRef]
17. Romozzi, M.; Di Tella, S.; Rollo, E.; Quintieri, P.; Silveri, M.C.; Vollono, C.; Calabresi, P. Theory of mind in migraine and medication-overuse headache: A cross-sectional study. *Front. Neurol.* **2022**, *13*, 968111. [CrossRef] [PubMed]
18. Ljubisavljevic, M.; Ignjatovic, A.; Djordjevic, V.; Pesic, M.H.; Ljubisavljevic, S. Depression, anxiety, stress, and health-related quality of life among patients with medication overuse headache in a tertiary headache center: A cross-sectional study. *J. Neuropsychiatry Clin. Neurosci.* **2021**, *33*, 132–143. [CrossRef] [PubMed]
19. Burish, M.J.; Pearson, S.M.; Shapiro, R.E.; Zhang, W.; Schor, L.I. Cluster headache is one of the most intensely painful human conditions: Results from the International Cluster Headache Questionnaire. *Headache* **2021**, *61*, 117–124. [CrossRef] [PubMed]
20. Liu, Q.; Zhang, Y.; Hu, C.; Yuan, D.; Wang, K.; Fan, W.; Pan, F.; Li, Q.; Wang, Y.; Tan, G. Therapy for psychiatric comorbidities in patients with episodic cluster headache: A prospective multicenter study. *J. Pain Res.* **2022**, *15*, 3245–3254. [CrossRef] [PubMed]
21. Andrasik, F.; Blanchard, E.B.; Arena, J.G.; Teders, S.J.; Teevan, R.C.; Rodichok, L.D. Psychological functioning in headache sufferers. *Psychosom. Med.* **1982**, *44*, 171–182. [CrossRef] [PubMed]
22. May, A.; Schulte, L.H. Chronic migraine: Risk factors, mechanisms, and treatment. *Nat. Rev. Neurol.* **2016**, *12*, 455–464. [CrossRef] [PubMed]

Disclaimer/Publisher's Note: The statements, opinions and data contained in all publications are solely those of the individual author(s) and contributor(s) and not of MDPI and/or the editor(s). MDPI and/or the editor(s) disclaim responsibility for any injury to people or property resulting from any ideas, methods, instructions or products referred to in the content.

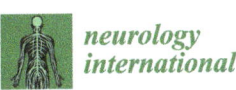

Article

Effects of Anti-CGRP Monoclonal Antibodies on Neurophysiological and Clinical Outcomes: A Combined Transcranial Magnetic Stimulation and Algometer Study

Paolo Manganotti [1,2], Manuela Deodato [1,2,*], Laura D'Acunto [1,2], Francesco Biaduzzini [1,2], Gabriele Garascia [1,2] and Antonio Granato [1,2]

[1] Department of Medical, Surgical and Health Sciences, University of Trieste, 34100 Trieste, Italy; pmanganotti@units.it (P.M.); laura.d.acun@gmail.com (L.D.); alterxx92@hotmail.it (F.B.); gabrielegarascia@gmail.com (G.G.); antonio_granato@hotmail.com (A.G.)
[2] Azienda Sanitaria Universitaria Giuliano Isontina (ASU GI), 34128 Trieste, Italy
* Correspondence: mdeodato@units.it

Citation: Manganotti, P.; Deodato, M.; D'Acunto, L.; Biaduzzini, F.; Garascia, G.; Granato, A. Effects of Anti-CGRP Monoclonal Antibodies on Neurophysiological and Clinical Outcomes: A Combined Transcranial Magnetic Stimulation and Algometer Study. *Neurol. Int.* 2024, *16*, 673–688. https://doi.org/10.3390/neurolint16040051

Academic Editor: Yasushi Shibata

Received: 17 May 2024
Revised: 16 June 2024
Accepted: 19 June 2024
Published: 22 June 2024

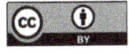

Copyright: © 2024 by the authors. Licensee MDPI, Basel, Switzerland. This article is an open access article distributed under the terms and conditions of the Creative Commons Attribution (CC BY) license (https://creativecommons.org/licenses/by/4.0/).

Abstract: Background: the aim of this study was to investigate the neurophysiological effect of anti-CGRP monoclonal antibodies on central and peripheral levels in migraine patients. Methods: An observational cohort study in patients with migraine was performed. All subjects underwent Single-Pulse and Paired-Pulse Transcranial Magnetic Stimulation, as well as a Pressure Pain Threshold assessment. The same protocol was repeated three and four months after the first injection of anti-CGRP monoclonal antibodies. Results: A total of 11 patients with a diagnosis of migraine and 11 healthy controls were enrolled. The main findings of this study are the significant effects of anti-CGRP mAb treatment on the TMS parameters of intracortical inhibition and the rise in the resting motor threshold in our group of patients affected by resistant migraine. The clinical effect of therapy on migraine is associated with the increase in short-interval intracortical inhibition (SICI), resting motor threshold (RMT), and Pressure Pain Threshold (PPT). In all patients, all clinical headache parameters improved significantly 3 months after the first injection of mAbs and the improvement was maintained at the 1-month follow-up. At baseline, migraineurs and HCs had significant differences in all TMS parameters and in PPT, while at follow-up assessment, no differences were observed on RMT, SICI, and PPT between the two groups. After anti-CGRP monoclonal antibody injection, a significant increase in the intracortical inhibition, in the motor threshold, and in the Pressure Pain Threshold in critical head areas was observed in patients with migraine, which was related to significant clinical benefits. Conclusions: Anti-CGRP monoclonal antibodies improved clinical and neurophysiological outcomes, reflecting a normalization of cortical excitability and peripheral and central sensitization. By directly acting on the thalamus or hypothalamus and indirectly on the trigeminocervical complex, treatment with anti-CGRP monoclonal antibodies may modulate central sensorimotor excitability and peripheral sensitization pain.

Keywords: migraine; cortical excitability; anti-CGRP monoclonal antibodies; transcranial magnetic stimulation; motor cortex; trigeminocervical complex

1. Introduction

Migraine represents one of the most severe and prevalent brain conditions [1]. Its physiopathology is characterized by two opposing processes, habituation and sensitization, that together determine the cycle of a migraine attack [2]. Indeed, migraine attacks present with two main phases, namely the prodromal and the headache phases. The prodromal phase is associated with a lack of habituation, which may be neuro-physiologically characterized by alterations both in cortical excitability and in intracortical circuits. The headache phase is associated with sensitization, possibly related to a reduction in Pressure Pain Threshold (PPT). Consequently, habituation and sensitization are considered fundamental in studying central and peripheral systems involved in migraine and in understanding the network modified by the treatments [2–4].

Extensive neurophysiological studies in migraineurs have recognized neurological lesions and damage [5,6], biomarkers associated with inflammation [7,8], and abnormal information processing and functional connectivity [9], involving habituation and sensitization opposing processes [4] that change during the migraine phases [10,11]. Habituation consists of a reduction in response to sensory stimulation, while sensitization consists of an increase in response to sensory stimulation. On the one hand, a lack of habituation leads to an abnormal state of cortical excitability characterized by an alteration, whose value stands between the threshold of motor/occipital cortex activation and that of inhibitory/excitatory intracortical circuits. On the other hand, sensitization leads to an abnormal state of responsiveness of central and peripheral neurons among the trigeminocervical complex and brain areas [2–4].

Transcranial Magnetic Stimulation (TMS) has been largely investigated in migraine patients [12,13]. Increases in cortical excitability and alterations in the inhibitory/excitatory intracortical circuits were largely reported in migraineurs [14,15]. On the other hand, sensitization at the peripheral level could be assessed with PPT. In particular, pressure algometry allows the evaluation of the sensitivity of tissues both over the muscles in the trigeminocervical area and over the muscles in the extra-trigeminocervical area [16–18].

The trigeminocervical complex seems to be at the center of the interplay between the central and peripheral structures involved in migraine, such as the intra- and extracranial blood vessels, upper cervical spinal cord, locus coeruleus, periaqueductal grey, hypothalamus, primary and secondary motor cortex, somatosensory and visual cortex, thalamus, insula, and amygdala [3,4]. The activation of the trigeminocervical complex connects peripheral events with central involvement through the release of different neuropeptides. Among these, the Calcitonin Gene-Related Peptide (CGRP) is considered the principal mediator of migraine. It is widely distributed in the central and peripheral nervous systems. Blood levels of CGRP are higher in migraine patients compared to healthy controls (HCs) both during the pain and the interictal phases; further, they are higher in Chronic Migraine (CM) compared to Episodic Migraine (EM) patients [19–21]. For this reason, the emerging treatment options against CGRP signaling have shown encouraging results in relieving migraine attacks.

Four monoclonal antibodies (mAbs) targeting the CGRP pathway have been approved for the prevention of migraine attacks in EM and CM in adults: erenumab, fremanezumab, galcanezumab, and eptinezumab. Fremanezumab, galcanezumab, and eptinezumab directly target CGRP, whereas erenumab acts as a blocker of CGRP receptors. Several studies have investigated the clinical effectiveness of anti-CGRP mAbs on headache frequency, duration, and intensity [22,23]. A comprehensive review of phase II–III RCTs involving the four anti-CGRP mAbs has shown that these molecules are significantly superior to placebo in both EM and CM [24]. Ongoing real-world studies are confirming these data, including refractory patients [25]. One study found a mild influence of erenumab 70 mg exclusively on trigeminal districts [26]. However, no previous studies have investigated whether the direct site of action of mAbs is exclusively peripheral or may also include central targets.

The main aim of this study was to investigate the effect of anti-CGRP mAbs on central and peripheral levels in migraine by the neurophysiological evaluation of cortical excitability and PPT. The secondary aim was to compare the neurophysiological outcomes with those of healthy subjects after mAb treatment.

2. Materials and Methods

This observational cohort study was performed in patients with migraine without aura according to the International Classification of Headache Disorders (ICHD-3) [27] criteria. This study was conducted in accordance with the Declaration of Helsinki and the project was approved by the relevant institutional review board and ethics committee (CEUR-2021-Os-246; ID 4174). Moreover, all patients signed the informed consent. Patients with migraine were enrolled at the tertiary Headache Centre of the Clinical Unit of Neurology from March 2021 to June 2021.

Patients were treated with anti-CGRP mAbs according to the AIFA (Italian Medicines Agency) criteria for anti-CGRP monoclonal antibody prescription (erenumab, galcanezumab, and fremanezumab; eptinezumab was not available in Italy). These criteria included the following: migraine diagnosis with more than 8 days per month of migraine in the last 3 months; MIDAS (Migraine Disability Assessment Score) > 11; and failure or contraindication of at least three classes of preventive drugs, including β-blockers, antiepileptics, antidepressants, and Onabotulinumtoxin-A. The exclusion criteria were as follows: patients <18 and >65 years old; pregnancy and breastfeeding; contraindications or low tolerance to TMS; other neurological or psychiatric disorders; cranial nerve impairment; cardiac implantable devices; current prophylactic treatments with antiepileptic drugs and/or benzodiazepines; other migraine prophylactic treatments in the past 3 months; and patients who did not provide their consent to this study. Failure of previous prophylaxes was defined as a treatment discontinuation due to unacceptable side-effects and/or to the absence of improvement in headache after a period of 6 weeks of therapy.

The type and doses of CGRP mAbs were determined according to the clinical evaluation of a headache expert and tailored on migraine patients' characteristics. The therapeutic doses subcutaneously administered were as follows: erenumab 140 mg/28 days dose; fremanezumab 225 mg/month dose; and galcanezumab 120 mg/month dose with a single loading dose of 240 mg. The control group included HCs recruited among resident doctors and health care practitioners between 18 and 65 years old who met the same exclusion criteria while not suffering from headache.

The migraine group was defined using the following frequency features: High-Frequency Episodic Migraine (HFEM) = 8–14 headache days per month, calculated as ≥ 8 to ≤ 14; CM $\geq$ 15 headache days per month for more than 3 months with at least 8 days with features of migraine headache (ICHD-3 criteria) [27].

2.1. Study Design

At baseline (t0), before starting anti-CGRP monoclonal antibody therapy, all patients underwent Single-Pulse (SP) and Paired-Pulse (PP)-TMS and PPT assessment. The same protocol was repeated three (t1) and four (t2) months after the first injection of anti-CGRP monoclonal antibodies. The control group underwent the same protocol with SP-TMS, PP-TMS, and PPT assessment only once (t0). All evaluations were performed during the pain-free periods (i.e., at least 3 days after the last day of migraine and 2 days before the following one) [28] and, for female patients, only in the late follicular phase (i.e., between the day following the end of the menstrual cycle and the day before the start of the ovulation) [29]. Furthermore, subjects should not have taken any medications in the 72 h before the TMS and PPT assessment [30]. The frequency of migraine, duration of attacks, and drug intake of each patient were collected in the headache diary and the MIDAS questionnaire was performed at t0 and t1.

2.2. Neurophysiological Parameters

2.2.1. Transcranial Magnetic Stimulation

SP and PP-TMS sessions were performed in line with the International Federation of Clinical Neurophysiology guidelines and well-established protocols adopted in previous studies to test the cortical excitability of migraine patients [31,32]. Subjects remained sitting in a quiet room, resting with open eyes. Stimuli were delivered by a stimulating figure-of-eight coil of a MagPro® magnetic stimulator (MagVenture Inc., Alpharetta, GA, USA) connected to an electromyographic device (Synergy®, Natus®, Middleton, WI, USA). The optimal site corresponding to the left motor cortex was identified by making patients wear a tight-fitting plastic swimming cap, in order to precisely elicit responses of the contralateral abductor pollicis brevis (APB) muscle in each subject [31]. The low frequency was set at 3 Hz and the high frequency was set at 10 kHz. The electromyographic signals were recorded using Ag-AgCl surface electrodes on the right hand, with a bandpass of 10 to 1000 Hz and a display gain ranging from 50 to 1000 µV/cm. The active (cathode) electrode was placed on the APB muscle, the reference electrode (anode) on the first proximal phalanx, and the ground electrode distally on the volar surface of the forearm. The background electromyographic activity was monitored and recorded to determine the state of muscle relaxation.

The following parameters were obtained for each patient:

1. The resting motor threshold (RMT), from SP-TMS, is defined as the minimum stimulation intensity required to produce a peak-to-peak motor-evoked potential (MEP) amplitude of ≥ 50 µV in at least five of ten stimulations.
2. A short-interval intracortical inhibition (SICI), from the PP-TMS session, evoked by delivering a subthreshold (80% RMT) Conditioning Stimulus (CS) followed by a suprathreshold (130% RMT) test stimulus (TS) at interstimulus intervals (ISIs) of 3 and 5 ms.
3. Intracortical facilitation (ICF), from the PP-TMS session, with the same CS (80% RMT) and TS (130% RMT) at longer ISIs of 10 ms, 15 ms, and 20 ms.
4. Eight MEPs were recorded from the SP-session, elicited by delivering a suprathreshold (130% RMT) TS.

Eight trials were recorded from the SP-TMS, while four trials were delivered for each ISI during the PP-TMS session. The amplitude of motor-evoked potentials (MEPs) elicited by single or paired magnetic stimuli was calculated peak-to-peak and then averaged for each stimulation intensity. From the PP-TMS session (SICI and ICF), the MEP variation was calculated as the mean percentage of the ratio between the MEP obtained by the conditioned stimulus and the basal MEP [15].

2.2.2. Pressure Pain Threshold

For PPT to be evaluated, the Somedic algometer was chosen for its reliability and validity [17,18,33]. The small surface of the Somedic algometer guaranteed an accurate assessment of the craniofacial muscles. The procedure was performed in accordance with Andersen's guidelines of the PPT assessment standardization over craniofacial muscles [33]. PPT was assessed bilaterally over five muscles of the trigeminocervical complex (i.e., masseter, temporalis, trapezius, sub-occipitalis, and procerus) and over one muscle far from this area (i.e., tensor fasciae latae). The first application was conducted on the wrist of each subject, so they could familiarize themselves with the procedure. Three consecutive measurements were carried out for each muscle, with a one-minute interval between each measurement and following the same order of application to the muscles. The increasing rate was approximately 30 kPa/s. When the feeling of pressure turned into pain, patients had to press the algometer stop button [33].

2.3. Headache Parameters

Each patient was given a headache diary for them to record the days of the month of migraine, the duration of pain, and the symptomatic drug intake. Patients were asked to take symptomatic medications only in case of severe headache with a limit of twice per week. At t1 and t2, patients who showed a $\geq 50\%$ reduction from baseline in the days of the month of migraine were considered responders, and those who showed a $\geq 75\%$ reduction were considered super-responders. Disability was evaluated with MIDAS.

2.4. Statistical Analysis

Data were analyzed with GraphPad InStat 3.06. The statistical significance level was a 95% (0.05). The Mann–Whitney Test was used to compare data of migraine patients with data of the HCs, while the Friedman Test (Nonparametric Repeated-Measures ANOVA) was used for establishing the differences among the three patient evaluations. The graphical representation of data was performed with GraphPad Prism 8.4.1.

3. Results

A total of 22 subjects were enrolled, 11 patients with migraine and 11 HCs. Migraineurs comprised 3 men and 8 women, with a mean age of 45 years (SD ± 13). At the time of enrollment, 6 patients met the CM criteria, while 5 patients suffered from HFEM (Table 1). The HC group consisted of 5 men and 6 women, with a mean age of 41 years (SD ± 13). No differences were found between the two groups at t1 in terms of age ($p = 0.4$).

3.1. Transcranial Magnetic Stimulation

3.1.1. SP-Protocol: Resting Motor Threshold

At t0, HCs had a mean RTM (68.6; SD ± 8.1) significantly higher (U = 91; $p = 0.04$) than that of migraineurs (59.2; SD ± 12.3), but the differences at t1 ($p = 0.5$) and t2 ($p = 0.8$) between the two groups were not significant. Indeed, at t1 and t2, RMT increased in the migraine group to 66 (SD ± 12.3) at t1 and to 70 (SD ± 15.8) at t3. Moreover, the Friedman Test revealed statistically significant differences ($X^2_F(2) = 9.000$; $p = 0.01$; Kendall's W = 0.8610) among the three evaluations (t0 vs. t1—6.000, ns $p > 0.05$; t0 vs. t2—12.000, * $p < 0.05$; t1 vs. t2—6.000, ns $p > 0.05$) (Figure 1) (Table 1).

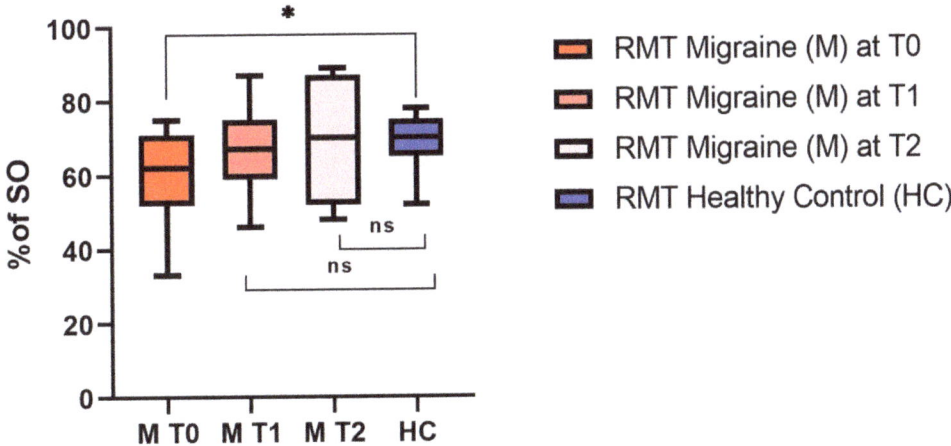

Figure 1. Resting motor threshold (rMT, % of stimulator output (SO)) of individuals with migraine at baseline (t0), at the end of 3 months of therapy with monoclonal antibodies (t1), and after one month of follow-up (t2) and resting motor threshold (rMT, % of stimulator output (SO)) of healthy controls. Mann–Whitney Test and Friedman Test (Nonparametric Repeated-Measures ANOVA): * $p < 0.05$.

Table 1. Demographic and clinical data of migraine group.

Patients	Gender	Age	Diagnosis	Previous Prophylactic Therapy	mAbs	MMDs t0	MMDs t1	MMDs t2	Duration t0	Duration t1	Duration t2	MDI t0	MDI t1	MDI t2	MIDAS t0	MIDAS t1
1	F	46	CM	Am; BoNTA; Tiz; Top	Er	20	5	6	163	24	47	20	12	7	124	28
2	F	22	CM	Am; BoNTA; Er; Flu; Prop; Top	Er	20	19	16	526	123	104	5	4	5	126	52
3	F	62	CM	Am; BoNTA; Flu; Prop; Top; Ven	Er	20	1	2	518	6	14	12	2	1	114	4
4	F	61	CM	Am; Flu; Prop; Top; VPA	Gal	15	5	4	105	30	14	25	4	3	120	19
5	M	41	HFEM	Am; BoNTA; Er; Flu; Prop; Top; VPA	Er	10	9	5	52	49	45	12	15	14	64	31
6	M	42	HFEM	Am; Flu; Top	Er	14	8	9	42	40	48	14	7	6	84	25
7	F	65	CM	Am; Preg	Er	18	11	7	92	70	29	24	11	8	114	32
8	F	47	HFEM	Am; Flu; Top	Fre	12	10	8	141	87	80	9	6	4	61	30
9	F	33	HFEM	Top	Er	12	6	3	45	14	6	12	10	3	86	6
10	M	49	CM	BoNTA; Met; Top;VPA	Fre	19	7	4	85	29	11	30	9	9	131	7
11	F	34	HFEM	Am; BoNTA; Top; VPA	Fre	12	6	5	37	15	8	15	6	7	78	2
Mean		45				15	7	6	164	44	36	15	7	6	100	21
(SD)		(±13)				(±3)	(±4)	(±3)	(±181)	(±35)	(±31)	(±7)	(±3)	(±3)	(±25)	(±15)
Median		46				15	7	5	92	30	29	12	7	6	114	25
(IQR)		(5.5–55)				(12–19.5)	(5.5–9.5)	(4–7.5)	(48.5–152)	(19.5–59.5)	(12.5–47.5)	(12–22)	(5–10.5)	(3.5–7.5)	(81–122)	(6.5–30.5)
Difference																
t0 vs. t1							$p \leq 0.01$			$p \leq 0.05$			$p = ns$			$p \leq 0.0001$	
t0 vs. t2							$p \leq 0.001$			$p \leq 0.01$			$p \leq 0.01$			-	
t1 vs. t2							$p = ns$			$p = ns$			$p = ns$				

Am: Amitriptyline; BoNTA: Onabotulinumtoxin-A; CM: Chronic Migraine; Er: erenumab 140 mg; Fre: fremanezumab; Flu: Flunarizine; Gal: galcanezumab; HFEM: High-Frequency Episodic Migraine; mAbs: monoclonal antibodies; Met: Metoprolol; MIDAS: Migraine Disability Assessment Score; MDI: Monthly Drug Intake; MMDs: Monthly Migraine Days; Preg: Pregabalin; Prop: Propranolol; Tiz: Tizanidine; Top: Topiramate; VPA: Valproic acid; Ven: Venlafaxine.

3.1.2. PP-Protocol of TMS: Intracortical Inhibition and Intracortical Facilitation

With regard to the PP-protocol of TMS, a significant difference was found between migraineurs and HCs only in the SICI at a 3 ms ISI only at baseline (t0) (U = 92; p = 0.04). Nevertheless, no significant differences were found between migraineurs and HCs at t1 (U = 86; p = 0.1) and at t2 (U = 67; p = 0.6). In particular, at t0, the amplitude of MEP at a 3 ms ISI was 0.3 (SD ± 0.5) for migraineurs and 0.05 (SD ± 0.03) for HCs. The SICI amplitude in migraineurs at a 3 ms ISI decreased at t1 (0.2 ± 0.2) and at t2 (0.1 ± 0.2). In addition, the Friedman Test showed statistically significant differences ($x^2_F(2)$ = 6.465; p = 0.03) among the three evaluations in the amplitude of SICI at a 3 ms ISI (t0 vs. t1 3.500, ns p > 0.05; t0 vs. t2 11.500, * p < 0.05; t1 vs. t2 8.000, ns p > 0.05). Moreover, no differences were found in the SICI amplitude at a 5 ISI and in the amplitude of intracortical facilitation (ICF) at 10, 15, and 20 ms ISIs between migraineurs and HCs, nor among the three evaluations (Figure 2a,b) (Table 2).

Transcranial Magnetic Stimulation Paired-Pulse protocol

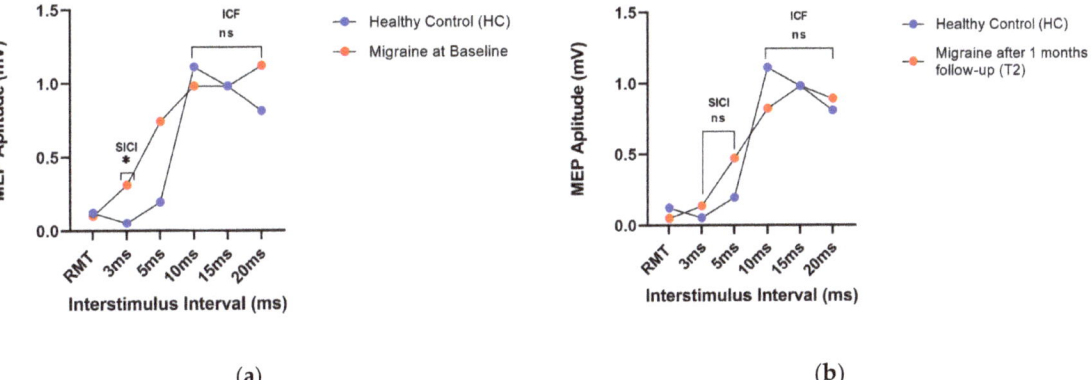

Figure 2. Transcranial Magnetic Stimulation (TMS) Paired-Pulse protocol: (**a**) TMS motor-evoked potentials (MEPs) at different interstimulus intervals (ISIs) of individuals with migraine at baseline (t0) and of healthy controls. Mann–Whitney Test and Friedman Test (Nonparametric Repeated-Measures ANOVA): * p < 0.05. (**b**) TMS motor-evoked potentials (MEPs) at different interstimulus intervals (ISIs) of individuals with migraine after one month of follow-up (t2) and of healthy controls. Mann–Whitney Test and Friedman Test (Nonparametric Repeated-Measures ANOVA).

Table 2. Paired-Pulse-TMS in migraine group at t0, t1, and t2 compared to healthy controls.

PP-TMS	M Mean (SD) Median (IQR)	HC Mean (SD) Median (IQR)	Differences t0 vs. t1 vs. t2	Differences M vs. HC
3 ms (SICI)	t0 0.3 (SD ± 0.5) 0.1 (0.1–0.25)	0.05 (SD ± 0.03) 0.05 (0.02–0.09)	t0 vs. t1: ns	$U = 92; p = 0.04$ *
	t1 0.2 (SD ± 0.2) 0.1 (0.35–0.25)		t0 vs. t2: $p < 0.05$ *	$U = 86; p = 0.1$
	t2 0.1 (SD ± 0.2) 0.04 (0.01–0.07)		t1 vs. t2: ns	$U = 67; p = 0.6$
5 ms (SICI)	t0 0.6 (SD ± 1.4) 0.1 (0.06–0.3)	0.1 (SD ± 0.1) 0.2 (0.01–0.3)	t0 vs. t1: ns	$U = 62; p = 0.9$
	t1 0.4 (SD ± 0.5) 0.2 (0.1–0.5)		t0 vs. t2: ns	$U = 72; p = 0.4$
	t2 0.4 (SD ± 0.5) 0.3 (0.06–0.85)		t1 vs. t2: ns	$U = 79; p = 0.2$
10 ms (ICF)	t0 0.9 (SD ± 1) 0.8 (0.1–1.3)	1.1 (SD ± 1) 1 (0.25–1.4)	t0 vs. t1: ns	$U = 73.5; p = 0.4$
	t1 1.2 (SD ± 1.1) 1 (0.5–1.9)		t0 vs. t2: ns	$U = 67.5; p = 0.6$
	t2 0.8 (SD ± 0.9) 0.5 (0.15–0.9)		t1 vs. t2: ns	$U = 75.5; p = 0.3$
15 ms (ICF)	t0 0.9 (SD ± 1.2) 0.5 (0.14–1.15)	0.9 (SD ± 0.9) 0.9 (0.2–1.4)	t0 vs. t1: ns	$U = 72.5; p = 0.4$
	t1 1.6 (SD ± 1.2) 1.7 (0.75–2.2)		t0 vs. t2: ns	$U = 82.5; p = 0.1$
	t2 1 (SD ± 0.9) 0.5 (0.35–1.3)		t1 vs. t2: ns	$U = 62.5; p = 0.9$
20 ms (ICF)	t0 1 (SD ± 1.2) 0.5 (0.19–1.3)	0.8 (SD ± 0.6) 0.5 (0.25–1.4)	t0 vs. t1: ns	$U = 61; p = 0.9$
	t1 1.4 (SD ± 1.2) 0.9 (0.55–1.9)		t0 vs. t2: ns	$U = 76.5; p = 0.3$
	t2 0.8 (SD ± 1) 0.3 (0.2–1.25)		t1 vs. t2: ns	$U = 63.5; p = 0.8$
RMT	t0 59.2 (SD ± 12.3) 62 (53.5–68)	68.6 (SD ± 8.1) 70 (65–75)	t0 vs. t1: $p < 0.05$ *	$U = 91; p = 0.04$ *
	t1 66 (SD ± 12.3) 67 (60.5–74)		t0 vs. t2: ns	$U = 69.5; p = 0.5$
	t2 70 (SD ± 15.8) 70 (57–84.5)		t1 vs. t2: ns	$U = 64.5; p = 0.8$

* $p < 0.05$. Friedman Test (Nonparametric Repeated-Measures ANOVA) (t0), after 3 months of therapy with monoclonal antibodies (t1), and after 1 month of follow-up (t2); Mann–Whitney test between migraineurs (M) and healthy controls (HCs). PP-TMS: Paired-Pulse Transcranial Magnetic Stimulation; SICI: short-interval intracortical inhibition; ICF: intracortical facilitation; RMT: resting motor threshold.

3.2. Pressure Pain Threshold

Migraine patients had a lower PPT compared to HCs in all muscles assessed except for the temporalis left and procerus. The PPT increased in all muscles at t1 and t2 and non-statistical differences were found between migraineurs and HCs at t0 and t2, respectively, in the Mann–Whitney Test. The Friedman Test revealed statistically significant differences among the three assessments in the sub-occipitalis left ($x^2{}_F(2) = 11.455$; $p = 0.002$; Kendall's W = 0.9990; t0 vs. t1—12.000, * $p < 0.05$; t0 vs. t2—15.000, ** $p < 0.01$; t1 vs. t2—3.000, ns $p > 0.05$) and in the trapezius right ($x^2{}_F(2) = 13.636$; $p = 0.0004$; Kendall's W = 1.0000; t0 vs. t1—15.000, ** $p < 0.01$; t0 vs. t2—15.000, ** $p < 0.01$; t1 vs. t2 0.000, ns $p > 0.05$). On the other hand, no differences were found among the three evaluations in the temporalis left ($x^2{}_F(2) = 0.7273$; $p = 0.7$; Kendall's W = 0.5620) and right ($x^2{}_F(2) = 0.7273$; $p = 0.7$; Kendall's W = 0.9990), in the sub-occipitalis right ($x^2{}_F(2) = 5.091$; $p = 0.08$; Kendall's W = 1.0000), in the masseter left ($x^2{}_F(2) = 0.1818$; $p = 0.9$; Kendall's W = 1.0000) and right ($x^2{}_F(2) = 4.545$; $p = 0.11$; Kendall's W = 1.0000), in the trapezius left ($x^2{}_F(2) = 5.091$; $p = 0.08$; Kendall's W = 1.0000), in the procerus ($x^2{}_F(2) = 5.163$; $p = 0.07$; Kendall's W = 0.9990), and in the tensor fasciae latae left ($x^2{}_F(2) = 1.273$; $p = 0.6$; Kendall's W = 1.0000) and right ($x^2{}_F(2) = 1.273$; $p = 0.6$; Kendall's W = 1.0000) (Table 3).

Table 3. Pressure Pain Threshold in migraine group at t0, t1, and t2 compared to healthy controls.

PPT	M Mean (SD) Median (IQR)	HC Mean (SD) Median (IQR)	Differences t0 vs. t1 vs. t2	Differences M vs. HC
Temporalis left	t0 250.6 (SD ± 118) 346.9 (258–443.5)	285.5 (SD ± 116) 260 (211–347.8)	t0 vs. t1: ns	U = 70; $p = 0.5$
	t1 285 (SD ± 138.8) 246.3 (209–325.6)		t0 vs. t2: ns	U = 65; $p = 0.7$
	t2 273.2 (SD ± 94.5) 237.1 (204.5–325.6)		t1 vs. t2: ns	U = 64; $p = 0.8$
Temporalis right	t0 251.7 (SD ± 108.2) 319.4 (233.9–404)	315.6 (SD ± 65.3) 328 (264.1–354.1)	t0 vs. t1: ns	U = 91; $p = 0.04$ *
	t1 270 (SD ± 81.7) 268.5 (222.7–292)		t0 vs. t2: ns	U = 84; $p = 0.1$
	t2 255 (SD ± 75.8) 242.3 (202.2–291.7)		t1 vs. t2: ns	U = 89; $p = 0.06$
Sub-occipitalis left	t0 257.2 (SD ± 109.8) 246.9 (195.3–334.4)	563.7 (SD ± 668.5) 314.6 (295.4–475.6)	t0 vs. t1: $p < 0.05$ *	U = 91; $p = 0.04$ *
	t1 345.3 (SD ± 77.1) 339.7 (279.3–377.2)		t0 vs. t2: $p < 0.01$ **	U = 73; $p = 0.4$
	t2 341.2 (SD ± 96.7) 340.3 (285.2–379.2)		t1 vs. t2: ns	U = 69; $p = 0.6$
Sub-occipitalis right	t0 241.4 (SD ± 109.5) 235.8 (172.4–310.8)	318.1 (SD ± 64.6) 299.2 (283.7–344.9)	t0 vs. t1: ns	U = 91; $p = 0.04$ *
	t1 309.2 (SD ± 84.2) 312.3 (249.9–379.5)		t0 vs. t2: ns	U = 65; $p = 0.7$
	t2 318.6 (SD ± 86.7) 326 (273.7–347.8)		t1 vs. t2: ns	U = 66; $p = 0.7$
Masseter left	t0 214.7 (SD ± 93.4) 207.1 (159.7–234.5)	257.9 (SD ± 41.5) 255.5 (232.6–266.6)	t0 vs. t1: ns	U = 91; $p = 0.04$ *
	t1 219.9 (SD ± 63.4) 209 (192.7–243.7)		t0 vs. t2: ns	U = 91; $p = 0.04$ *
	t2 232.9 (SD ± 86.7) 230.6 (182.2–249.9)		t1 vs. t2: ns	U = 89; $p = 0.06$

Table 3. Cont.

PPT	M Mean (SD) Median (IQR)	HC Mean (SD) Median (IQR)	Differences t0 vs. t1 vs. t2	Differences M vs. HC
Masseter right	t0 171.2 (SD ± 59.3) 170.3 (119.8–220.1)	255.4 (SD ± 68.7) 235.2 (211–305.4)	t0 vs. t1: ns	U = 99; p = 0.01 *
	t1 184.6 (SD ± 46.6) 180.3 (148.6–194.6)		t0 vs. t2: ns	U = 103; p = 0.004 *
	t2 218.2 (SD ± 79.6) 209.1 (166.5–225.1)		t1 vs. t2: ns	U = 85; p = 0.1
Trapezius left	t0 334.8 (SD ± 146.4) 346.9 (258–443.5)	509.1 (SD ± 180.2) 471 (369.1–597)	t0 vs. t1: ns	U = 93; p = 0.03 *
	t1 398.1 (SD ± 114.1) 369.5 (322.4–463.8)		t0 vs. t2: p < 0.05 *	U = 83; p = 0.1
	t2 423.11 (SD ± 145.7) 369.9 (324.9–509.4)		t1 vs. t2: ns	U = 78; p = 0.2
Trapezius right	t0 321.7 (SD ± 125.2) 319.4 (233.9–404)	522.8 (SD ± 171.9) 499.8 (409.9–600)	t0 vs. t1: p < 0.01 **	U = 100; p = 0.008 *
	t1 462.5 (SD ± 104.9) 479.5 (395.6–543.1)		t0 vs. t2: p < 0.01 **	U = 70; p = 0.5
	t2 473.6 (SD ± 203.5) 454.7 (318.1–616.7)		t1 vs. t2: ns	U = 70; p = 0.5
Procerus	t0 250.7 (SD ± 82.3) 246.9 (204.1–317.5)	287.4 (SD ± 83.6) 285.5 (230.3–343.5)	t0 vs. t1: ns	U = 74; p = 0.4
	t1 308.7 (SD ± 75.4) 294 (275–338.1)		t0 vs. t2: ns	U = 68; p = 0.6
	t2 328 (SD ± 55.9) 310.3 (280.3–382.5)		t1 vs. t2: ns	U = 67; p = 0.6
Tensor fasciae latae left	t0 490.8 (SD ± 238.5) 484.8 (339.4–563.1)	667.7 (SD ± 182.3) 642.9 (574.9–768.7)	t0 vs. t1: ns	U = 92; p = 0.04 *
	t1 560.2 (SD ± 217.6) 494.5 (409–731.1)		t0 vs. t2: ns	U = 79; p = 0.2
	t2 590.1 (SD ± 255.7) 510.2 (418.7–719.6)		t1 vs. t2: ns	U = 79; p = 0.2
Tensor fasciae latae right	t0 486.6 (SD ± 235.2) 463.2 (259.3–651.4)	1283.9 (SD ± 1891.8) 710.6 (584.5–917.6)	t0 vs. t1: ns	U = 95; p = 0.02 *
	t1 558.2 (SD ± 235.5) 495.8 (401.4–730.4)		t0 vs. t2: ns	U = 89; p = 0.06
	t2 567.3 (SD ± 260.5) 658.5 (354.7–682)		t1 vs. t2: ns	U = 85; p = 0.1

* p < 0.05; ** p < 0.01. Friedman Test (Nonparametric Repeated-Measures ANOVA) (t0), after 3 months of therapy with monoclonal antibodies (t1), and after 1 month of follow-up (t2); Mann–Whitney Test between migraineurs (M) and healthy controls (HCs). PPT: Pressure Pain Threshold.

3.3. Headache Parameters

All headache parameters improved at t1 and t2 (Table 1). In particular, the mean MMDs decreased from 15 (SD ± 3) days at t0 to 7 (SD ± 4) at t1 and to 6 (SD ± 3) at t2. The Friedman Test found statistically significant differences among the three evaluations ($x^2{}_F(2)$ = 17.636; $p \leq 0.0001$; Kendall's W = 0.4671; t0 vs. t1 14.000, * p < 0.01; t0 vs. t2 19.000 *** p < 0.001; t1 vs. t2 5.000, ns p > 0.05). At t1, 6 patients were responders (of which 2 were super-responders), and at t2, 8 patients were responders (of which 2 were super-responders). The average duration of attacks significantly decreased from 164 h (SD ± 181) at t0 to 44 h (SD ± 35) at t1 and to 36 h (SD ± 31) at t2. Furthermore, the variance among the three assessments was statistically significant ($x^2{}_F(2)$ = 14.364; p = 0.0002; Kendall's W = 0.6712; t0 vs. t1 13.000, ns p > 0.05; t0 vs. t2 17.000, ** p < 0.01; t1 vs. t2 4.000, ns p > 0.05).

Mean Monthly Drug Intake decreased from 15 (SD ± 7) at t0 to 7 (SD ± 3) at t1 and to 6 (SD ± 3) at t2. Moreover, the variance shown by the Friedman Test was statistically significant ($x^2{}_F(2) = 11.762$; $p = 0.002$; Kendall's W = 0.6290; t0 vs. t1 10.000, ns $p > 0.05$; t0 vs. t2 15.500, ** $p < 0.01$; t1 vs. t2 5.500, ns $p > 0.05$). Lastly, the disability related to headache assessed with the MIDAS questionnaire significantly reduced from 100 (SD ± 25) to 21 (SD ± 15) points ($p = 0.001$, Wilcoxon matched-pairs).

4. Discussion

The main findings of this study are the significant effects of anti-CGRP mAb treatment on the TMS parameters of intracortical inhibition and the rise in the resting motor threshold in our group of patients affected by resistant migraine. The clinical effect of therapy on migraine is associated with the increase in short-interval intracortical inhibition (SICI), resting motor threshold (RMT), and Pressure Pain Threshold (PPT). In all patients, all clinical headache parameters improved significantly 3 months after the first injection of mAbs and the improvement was maintained at the 1-month follow-up. At baseline, migraineurs and HCs had significant differences in all TMS parameters and in PPT, while at follow-up assessment, no differences were observed on RMT, SICI, and PPT between the two groups.

RMT reflects different aspects of brain circuit excitability investigated by SS-TMS [14,34,35]. We found that RMT significantly increased in the migraine group after anti-CGRP mAb treatment, reaching the same values of HCs. These observations may suggest that anti-CGRP mAbs may act not only peripherally but also at a central level, probably on cortico-cortical axons excitability or on fast synaptic transmission. Recent studies suggest that anti-CGRP mAbs do not penetrate the blood–brain barrier. They may exert an indirect effect on the trigeminocervical complex, on the meningeal vessels, or on the hypothalamus [20,21]. The trigeminocervical complex represents the main actor of an interplay between central and peripheral structures [2–4]. Thanks to these connections, anti-CGRP mAbs may also have a central effect. In fact, peripheral sensitization of the trigeminocervical complex leads to increased painful stimulation of the thalamus and consequently to central sensitization [20]. Furthermore, the hypothalamus plays an important role both in migraine pathogenesis and in descending pain inhibition [36,37]. The CGRP receptor is expressed also at the hypothalamic level, where the capillary endothelium is fenestrated. Consequently, authors have supposed a central effect of anti-CGRP mAbs on migraine [38,39]. As already reported with some symptomatic medication, in particular triptans [30,40], the improvement in migraine after anti-CGRP mAb treatment could be related to a normalization of cortical excitability and pain perception. The increase in motor threshold in sensory motor areas may be an indirect epiphenomenon of action of anti-CGRP mAbs on the trigeminocervical complex and on the hypothalamus.

SICI and ICF allow the assessment of the GABAergic inhibitory circuits and the glutamatergic excitatory pathways of neurotransmission, respectively [34,35,41]. Neurophysiological studies in migraine evidenced a higher reduction in SICI, reflecting the lack of habituation during stimulus repetition, and a more pronounced ICF, reflecting sensitization during stimulus repetition compared with HCs [14,15,42]. No previous studies investigated SICI and ICF before and after anti-CGRP mAb treatment. Our results highlighted significant differences between migraineurs and HCs in SICI only at a 3 ms ISI, but not at a 5 ms ISI, while no differences were found at 10 ms, 15 ms, or 20 ms of ICF. One unexpected finding was that at the end of the 4 months of anti-CGRP mAbs, no differences were found between migraineurs and HCs in SICI at a 3 ms ISI, which may be related to a normalizing effect on inhibitory circuits mediated by GABAergic neurotransmission. The increase in intracortical inhibition, associated with the rise in motor threshold, suggests a combined and probably indirect effect of anti-CGRP mABs on GABAergic neurotransmission and cortico-cortical axon excitability, which are usually abnormal in migraine. Consequently, it could be supposed that anti-CGRP mAbs may act directly or indirectly on the central nervous system even in the case of a lack of habituation and of sensitization. Moreover, the lack of habituation depends on thalamocortical dysrhythmia. The response of the thalamus to inputs of the trigeminocervical complex is mediated by CGRP antagonists, which block the release of CGRP in areas involved in migraine through the inhibition of neurogenic inflammation [22–26]. Understanding whether long-term treatment with monoclonal antibodies would result in a normalization of SICI also at a 5 ms ISI would be compelling, as well as whether this normalization would last over time.

We found a significantly reduced PPT in almost all points of the craniocervical regions and also in the extra-cephalic regions. Several pieces of research highlighted a lower PPT in migraineurs compared to HCs both in the trigeminocervical complex and throughout the body [18,33,43]. These parameters have never been studied in patients with migraine after mAb treatment. One study assessed PPT in CM after Onabotulinumtoxin-A (BoNT-A), physical therapy, and their combination [11]. Although each treatment increased PPT, the combined approach was more effective than the respective monotherapies. Different pharmacological and non-pharmacological therapies target sub-occipitalis muscles in migraine due to their anatomical connections [17,18,33]. Similarly to BoNT-A in monotherapy, anti-CGRP mAbs in monotherapy increased PPT bilaterally in the sub-occipitalis muscles, too [18]. The sub-occipitalis muscles are innervated both by the C1 nerve and by the greater occipital nerve. Particularly, the rectus capitis posterior is anatomically linked to the dura mater, which in turn is innervated by the ophthalmic division of the trigeminal nerve, too [44]. The increase in PPT over craniocervical and extracervical regions suggests a pain modulation effect of anti-CGRP mAbs, which is also related to the improvement in headache parameters [21]. In fact, our patients reported a progressive and significant reduction in MMDs, duration of attacks, symptomatic drug intake, and MIDAS. At t2, 5 out of 8 responder patients were super-responders. This high rate of responders reflects what has already been found in meta-analyses by evaluating the efficacy and tolerability of anti-CGRP mAbs in the preventive treatment of EM and CM [45,46].

Our neurophysiological outcomes on RMT, SICI, and PPT corroborate the hypothesis that anti-CGRP mAbs may directly or indirectly normalize cortical excitability and PPT through a reduction in peripheral and central sensitization. Despite these promising results, further studies are needed to establish whether anti-CGRP mAbs may also exert an effect on the lack of habituation. The exact site and mechanism of action of this targeted therapy are still debated. Recent studies reported a possible central effect of erenumab and galcanezumab; in fact, a decrease in hypothalamic activation was found among patients treated with these two mAbs [47]. On such a basis, our findings suggest some hypotheses on functioning: (1) an indirect peripheral modulation through trigeminal afferents fibers leads to a normalization of cortical excitability and PPT; (2) a direct central modulation through the thalamus and hypothalamus influences pain perception and central sensitization; and (3) an indirect central effect through the reduction in analgesic intake, in particular triptans, influences cortical excitability and pain perception [30,37,40].

Our study had some limitations. First, the small sample size did not allow a stratification between HFEM and CM, nor between responders and partial responders, nor among the different anti-CGRP mAbs used. However, our aim was to evaluate the neurophysiological effect of monoclonal antibodies on central and peripheral outcomes, since the effectiveness on clinical parameters had already been demonstrated. Second, a long-term follow-up is necessary to determine whether early results last over time. Third, the guidelines allow the consumption of symptomatic medications in the case of severe migraine attack, but this intake may bias the results. Despite these limitations, the study presented three strong points: (1) for the first time, the cortical excitability was studied with TMS after anti-CGRP mAb treatment; (2) for the first time, the changes in PPT were assessed with a specific algometer after anti-CGRP mAb treatment; and (3) for the first time, the neurophysiological outcomes on cortical excitability and PPT between migraineurs and HCs before and after anti-CGRP mAb treatment were compared.

5. Conclusions

This study evidences an abnormal cortical excitability in migraineurs, reflected by a lower RMT and SICI, as well as hyperalgesia, reflected by a lower PPT in the cephalic and extra-cephalic muscles, compared to HCs. Despite the site and mechanism of action still being uncertain, anti-CGRP mABs seem to be able to modulate the central and peripheral sensitization to pain both indirectly through the trigeminocervical complex and directly through the thalamus or hypothalamus. Lastly, this study highlights the clinical and neurophysiological effects of anti-CGRP monoclonal antibodies in migraine. In the future, larger randomized controlled trials may shed light on the possible responses to each anti-CGRP mAb and their effect on the habituation phenomenon.

Author Contributions: Conception, P.M., A.G. and M.D.; methodology, P.M., M.D. and A.G.; software, M.D., L.D., F.B. and G.G.; validation, P.M., A.G. and M.D.; formal analysis, P.M., A.G. and M.D.; investigation, P.M., M.D., L.D., F.B., G.G. and A.G.; resources, P.M., A.G. and M.D.; data curation, M.D., L.D., F.B. and G.G.; writing—original draft preparation, M.D., L.D., F.B. and G.G.; writing—review and editing, P.M., M.D., L.D., F.B., G.G. and A.G.; visualization, P.M., A.G. and M.D.; supervision, P.M. and A.G.; project administration, P.M., A.G. and M.D. All authors have read and agreed to the published version of the manuscript.

Funding: This research received no external funding.

Institutional Review Board Statement: This study was conducted in accordance with the Declaration of Helsinki and approved by the Institutional Review Board of Comitato Etico Unico Regionale (CEUR) (CEUR-2021-Os-246; ID 4174).

Informed Consent Statement: Informed consent was obtained from all subjects involved in the study and written informed consent has been obtained from the patient(s) to publish this paper.

Data Availability Statement: The principal author takes full responsibility for the data presented in this study, analysis of the data, conclusions, and conduct of the research. The dataset page containing authors' details analyzed during the current study are available from the corresponding author on reasonable request.

Acknowledgments: The authors are thankful to the people with migraine and the healthy controls for their participation.

Conflicts of Interest: The authors declare no conflicts of interest.

Abbreviation

anti-CGRP mAbs	Anti-Calcitonin Gene-Related Peptide monoclonal Antibodies
BoNTA	Onabotulinumtoxin-A
CGRP	Calcitonin Gene-Related Peptide
CSP	Cortical Silent Period
CM	Chronic Migraine
EM	Episodic Migraine
FDA	Food and Drug Administration
HF-EM	High-Frequency Episodic Migraine
ICHD-3	International Classification of Headache Disorders, Third Edition
ISI	interstimulus interval
ICF	intracortical facilitation
LICI	long-interval intracortical inhibition
LF-EM	Low-Frequency Episodic Migraine
MOH	Medication Overuse Headache
MEP	motor-evoked potential
NSAIDs	Nonsteroidal Anti-Inflammatory Drugs

PPT	Pressure Pain Threshold
PP-TMS	Paired-Pulse Transcranial Magnetic Stimulation
RCT	Randomized Control Trial
RMT	resting motor threshold
SICI	short-interval intracortical inhibition
SP-TMS	Single-Pulse Transcranial Magnetic Stimulation
TMS	Transcranial Magnetic Stimulation

References

1. Di Cola, F.S.; Bolchini, M.; Caratozzolo, S.; Ceccardi, G.; Cortinovis, M.; Liberini, P.; Rao, R.; Padovani, A. Migraine Disability Improvement during Treatment with Galcanezumab in Patients with Chronic and High Frequency Episodic Migraine. *Neurol. Int.* **2023**, *15*, 273–284. [CrossRef] [PubMed]
2. Coppola, G.; Di Lorenzo, C.; Schoenen, J.; Pierelli, F. Habituation and sensitization in primary headaches. *J. Headache Pain* **2013**, *14*, 65. [CrossRef] [PubMed]
3. Charles, A. The pathophysiology of migraine: Implications for clinical management. *Lancet Neurol.* **2018**, *17*, 174–182. [CrossRef] [PubMed]
4. Goadsby, P.J.; Holland, P.R.; Martins-Oliveira, M.; Hoffmann, J.; Schankin, C.; Akerman, S. Pathophysiology of Migraine: A Disorder of Sensory Processing. *Physiol. Rev.* **2017**, *97*, 553–622. [CrossRef] [PubMed]
5. Shibata, Y.; Ishiyama, S. Neurite Damage in Patients with Migraine. *Neurol. Int.* **2024**, *16*, 299–311. [CrossRef] [PubMed]
6. Shibata, Y.; Goto, M.; Ishiyama, S. Analysis of Migraine Pathophysiology by Magnetic Resonance Imaging. *OBM Neurobiol.* **2021**, *6*, 115. [CrossRef]
7. Pleș, H.; Florian, I.-A.; Timis, T.-L.; Covache-Busuioc, R.-A.; Glavan, L.-A.; Dumitrascu, D.-I.; Popa, A.A.; Bordeianu, A.; Ciurea, A.V. Migraine: Advances in the Pathogenesis and Treatment. *Neurol. Int.* **2023**, *15*, 1052–1105. [CrossRef] [PubMed]
8. Shibata, Y. Migraine Pathophysiology Revisited: Proposal of a New Molecular Theory of Migraine Pathophysiology and Headache Diagnostic Criteria. *Int. J. Mol. Sci.* **2022**, *23*, 13002. [CrossRef] [PubMed]
9. Ishiyama, S.; Shibata, Y.; Ayuzawa, S.; Matsushita, A.; Matsumura, A.; Ishikawa, E. The Modifying of Functional Connectivity Induced by Peripheral Nerve Field Stimulation using Electroacupuncture for Migraine: A Prospective Clinical Study. *Pain Med.* **2022**, *23*, 1560–1569. [CrossRef]
10. Finocchi, C.; Di Antonio, S.; Castaldo, M.; Ponzano, M.; Bovis, F.; Villafañe, J.H.; Torelli, P.; Arendt-Nielsen, L. Increase pain sensitivity during the four phases of the migraine cycle in patients with episodic migraine. *Neurol. Sci.* **2022**, *43*, 5773–5775. [CrossRef]
11. Di Antonio, S.; Arendt-Nielsen, L.; Ponzano, M.; Bovis, F.; Torelli, P.; Finocchi, C.; Castaldo, M. Trigeminocervical pain sensitivity during the migraine cycle depends on headache frequency. *Neurol. Sci.* **2023**, *44*, 4021–4032. [CrossRef]
12. Brigo, F.; Storti, M.; Tezzon, F.; Manganotti, P.; Nardone, R. Primary visual cortex excitability in migraine: A systematic review with meta-analysis. *Neurol. Sci.* **2012**, *34*, 819–830. [CrossRef]
13. Badawy, R.A.B.; Loetscher, T.; Macdonell, R.A.L.; Brodtmann, A. Cortical excitability and neurology: Insights into the pathophysiology. *Funct. Neurol.* **2012**, *27*, 131–145.
14. Neverdahl, J.; Omland, P.; Uglem, M.; Engstrøm, M.; Sand, T. Reduced motor cortical inhibition in migraine: A blinded transcranial magnetic stimulation study. *Clin. Neurophysiol.* **2017**, *128*, 2411–2418. [CrossRef] [PubMed]
15. Deodato, M.; Granato, A.; Martini, M.; Stella, A.B.; Galmonte, A.; Murena, L.; Manganotti, P. Neurophysiological and Clinical Outcomes in Episodic Migraine Without Aura: A Cross-Sectional Study. *J. Clin. Neurophysiol.* **2024**, *41*, 388–395. [CrossRef]
16. Graven-Nielsen, T.; Vaegter, H.B.; Finocchietti, S.; Handberg, G.; Arendt-Nielsen, L. Assessment of musculoskeletal pain sensitivity and temporal summation by cuff pressure algometry: A reliability study. *Pain* **2015**, *156*, 2193–2202. [CrossRef] [PubMed]
17. Deodato, M.; Granato, A.; Borgino, C.; Galmonte, A.; Manganotti, P. Instrumental assessment of physiotherapy and onabolulinumtoxin-A on cervical and headache parameters in chronic migraine. *Neurol. Sci.* **2021**, *43*, 2021–2029. [CrossRef] [PubMed]
18. Deodato, M.; Granato, A.; Ceschin, M.; Galmonte, A.; Manganotti, P. Algometer Assessment of Pressure Pain Threshold After Onabotulinumtoxin-A and Physical Therapy Treatments in Patients With Chronic Migraine: An Observational Study. *Front. Pain Res.* **2022**, *3*, 770397. [CrossRef]
19. Edvinsson, L. The Trigeminovascular Pathway: Role of CGRP and CGRP Receptors in Migraine. *Headache J. Head Face Pain* **2017**, *57*, 47–55. [CrossRef]
20. Iyengar, S.; Johnson, K.W.; Ossipov, M.H.; Aurora, S.K. CGRP and the Trigeminal System in Migraine. *Headache J. Head Face Pain* **2019**, *59*, 659–681. [CrossRef]
21. Benedicter, N.; Messlinger, K.; Vogler, B.; Mackenzie, K.D.; Stratton, J.; Friedrich, N.; Dux, M. Semi-Automated Recording of Facial Sensitivity in Rat Demonstrates Antinociceptive Effects of the Anti-CGRP Antibody Fremanezumab. *Neurol. Int.* **2023**, *15*, 622–637. [CrossRef] [PubMed]

22. Tepper, S.; Ashina, M.; Reuter, U.; Brandes, J.L.; Doležil, D.; Silberstein, S.; Winner, P.; Leonardi, D.; Mikol, D.; Lenz, R. Safety and efficacy of erenumab for preventive treatment of chronic migraine: A randomised, double-blind, placebo-controlled phase 2 trial. *Lancet Neurol.* **2017**, *16*, 425–434. [CrossRef]
23. Zhu, C.; Guan, J.B.; Xiao, H.; Luo, W.; Tong, R. Erenumab safety and efficacy in migraine: A systematic review and meta-analysis of randomized clinical trials. *Medicine* **2019**, *98*, e18483. [CrossRef]
24. Dodick, D.W. CGRP ligand and receptor monoclonal antibodies for migraine prevention: Evidence review and clinical implications. *Cephalalgia* **2019**, *39*, 445–458. [CrossRef]
25. Lambru, G.; Hill, B.; Murphy, M.; Tylova, I.; Andreou, A.P. A prospective real-world analysis of erenumab in refractory chronic migraine. *J. Headache Pain* **2020**, *21*, 61. [CrossRef] [PubMed]
26. De Tommaso, M.; Delussi, M.; Gentile, E.; Ricci, K.; Quitadamo, S.G.; Libro, G. Effect of single dose Erenumab on cortical responses evoked by cutaneous a-delta fibers: A pilot study in migraine patients. *Cephalalgia* **2021**, *41*, 1004–1014. [CrossRef]
27. Arnold, M. Headache Classification Committee of the International Headache Society (IHS) The International Classification of Headache Disorders. *Cephalalgia* **2018**, *38*, 1–211.
28. Peng, K.-P.; May, A. Quantitative sensory testing in migraine patients must be phase-specific. *Pain* **2018**, *159*, 2414–2416. [CrossRef]
29. Delaruelle, Z.; on behalf of the European Headache Federation School of Advanced Studies (EHF-SAS); Ivanova, T.A.; Khan, S.; Negro, A.; Ornello, R.; Raffaelli, B.; Terrin, A.; Mitsikostas, D.D.; Reuter, U. Male and female sex hormones in primary headaches. *J. Headache Pain* **2018**, *19*, 117. [CrossRef]
30. Ziemann, U.; Reis, J.; Schwenkreis, P.; Rosanova, M.; Strafella, A.; Badawy, R.; Müller-Dahlhaus, F. TMS and drugs revisited 2014. *Clin. Neurophysiol.* **2015**, *126*, 1847–1868. [CrossRef]
31. Cosentino, G.; Di Marco, S.; Ferlisi, S.; Valentino, F.; Capitano, W.M.; Fierro, B.; Brighina, F. Intracortical facilitation within the migraine motor cortex depends on the stimulation intensity. A paired-pulse TMS study. *J. Headache Pain* **2018**, *19*, 65. [CrossRef] [PubMed]
32. Rossi, S.; Antal, A.; Bestmann, S.; Bikson, M.; Brewer, C.; Brockmöller, J.; Carpenter, L.L.; Cincotta, M.; Chen, R.; Daskalakis, J.D.; et al. Safety and recommendations for TMS use in healthy subjects and patient populations, with updates on training, ethical and regulatory issues: Expert Guidelines. *Clin. Neurophysiol.* **2020**, *132*, 269–306. [CrossRef] [PubMed]
33. Andersen, S.; Petersen, M.W.; Svendsen, A.S.; Gazerani, P. Pressure pain thresholds assessed over temporalis, masseter, and frontalis muscles in healthy individuals, patients with tension-type headache, and those with migraine—A systematic review. *Pain* **2015**, *156*, 1409–1423. [CrossRef] [PubMed]
34. Lefaucheur, J.-P. Transcranial magnetic stimulation. *Handb. Clin. Neurol.* **2019**, *160*, 559–580. [PubMed]
35. Manganotti, P.; Michelutti, M.; Furlanis, G.; Deodato, M.; Stella, A.B. Deficient GABABergic and glutamatergic excitability in the motor cortex of patients with long-COVID and cognitive impairment. *Clin. Neurophysiol.* **2023**, *151*, 83–91. [CrossRef] [PubMed]
36. Schulte, L.H.; Allers, A.; May, A. Hypothalamus as a mediator of chronic migraine. *Neurology* **2017**, *88*, 2011–2016. [CrossRef] [PubMed]
37. Coppola, G.; Di Renzo, A.; Petolicchio, B.; Tinelli, E.; Di Lorenzo, C.; Serrao, M.; Calistri, V.; Tardioli, S.; Cartocci, G.; Parisi, V.; et al. Increased neural connectivity between the hypothalamus and cortical resting-state functional networks in chronic migraine. *J. Neurol.* **2019**, *267*, 185–191. [CrossRef] [PubMed]
38. Iannone, L.F.; De Cesaris, F.; Ferrari, A.; Benemei, S.; Fattori, D.; Chiarugi, A. Effectiveness of anti-CGRP monoclonal antibodies on central symptoms of migraine. *Cephalalgia* **2022**, *42*, 1323–1330. [CrossRef] [PubMed]
39. Szabo, E.; Ashina, S.; Melo-Carrillo, A.; Bolo, N.R.; Borsook, D.; Burstein, R. Peripherally acting anti-CGRP monoclonal antibodies alter cortical gray matter thickness in migraine patients: A prospective cohort study. *NeuroImage Clin.* **2023**, *40*, 103531. [CrossRef]
40. Cortese, F.; Pierelli, F.; Pauri, F.; Di Lorenzo, C.; Lepre, C.; Malavolta, G.; Merluzzo, C.; Parisi, V.; Ambrosini, A.; Serrao, M.; et al. Withdrawal from acute medication normalises short-term cortical synaptic potentiation in medication overuse headache. *Neurol. Sci.* **2019**, *40*, 963–969. [CrossRef]
41. Chen, R.; Tam, A.; Bütefisch, C.; Corwell, B.; Ziemann, U.; Rothwell, J.C.; Cohen, L.G.; Rozand, V.; Senefeld, J.W.; Sundberg, C.W.; et al. Intracortical Inhibition and Facilitation in Different Representations of the Human Motor Cortex. *J. Neurophysiol.* **1998**, *80*, 2870–2881. [CrossRef] [PubMed]
42. Siniatchkin, M.; Kröner-Herwig, B.; Kocabiyik, E.; Rothenberger, A. Intracortical Inhibition and Facilitation in Migraine—A Transcranial Magnetic Stimulation Study. *Headache J. Head Face Pain* **2007**, *47*, 364–370. [CrossRef] [PubMed]
43. Barón, J.; Ruiz, M.; Palacios-Ceña, M.; Madeleine, P.; Guerrero, Á.L.; Arendt-Nielsen, L.; Fernández-De-Las-Peñas, C. Differences in Topographical Pressure Pain Sensitivity Maps of the Scalp Between Patients With Migraine and Healthy Controls. *Headache J. Head Face Pain* **2016**, *57*, 226–235. [CrossRef] [PubMed]
44. Noseda, R.; Melo-Carrillo, A.; Nir, R.-R.; Strassman, A.M.; Burstein, R. Non-Trigeminal Nociceptive Innervation of the Posterior Dura: Implications to Occipital Headache. *J. Neurosci.* **2019**, *39*, 1867–1880. [CrossRef] [PubMed]
45. Han, L.; Liu, Y.; Xiong, H.; Hong, P. CGRP monoclonal antibody for preventive treatment of chronic migraine: An update of meta-analysis. *Brain Behav.* **2019**, *9*, e01215. [CrossRef]

46. Alasad, Y.W.; Asha, M.Z. Monoclonal antibodies as a preventive therapy for migraine: A meta-analysis. *Clin. Neurol. Neurosurg.* **2020**, *195*, 105900. [CrossRef]
47. Ziegeler, C.; Mehnert, J.; Asmussen, K.; May, A. Central effects of erenumab in migraine patients: An event-related functional imaging study. *Neurology* **2020**, *95*, e2794–e2802. [CrossRef]

Disclaimer/Publisher's Note: The statements, opinions and data contained in all publications are solely those of the individual author(s) and contributor(s) and not of MDPI and/or the editor(s). MDPI and/or the editor(s) disclaim responsibility for any injury to people or property resulting from any ideas, methods, instructions or products referred to in the content.

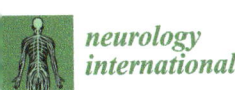

Article

Efficacy of Lasmiditan as a Secondary Treatment for Migraine Attacks after Unsuccessful Treatment with a Triptan

Yasushi Shibata [1,*], Hiroshige Sato [2], Akiko Sato [3] and Yoichi Harada [4]

1. Department of Neurosurgery, Mito Medical Center, University of Tsukuba, Mito 310-0015, Japan
2. Department of Neurosurgery, Sato Clinic of Internal Medicine and Neurosurgery, Moriya 302-0117, Japan
3. Department of Neurology, Sato Clinic of Internal Medicine and Neurosurgery, Moriya 302-0117, Japan; hiroshigesato@gmail.com
4. Department of Neurosurgery, Mito Brain Heart Center, Mito 310-0004, Japan; harada-mbhc_neuro@mito-bhc.com
* Correspondence: yshibata@md.tsukuba.ac.jp

Abstract: The combined use of lasmiditan and triptan is unexplored in medical literature. This study aimed to investigate whether the intake of lasmiditan following triptan improves migraine pain. Following triptan intake, if headache relief was less than 50% at 1 h, patients took 50 mg of lasmiditan within 2 h of migraine onset. Patients recorded headache intensity and adverse events (AEs) caused by lasmiditan at 1, 2, and 4 h after the intake of an additional 50 mg of lasmiditan. A significant reduction in pain scale was observed post 50 mg lasmiditan intake ($p < 0.001$, t-test). Pain relief was reported for 32 migraine attacks (80%) at 1 h after additional lasmiditan intake. Although AEs were observed in 63% of the patients who took an additional lasmiditan, most were mild and resolved 1 h after lasmiditan intake. Our study revealed the significant headache relief provided by an additional lasmiditan for patients who did not achieve satisfactory results following initial triptan intake for treating migraine. The AEs associated with this treatment strategy were mild and lasted for a short time. This study suggested that the combination of triptan and lasmiditan is promising for the treatment of migraine and should be studied in a randomized placebo-controlled trial.

Keywords: migraine; triptan; lasmiditan; step care

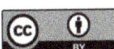

1. Introduction

The Global Burden of Disease considers migraines one of the most prevalent and disabling burdens worldwide, especially among the working population. Because of their recurrent nature, long duration, and adverse effect on the quality of life, migraines were internationally ranked second with regard to the years lived with disabilities by the Global Burden of Disease study in 2016 [1].

The neurophysiology of headaches indicates that the neuro-fibers, namely C-fibers and A-delta (Aδ) fibers, play a significant role in the perception of headaches. Specifically, it is postulated that stimulation of C-fibers causes slow building aching, throbbing, or burning headaches, whereas stimulation of the Aδ fiber causes sharp and painful headaches [2]. The sensory neurons, C-fibers and Aδ fibers, are found in the trigeminal ganglion and nerve terminals [2]. Calcitonin gene-related peptides (CGRPs) have recently been discovered to stimulate the trigeminal fibers [2,3]. Unmyelinated C-fiber sensory nerves are characterized by high CGRP expression, while myelinated Aδ-sensory nerves that are found in the peripheral nervous system have a high concentration of CGRP receptors. During the onset of a migraine, CGRP is released from the C-fiber of the trigeminal nerve ganglion and the trigeminal nerve terminal. This release subsequently stimulates the Aδ fiber, leading to the individual experiencing sharp, painful migraine headaches [3,4].

Triptans are 5-HT$_{1B}$ and 5-HT$_{1D}$ receptor agonists, and 5-HT$_{1D}$ receptors are found at the Aδ-neurofiber terminal and commonly prescribed as migraine-specific abortive medications [5]. Nonsteroidal anti-inflammatory drugs (NSAIDs) and nonspecific analgesia are only effective for treating mild headaches and migraine attacks. It is not uncommon for a migraine attack to remain unabated with a single tablet of triptan, which leads to the cycling of triptans or NSAIDs, which not only leads to a failure in controlling headaches associated with migraine attacks, but continuous intake of both triptans as well as NSAIDs can also result in medication overuse headache (MOH). NSAIDs are easily available to patients as over-the-counter medications and do not require a prescription, whereas triptans require a prescription. Therefore, NSAIDs are more commonly associated with MOH [5]. This conundrum has inspired medical researchers to search for a new specific medication that will be more selective in migraine treatment and will reduce the risk of MOHs for patients already suffering from an acute migraine attack.

Lasmiditan, a 5-HT$_{1F}$ receptor agonist, is a recently developed drug for treating acute migraines [6]. The 5-HT$_{1F}$ receptor is present at C-fiber as well as Aδ-fiber terminals. Positive stimulation of the 5-HT$_{1F}$ receptor on the C-fiber terminal by the drug inhibits CGRP release from the C-fiber terminal. In addition, the drug's positive stimulation of the 5-HT$_{1F}$ receptor on the Aδ-fiber terminal inhibits pain signal transmission from the Aδ-fibers.

Both triptan and lasmiditan have exhibited high efficacies for the treatment of migraine attacks with varying intensity; however, triptans are contraindicated for some patients, such as those diagnosed with cardiovascular diseases, cerebrovascular diseases, hemiplegic migraines, and migraines with brainstem aura. Lasmiditan is a good medical alternative for these patients. In addition, the time of administration of triptans plays a crucial role in their efficacy. Treatment with triptans needs to be initiated as early as possible after the onset of a migraine attack, as a late intake of triptans has been observed to be ineffective [7]. In contrast, the efficacy of lasmiditan is independent of the time of migraine onset [8]. In addition, lasmiditan has been shown to be effective in treating acute migraine attacks in patients whose symptoms could not be abated by triptans [9].

Currently, lasmiditan is commercially available at two doses (50 and 100 mg), and its efficacy and associated adverse events (AEs) have been observed to be dose-dependent [10]. Although Japanese pharmaceuticals recommend the standard and starting dose of lasmiditan to be 100 mg [11], this dosage has been associated with frequent AEs. The severity of AEs (dizziness and drowsiness) has resulted in discontinuation of treatment and hesitation among patients to continue with the treatment. In the United States, the recommended dose of lasmiditan is 50, 100, or 200 mg [12].

Lasmiditan and triptan have different mechanisms of action, because of which the combination of these two different classes of drugs could be compensatory or synergistic. The combined use of lasmiditan and triptan has not yet been reported in the medical literature.

The aim of this study was to investigate whether the acute treatment protocol involving sequential intake of lasmiditan after prior intake of triptan would result in better resolution of migraine pain. Patients whose acute migraine attacks were previously treated unsuccessfully with a single tablet of triptan were included in this study. Our secondary goal was to investigate the AEs associated with the administration of an additional 50 mg of lasmiditan for patients with persistent migraines even after taking triptans (Lasmiditan Addition for the Patients after Poor Results of Triptan: LAPPORT). In this study, we selected 50 mg as the additional lasmiditan dose because the AEs of lasmiditan are dose-dependent. Our hypothesis is that an additional 50 mg of lasmiditan is effective and safe for the patients for whom one tablet of triptan is not effective enough.

2. Patients and Methods

2.1. Patients

The patients participating in this study had been previously diagnosed with migraines by board-certified headache specialists. The participating patients had no previous exposure to lasmiditan before their participation in this study. Only patients who had taken a single tablet of triptan (zolmitriptan, rizatriptan, or eletriptan) and self-reported unsatisfactory results were included in this study. All patients were Japanese and had no vascular disease, severe depression, or chronic pain conditions such as fibromyalgia.

2.2. Methods

The outcomes of this study were headache intensity evaluated using the numerical rating scale (NRS) and any AEs at 1, 2, and 4 h after taking an additional 50 mg of lasmiditan.

The following intake instructions were given to participants:

(1) At the onset of a migraine attack, ingest a single tablet of triptan within 30 min after the initiation of the migraine attack. (2) At 1 h following the intake of triptan, if headache relief is less than 50%, proceed to take lasmiditan 50 mg. (3) Patients were required to record headache intensity and any AEs on paper caused by lasmiditan at 1, 2, and 4 h after taking an additional 50 mg of lasmiditan. Pain relief was defined as an improvement in NRS by more than 2 points, and a pain-free condition was defined as an NRS value of less than 2. We instructed the participants not to consume more than one tablet of triptan and lasmiditan each on the same day.

Three facilities, including two community hospitals and one private clinic, participated in this study, and study approval was granted by the institutional review boards at each participating facility. Ethical approval number from the ethical committee in Mito Kyodo General Hospital is No. 22-53.

This study was conducted at out-patient clinics in these three facilities.

This study had been registered in the public database of the University Hospital Medical Information Network (UMIN) as a clinical trial prior to the initiation of the study (UMIN ID UMIN000050092).

2.3. Statistical Analysis

Statistical analysis for paired groups was conducted using a two-tailed *t*-test program on SPSS version 28.00 (IBM, Tokyo, Japan). A *p* value of <0.05 was considered statistically significant.

3. Results

Twenty-four patients participated in the study (Figure 1). Two patients were excluded because they did not take the lasmiditan tablet as per the protocol. One patient did not return for follow-up. Among the 21 patients who took additional lasmiditan and completed the reports, 1 patient violated the protocol and did not take additional lasmiditan at the designated time periods.

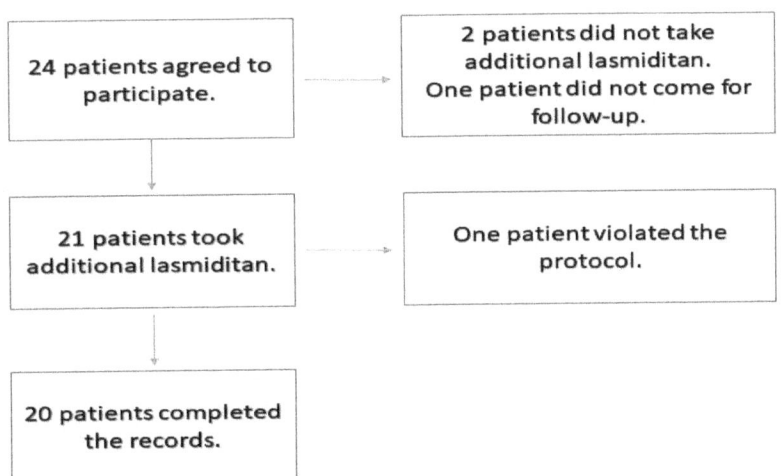

Figure 1. Flowchart indicating patient selection.

The final number of participants remaining in the study, whose results were recorded, was 20. There were 4 males and 16 females in this group. The ages of the participants ranged from 14 years to 62 years, with the mean age being 43.1 years. A total of 40 migraine attacks were treated and recorded in the study. Eleven patients used this treatment protocol only once. Four patients used it twice, two patients used it three times, and three patients used it five times.

Among the 40 migraine attacks that were treated and recorded in the study, the records for the 2 h post-lasmiditan intake were partially missing for 12 migraine attacks in four patients since they fell asleep. For these patients, records obtained until one hour after lasmiditan intake were included in the analysis.

Figure 2 depicts the results for NRS for all 40 migraine attacks. A significant reduction in NRS was observed following the intake of lasmiditan 50 mg ($p < 0.001$, t-test). Pain relief, defined as an improvement in NRS by more than 2 points, was reported for 32 migraine attacks (80%) at one hour and for 24 migraine attacks (86%) at two hours after additional lasmiditan intake (Figure 3).

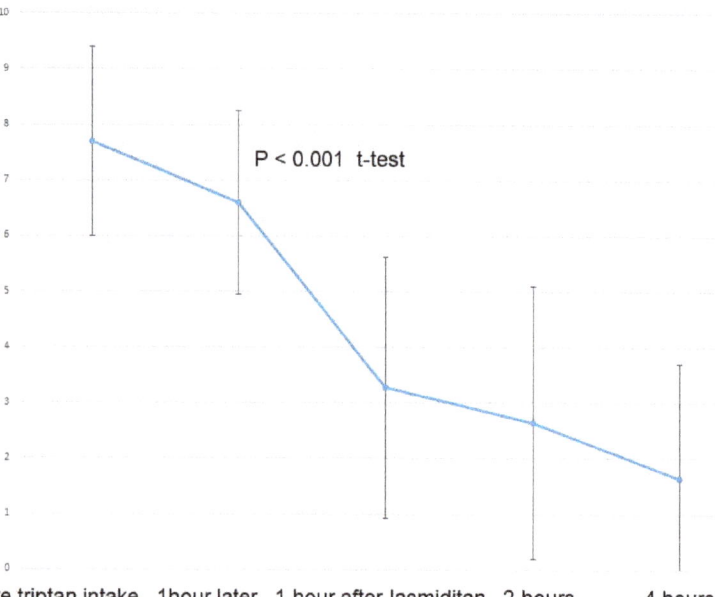

Figure 2. Results of the NRS for all 40 migraine attacks (NRS: numerical rating scale).

Relief from pain status (pain-free), defined as an NRS value of less than 2, was reported for 17 migraine attacks (43%) at one hour and for 16 migraine attacks (57%) at two hours following additional lasmiditan intakes (Figure 3).

The AEs, which were mostly dizziness and drowsiness, were observed in 25 migraine attacks (63%) at one hour after additional lasmiditan intake (Figure 3). However, a reduction in these AEs was observed in six migraine attacks (21%), two hours following additional lasmiditan intake. No same-day migraine headache recurrence was observed in our study population.

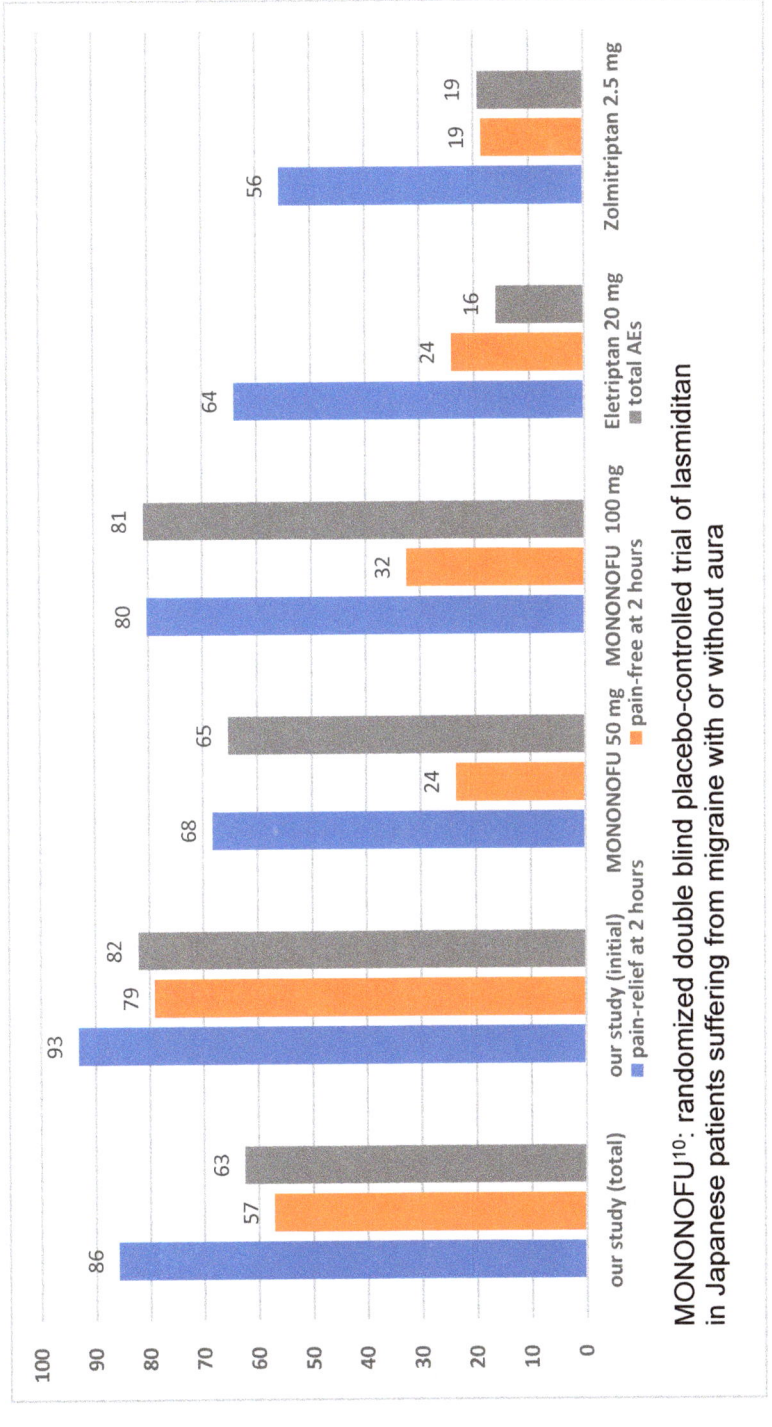

Figure 3. Results of pain-relief, pain-free, and total AE rates (%) (AEs: adverse events).

The results of 17 migraine attacks that were initially treated with this protocol were also analyzed, and a significant reduction in NRS was observed ($p < 0.001$, t-test) after the intake of 50 mg lasmiditan (Figure 4). Pain relief, defined as a reduction in NRS by 2 points, was achieved in 16 migraine attacks (94%) at one hour and in 13 migraine attacks (93%) at two hours following additional lasmiditan intakes (Figure 3). Pain-free status, defined as an NRS less than 2, was observed in nine migraine attacks (53%) at one hour and 11 migraine attacks (79%) at two hours after additional lasmiditan intakes. The AEs, mostly dizziness and drowsiness, were observed in 14 migraine attacks (82%) at one hour after additional lasmiditan intake. However, a reduction in these AEs was observed for 5 of the 14 migraine attacks (36%) at two hours after the additional lasmiditan intake.

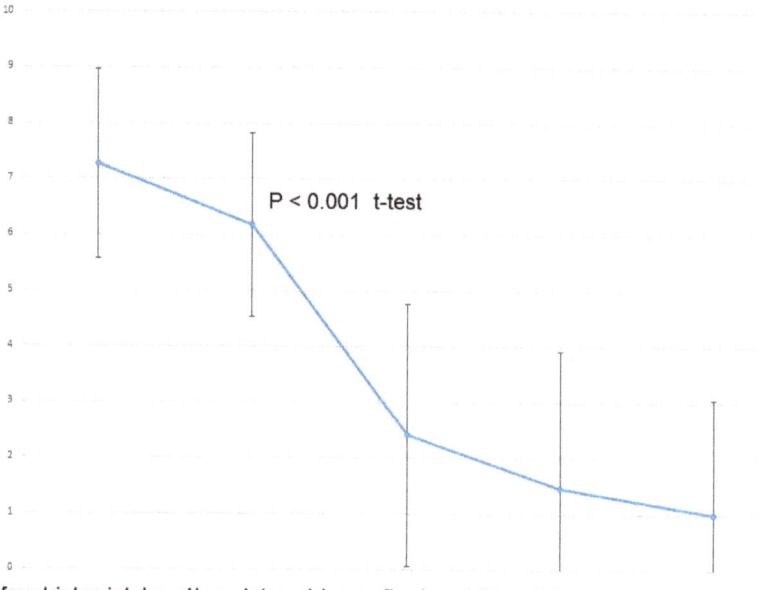

Figure 4. NRS results for 18 migraine attacks initially treated with lasmiditan.

4. Discussion

The results of this study indicate that participants who continued to experience migraine even after taking a triptan benefited from the intake of lasmiditan 50 mg, leading to a significant improvement in headache severity. Although AEs were observed in 63% of the patients who took an additional 50 mg of lasmiditan, most were mild and resolved 1 h after lasmiditan intake.

In a phase 2 randomized placebo-controlled study, MONONOFU, the acute treatment of migraine in Japanese patients with Lasmiditan, was investigated [8]. Pain-relief rates observed 2 h post-dose were 55.0% for the placebo, 68.2% for lasmiditan 50 mg, 80.2% for lasmiditan 100 mg, and 78.2% for lasmiditan 200 mg. Pain-free rates observed 2 h post-dose were 16.6% for placebo, 23.5% for lasmiditan 50 mg, 32.4% for lasmiditan 100 mg, and 40.8% for lasmiditan 200 mg (Figure 3). Pain-free rates observed after administration of lasmiditan 50 mg were not significantly different from those of placebo. However, as the sample size for this study was small, calculations to ensure a certain statistical power in comparison with placebo could not be achieved. Pain-free and pain-relief rates showed significant improvement compared with those obtained with a placebo. In our study, 80% of patients achieved pain relief, defined as an improvement in the NRS of more than 2 points, at 1 h and 86% at 2 h after additional lasmiditan intake. Pain-free status, defined as a NRS of less than 2, was achieved by 43% of patients at 1 h and 57% at 2 h after additional lasmiditan intake. In the MONONOFU study, migraine severity was recorded using a 4-point headache severity rating scale, whereas the NRS was used to rate headache pain in our study. This complicates the comparison of the results obtained in this study with those obtained in the MONONOFU study [8]. Conversely, our study suggests better headache elimination with an additional 50 mg of lasmiditan.

A prospective study for Japanese migraine patients showed a headache response rate of 64% at 2 h post-dose for eletriptan 20 mg. The pain-free rate at 2 h post-dose for eletriptan 20 mg was 24%, and total AEs rates were 16.3% [13]. Another prospective study for Japanese migraine patients showed a headache response rate of 55.6% at 2 h post-dose for zolmitriptan 2.5 mg; the pain-free rate at 2 h post-dose for zolmitriptan 2.5 mg was 18.5%, and total AEs rates were 19.2% [14]. Our results showed better pain relief and were pain-free compared with these triptan studies (Figure 3), even though our study population had poor initial triptan intake results.

In global phase 3 studies (SAMURAI and SPARTAN), 14%–15% of participants experienced headache recurrence after lasmiditan intake [10,15]. In the MONONOFU study, sustained pain-free rates at 24 and 48 h were 14.9% for lasmiditan 50 mg and around 20% for lasmiditan 100 mg [8]. A significant proportion of the patients reported migraine headache recurrence on the same day. No migraine headache recurrence on the same day was observed in our study population. So our results suggest that better control of migraine headaches may be obtained using our treatment protocol.

AEs were also found to be dose-dependent in the MONONOFU study. The most common AEs were dizziness, fatigue, paresthesia, and sedation [12]. Patients should be advised not to drive or operate machinery until at least 8 h after taking lasmiditan. Our study found similar rates of AEs with the MONOFOFU study at lasmiditan doses of 50 mg. A higher treatment-emergent rate of AEs was reported in the MONONOFU study compared to other global phase 3 studies [8,15,16]. The cause of this difference can most likely be attributed to the differences in data collection methods, informed consent methods, and the body mass indices of Japanese participants in comparison with non-Asian population participants [8,15]. The mean body mass index of the participants in the MONONOFU study was 22.6 kg/m^2, and the mean body mass indices of the global phase 3 studies were from 30 to 31 kg/m^2.

Our study analyzed the results for headache relief observed in migraine attacks treated with a secondary treatment of 50 mg lasmiditan after unsatisfactory results observed with triptan. The number of migraine attacks reported in this study varied for each patient. The patients with favorable effects of additional lasmiditan might have recorded more migraine attacks in this study. In addition, repeat intake of lasmiditan is effective in reducing the AEs caused by lasmiditan [9]. To prevent these factors from introducing a bias in our study results, we conducted a separate analysis that included patients who took additional lasmiditan for the first time using this treatment protocol for migraine headaches. Our analyses revealed higher rates of headache relief, pain-free patients and a higher incidence of AEs for the patients who took additional lasmiditan for the first time in this study. These results indicate a reduced incidence of AEs with repeat intake of Lasmiditan, as anticipated. An important finding from this study is that the clinical effects of lasmiditan were observed from the first intake of lasmiditan, confirming its efficacy as an anti-migraine medication.

Based on the results obtained, we would recommend a step-care treatment consisting of an initial triptan, followed by lasmiditan if needed, for treating the symptoms of migraines. The Disability in Strategies of Care study investigated stratified care (a strategy of rigid, predetermined medications to give an ailing patient with no rescue measures) versus step-care strategies for treating acute migraine attacks [17]. In this randomized, controlled, parallel-group clinical trial, three strategies were compared. In accordance with this stratified care program, grade II patients based on the Migraine Disability Assessment Scale (MIDAS) would be treated with aspirin plus metoclopramide, and patients with MIDAS grades III and IV would be treated with zolmitriptan. MIDAS is a self-assessment questionnaire aimed at measuring the impact of headaches. MIDAS grades II, III, and IV define mild, moderate, and severe disabilities. In the step-care plan, across attacks, initial treatment was aspirin plus metoclopramide. Patients who did not achieve satisfactory results in at least two of the first three attacks are switched to zolmitriptan. In step care within attacks, initial treatment was aspirin and metoclopramide. Patients not responding to this treatment after two hours at the beginning of each attack were shifted to zolmitriptan. As the results indicated, stratified care provided significantly better clinical outcomes compared with step-care strategies within or across attacks, as indicated by headache response and disability time. In these step-care strategies, aspirin plus metoclopramide were used as initial treatment agents. In the step-care strategy within attacks, triptan was not administered within 2 h of each attack. However, our study used triptan as an initial medication. For step-care within attacks, lasmiditan was taken within 1.5 h after the initiation of a migraine attack. We believe that migraine-specific medication should be administered as early as possible. Our study results indicated recommending a step-care treatment consisting of an initial triptan followed by lasmiditan if needed for the acute treatment of migraine. The treatment strategy for a migraine should be tailor-made for each migraine attack, not each migraine patient, because every migraine patient has various migraine attacks.

Although easy access and the cost of aspirin and NSAIDs are the major factors based on which it is recommended as the first medication treatment for migraines, it is associated with several AEs, making it inferior as an abortive treatment. We believe that migraine-specific drugs should be used to treat migraine attacks instead of abortive treatments. Rothrock recommended different therapies for acute migraine treatment since the symptoms of a migraine attack might vary across attacks [18]. He proposed additional rescue therapy despite initial treatment as "stratified" care. We believe that this additional therapeutic strategy is referred to as step care. From the point of view of shared decision making and patient education about self-medication, this treatment strategy is beneficial, and rapport will be obtained.

As an acute medication for migraine attacks, triptans are commercially available in most developed countries. The benefits of triptans are their long history and experiences in clinical applications, the availability of several brands, and the availability of drugs in various forms, including hard tablets, orally disintegrating tablets, subcutaneous injections, and nasal sprays. Gepants, such as rimegapant, are new oral CGRP antagonists used for acute treatment as well as the prevention of migraine attacks. While gepants are commercially available in some countries, all gepants are currently under clinical trials in Japan. A prior meta-analysis has indicated favorable outcomes in terms of pain freedom and pain relief 2 h after the intake of gepants [19].

Our study had some limitations. This was a single-arm study and did not involve comparison with a placebo or other medications. Furthermore, triptans may not be effective within 1 h after consumption. The effect of additional lasmiditan in our study may partially reflect the late effect of triptans. However, in our study, only patients who had experienced frequent unsatisfactory effects of triptans were included. Whether the results of this study can be generalized to all patients remains unclear. In the future, we plan to conduct a study that compares the efficacy of patients receiving lasmiditan as a second-line drug in comparison to patients receiving a placebo. Since our study was a single-armed study, the cost benefits of our treatment strategy were not evaluated. This aspect will also be analyzed in future studies. Since the study population was small, various sub-analyses, including migraine types, disease durations, concomitant prophylactic medications, triptan brand, and MIDAS class, were not possible. However, most patients in our study needed frequent intake of triptans, and standard dosing recommendations for triptans were not enough. Having large-scale data can provide the answers to these questions. Our study population was limited to migraine patients who had some experience with triptans. Most of these patients had not experienced any severe AEs from triptans. Our study result may not be applicable for the patients who did not have a history of triptan intake. Some patients could not record their headache information and AEs after two hours of additional lasmiditan intake. Long-term effects and AEs beyond two hours following additional lasmiditan intake need to be clarified in future studies. Our study used NRS for self-evaluating headaches. Some clinical trials used a 4-point pain scale [8–10,20]. Therefore, comparing our study with these studies may be difficult. However, we believe that an 11-point NRS is more sensitive than a 4-point scale. Gepants are not commercially available in Japan; hence, the clinical effects of gepants could not be evaluated. In future studies, combination or sequential studies of these acute medications or migraine-specific drugs should be studied.

5. Conclusions

Our study indicated the significant headache relief provided by an additional 50 mg dose of lasmiditan for patients who did not achieve satisfactory results following initial triptan intake for treating migraine attacks. The AEs associated with this treatment strategy were mild and short-term. Our open-label study suggested that the combination of triptan and lasmiditan is promising and should be studied in a randomized, placebo-controlled trial. We should apply step care rather than stratified care for treating each migraine attack, not for each patient. From the point of view of shared decision making and patient education regarding self-medication, this treatment strategy is beneficial, and rapport will be obtained.

Author Contributions: Conceptualization, Y.S.; methodology, Y.S.; formal analysis, Y.S.; investigation, Y.S.; data curation, Y.S., H.S., A.S. and Y.H.; writing—original draft preparation, Y.S.; writing—review and editing, Y.S. All authors have read and agreed to the published version of the manuscript.

Funding: This research received no external funding.

Institutional Review Board Statement: The study was conducted in accordance with the Declaration of Helsinki, and approved by the Ethics Committee of Mito Kyodo General Hospital (protocol code no. 22-53).

Informed Consent Statement: Informed consent was obtained from all subjects involved in the study.

Data Availability Statement: The raw data supporting the conclusions of this article will be made available by the authors on request.

Conflicts of Interest: The authors declare no conflicts of interest.

References

1. Vos, T.; Abajobir, A.A.; Abate, K.H.; Abbafati, C.; Abbas, K.M.; Abd-Allah, F.; Abdulkader, R.S.; Abdulle, A.M.; Abebo, T.A.; Abera, S.F.; et al. Global, regional, and national incidence, prevalence, and years lived with disability for 328 diseases and injuries for 195 countries, 1990–2016: A systematic analysis for the Global Burden of Disease Study 2016. *Lancet* **2017**, *390*, 1211–1259. [CrossRef] [PubMed]
2. Eftekhari, S.; Warfvinge, K.; Blixt, F.W.; Edvinsson, L. Differentiation of Nerve Fibers Storing CGRP and CGRP Receptors in the Peripheral Trigeminovascular System. *J. Pain* **2013**, *14*, 1289–1303. [CrossRef] [PubMed]
3. Lassen, L.H.; Haderslev, P.A.; Jacobsen, V.B.; Iversen, H.K.; Sperling, B.; Olesen, J. Cgrp May Play A Causative Role in Migraine. *Cephalalgia* **2002**, *22*, 54–61. [CrossRef] [PubMed]
4. Shibata, Y. Migraine Pathophysiology Revisited: Proposal of a New Molecular Theory of Migraine Pathophysiology and Headache Diagnostic Criteria. *Int. J. Mol. Sci.* **2022**, *23*, 13002. [CrossRef] [PubMed]
5. Thorlund, K.; Sun-Edelstein, C.; Druyts, E.; Kanters, S.; Ebrahim, S.; Bhambri, R.; Ramos, E.; Mills, E.J.; Lanteri-Minet, M.; Tepper, S. Risk of medication overuse headache across classes of treatments for acute migraine. *J. Headache Pain* **2016**, *17*, 107. [CrossRef] [PubMed]
6. Clemow, D.B.; Johnson, K.W.; Hochstetler, H.M.; Ossipov, M.H.; Hake, A.M.; Blumenfeld, A.M. Lasmiditan mechanism of action—Review of a selective 5-HT1F agonist. *J. Headache Pain* **2020**, *21*, 71. [CrossRef] [PubMed]
7. Kelley, N.E.; Tepper, D.E. Rescue Therapy for Acute Migraine, Part 1: Triptans, Dihydroergotamine, and Magnesium. *Headache J. Head Face Pain* **2012**, *52*, 114–128. [CrossRef] [PubMed]
8. Sakai, F.; Takeshima, T.; Homma, G.; Tanji, Y.; Katagiri, H.; Komori, M. Phase 2 randomized placebo-controlled study of lasmiditan for the acute treatment of migraine in Japanese patients. *Headache J. Head Face Pain* **2021**, *61*, 755–765. [CrossRef]
9. Ashina, M.; Reuter, U.; Smith, T.; Krikke-Workel, J.; Klise, S.R.; Bragg, S.; Doty, E.G.; Dowsett, S.A.; Lin, Q.; Krege, J.H. Randomized, controlled trial of lasmiditan over four migraine attacks: Findings from the CENTURION study. *Cephalalgia* **2021**, *41*, 294–304. [CrossRef]

10. Goadsby, P.J.; Wietecha, L.; Dennehy, E.B.; Kuca, B.; Case, M.G.; Aurora, S.K.; Gaul, C. Phase 3 randomized, placebo-controlled, double-blind study of lasmiditan for acute treatment of migraine. *Brain* **2019**, *142*, 1894–1904. [CrossRef] [PubMed]
11. PMDA. *Reyvow Drug Information*; Pharmacenuticals and Medical Devices Agency: Tokyo, Japan, 2022. (In Japanese)
12. FDA US. *Highlights of Prescribing Information*; U.S. Food & Drug Administration: White Oak, MD, USA, 2022.
13. Fukuuchi, Y. Efficacy and Safety of Eletriptan 20 Mg, 40 Mg and 80 Mg in Japanese Migraineurs. *Cephalalgia* **2002**, *22*, 416–423. [CrossRef] [PubMed]
14. Sakai, F.; Iwata, M.; Tashiro, K.; Itoyama, Y.; Tsuji, S.; Fukuuchi, Y.; Sobue, G.; Nakashima, K.; Morimatsu, M. Zolmitriptan is Effective and Well Tolerated in Japanese Patients with Migraine: A Dose-Response Study. *Cephalalgia* **2002**, *22*, 376–383. [CrossRef] [PubMed]
15. Kuca, B.; Silberstein, S.D.; Wietecha, L.; Berg, P.H.; Dozier, G.; Lipton, R.B. Lasmiditan is an effective acute treatment for migraine. *Neurology* **2018**, *91*, e2222–e2232. [CrossRef]
16. Vila-Pueyo, M. Targeted 5-HT1F Therapies for Migraine. *Neurotherapeutics* **2018**, *15*, 291–303. [CrossRef]
17. Lipton, R.B.; Stewart, W.F.; Stone, A.M.; Láinez, M.J.A.; Sawyer, J.P.C. Stratified Care vs Step Care Strategies for MigraineThe Disability in Strategies of Care (DISC) Study:A Randomized Trial. *JAMA* **2000**, *284*, 2599–2605. [CrossRef]
18. Rothrock, J.F. Acute Migraine Treatment: "Stratified" Care. *Headache J. Head Face Pain* **2012**, *52*, 193. [CrossRef] [PubMed]
19. Yang, C.P.; Liang, C.S.; Chang, C.M.; Yang, C.C.; Shih, P.H.; Yau, Y.C.; Tang, K.T.; Wang, S.J. Comparison of New Pharmacologic Agents With Triptans for Treatment of Migraine: A Systematic Review and Meta-analysis. *JAMA Netw. Open* **2021**, *4*, e2128544. [CrossRef] [PubMed]
20. Knievel, K.; Buchanan, A.S.; Lombard, L.; Baygani, S.; Raskin, J.; Krege, J.H.; Loo, L.S.; Komori, M.; Tobin, J. Lasmiditan for the acute treatment of migraine: Subgroup analyses by prior response to triptans. *Cephalalgia* **2019**, *40*, 19–27. [CrossRef] [PubMed]

Disclaimer/Publisher's Note: The statements, opinions and data contained in all publications are solely those of the individual author(s) and contributor(s) and not of MDPI and/or the editor(s). MDPI and/or the editor(s) disclaim responsibility for any injury to people or property resulting from any ideas, methods, instructions or products referred to in the content.

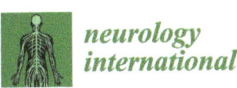

Article

Effectiveness of Switching CGRP Monoclonal Antibodies in Non-Responder Patients in the UAE: A Retrospective Study

Reem Suliman *, Vanessa Santos, Ibrahim Al Qaisi, Batool Aldaher, Ahmed Al Fardan, Hajir Al Barrawy, Yazan Bader, Jonna Lyn Supena, Kathrina Alejandro and Taoufik Alsaadi *

American Center for Psychiatry and Neurology, Abu Dhabi P.O. Box 108699, United Arab Emirates; batool.c.2014@gmail.com (B.A.)
* Correspondence: rk.suliman16@gmail.com (R.S.); talsaadi@live.ca (T.A.)

Abstract: Calcitonin gene-related peptide monoclonal antibodies (CGRP mAbs) have shown promising effectiveness in migraine management compared to other preventative treatment options. Many questions remain regarding switching between antibody classes as a treatment option in patients with migraine headaches. This preliminary retrospective real-world study explored the treatment response of patients who switched between CGRP mAb classes due to lack of efficacy or poor tolerability. A total of 53 patients with migraine headache switched between three of the CGRP mAbs types due to lack of efficacy of the original prescribed CGRP mAbs, specifically eptinezumab, erenumab, and galcanezumab. Fremanezumab was not included due to unavailability in the UAE. Galcanezumab and eptinezumab target the CGRP ligand (CGRP/L), while erenumab targets CGRP receptors (CGRP/R). The analysis of efficacy demonstrated that some improvements were seen in both class switch cohorts (CGRP/R to CGRP/L and CGRP/L to CGRP/R). The safety of switching between CGRP classes was well observed, as any adverse events presented before the class switch did not lead to the discontinuation of treatment following the later switch. The findings of this study suggest that switching between different classes of CGRP mAbs is a potentially safe and clinically viable practice that may have some applications for those experiencing side effects on their current CGRP mAb or those witnessing suboptimal response.

Keywords: CGRP monoclonal antibodies; effectiveness; migraine; treatment; switching

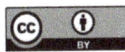

1. Introduction

Migraine is a neurological disorder experienced by an estimated global point prevalence range of 14,107 cases per 100,000 [1]. According to the 2019 Global Burden of Disease Study, migraine is the second most common non-fatal disease in terms of "years lived with disability" [2]. Those suffering from migraine experience a significant impact on their ability to maintain their productivity and relationships, mandating continuous efforts to better understand its pathophysiology and optimal treatment options [3]. Although the precise mechanism of migraine remains unknown, recent findings suggest the calcitonin gene-related peptide (CGRP) plays an integral role [4]. Responsible for nociception within the trigeminal ganglion, CGRP represents a major point of interest in the development of migraine prophylactic medication. Thus, numerous studies have emerged within the past decade investigating the effectiveness of monoclonal antibodies (mAbs) as CGRP receptor antagonists in migraine treatment [5].

Older treatment options for migraine prevention have not been very successful in alleviating the personal and economic burden of migraine [6]. A major reason for the lack of success is their limited tolerability and patient adherence [7]. Antiepileptics, beta-blockers, and antidepressants are examples of these medications. Furthermore, these medications have not been very effective in treating migraine headaches and reducing migraine burden [7].

On the other hand, mAbs result in better treatment outcomes and, due to their long half-lives, they can be dosed at long intervals, which can be a preferable option for some patients [8]. Less frequent dosing can minimize the burden on the patient and assures better treatment adherence. Presently, a small collection of monoclonal antibody medications has been approved for the preventative treatment of episodic and chronic migraine by the U.S. Food and Drug Administration (FDA). Such monoclonal antibodies include galcanezumab, eptinezumab, and fremanezumab, which target the CGRP ligand, and erenumab, which targets CGRP receptors, as shown in Table 1 [4].

Table 1. CGRP targeting drugs.

Drug	Mechanism	Indication	Dosing	FDA Approved	Availability in the UAE
Erenumab	Blocks CGRP receptor	Prophylactic	Monthly, subcutaneous	2018	Yes
Eptinezumab	Binds to CGRP ligand	Prophylactic	Quarterly, intravenous	2020	Yes
Galcanezumab	Binds to CGRP ligand	Prophylactic	Monthly, subcutaneous	2018	Yes
Fremanezumab	Binds to CGRP ligand	Prophylactic	Monthly or quarterly, subcutaneous, but intravenous load for cluster headache	2018	No

Recent studies examining the usage of erenumab suggest that it can effectively reduce migraine frequency and improve quality of life [9]. In a similar study assessing the efficacy and tolerability of erenumab among 418 patients, 168 (69.7%) reported that the benefits of erenumab outweighed any potential drawbacks [10]. Episodic migraine patients with at least one previous preventative treatment failure (PPTF) exhibited significantly greater gains in efficacy compared to placebo [11]. Among the aforementioned mAbs, Eptinemzumab stands out as the sole drug capable of intravenous administration, allowing for a rapid onset of action [12]. This unique quality allows for quicker headache pain relief [13] and reduced monthly migraine days compared to placebo [14]. The existing literature on CGRP monoclonal antibodies (CGRP mAbs) suggests high patient tolerability; discontinuation is most commonly attributed to lack of efficacy rather than adverse effects [15]. Despite a lack of major differences in efficacy across clinical trials, a few case studies found that some patients with suboptimal response to one mAb had managed to successfully switch to another one with noted significant improvements [16–19]. One real-world analysis study demonstrated that one-third of erenumab non-responders achieved >30% response after switching to another CGRP mAb [20]. In the aforementioned analysis, the focus was on switching from erenumab to either galcanezumab or fremanezumab. This was based on the fact that erenumab was approved first in Europe.

These findings warrant further investigation into the efficacy and safety of switching between CGRP mAb classes. Therefore, this study investigated the treatment effectiveness, tolerability, and adherence of migraine patients in the United Arab Emirates (UAE) following a switch from a PPTF to another mAb. The primary objective was to retrospectively assess the reduction in the frequency of monthly migraines headache days and determine the efficacy of the second preventative therapy following the switch from a previously failed CGRP mAb. Additionally, the study sought to evaluate the tolerability of this therapy and report any potential adverse reactions. This study will serve as an integral step toward advancing our understanding of migraine treatment. It shall also represent the first study of its kind by focusing on an underrepresented population in clinical research.

2. Patients and Methods

This was a retrospective, real-world exploratory study. Data used were gathered from one site, namely the American Center for Psychiatry and Neurology (ACPN), Abu Dhabi, UAE. A total of 391 patients with episodic migraine (EM) or chronic migraine (CM) who had received at least one dose of GCGRP/R mAb (erenumab) or CGRP/L mAb (eptinezumab or galcanezumab) were reviewed for eligibility to be included in the study. Fremanezumab is currently not available in the UAE and was therefore not included in the analysis.

Data were gathered from patients' clinical records, which contain all the required demographic information as well as information relating to diagnosis, medication history, Monthly Migraine Day (MMD) at baseline, visual pain scores, and follow-up visits. Additionally, patient satisfaction with medication was documented in their clinical records. Patients were asked to keep a record of attacks and symptoms in their headache diaries. Efficacy of the prescribed treatment was evaluated by measuring the change in MMDs between visits. Safety was also assessed; this was achieved by monitoring adverse events.

Follow-up visits were scheduled monthly or as deemed necessary, which is a standard protocol at our site for all patients initiating treatment with mAbs. Patients were assessed on their baseline frequency of MMDs and subsequent thorough discussions with treating physician on which mAb would be most effective, addressing each patient's specific needs. If the current medication did not result in any meaningful reduction in MMDs, an option to switch to another mAb was offered to the patient. The intensity of the headache was also recorded using a visual scale pain, a measurement which was conducted by the treating physician.

The retrospective analysis mainly focused on two main periods. The first period included data from patients treated with a specific CGRP mAb, while the second period involved data from patients who switched to another anti-CGRP mAb. Switching was mainly due to lack of efficacy; it was ensured that patients included in the analysis completed at least 3 months of treatment before switching. Evaluating efficacy after a minimum of 3 consecutive months of treatment was adopted based on the EHF and our local guidelines [21,22]. During each phase, patients' MMDs were assessed at 3 stages prior to and following their medication switch: at least one month before the first injection (baseline), at a 3-month follow-up, and at a 6-month follow-up.

This study was conducted in accordance with the Helsinki Declaration of 1964 and is consistent with Good Clinical Practice (GCP) guidelines. All ethical guidelines, health authority regulations, and data privacy laws were adhered to. Prior to the start of the study, all relevant approvals were obtained from the ACPN's Institutional Review Board (IRB), and a waiver of informed consent from the corresponding ethics committee was obtained. To ensure transparency and accuracy, all authors were provided access to the study data.

Records from the ACPN's nursing department were gathered, and all patients who had been administered one mAb were screened and identified (Figure 1). Data included patients from January 2018 up to September 2022 who were adults (≥18 years) and who had a diagnosis of either EM or CM, as per the International Classification of Headache Disorders (ICHD-3) criteria [23]. Data were shared independent of treatment effects or cause for the CGRP mAb switch.

Patients were included in the analysis if they (i) switched between two of the previously mentioned CGRP mAbs (switchers), (ii) received at least three doses of the first CGRP mAb, and maintained treatment for a minimum of 6 months after switching. Those who demonstrated a meaningful response (which is defined as more than a 50% reduction in MMDs for EM and more than 30% for CM) and were satisfied concerning their treatment remained on their current preventative treatment and were thus not included in the effectiveness analysis. Patients were categorized according to their switching profiles. The three profiles represented were as follows: CGRP/R mAb to GCRP/L mAb, CGRP/L to CGRP/R, or CGRP/L to another CGRP/L mAb (Figure 1).

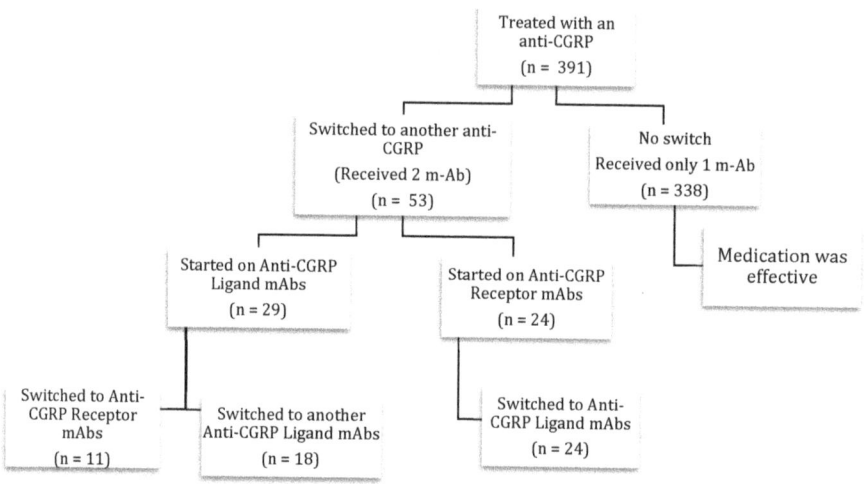

Figure 1. Flowchart of patients.

The number of MMDs was extracted from the headache diaries, as documented on the patients' electronic medical records (EMRs). Due to the non-standardized headache diaries and the varying details of documentation of headache characteristics and accompanying symptoms during each headache attack, reliable differentiation between headache and migraine days was not possible. The primary endpoint was the absolute change from baseline in MMD response rate (>25%, >50%, >75%, and 100% reduction in MMDs) for each category of the switchers. As per the methodology outlined by Kaltseis et al. in 2023, patients who demonstrated a positive response to treatment were classified as responders [24]. This was determined by a minimum reduction of 50% in MMDs for EM or a minimum reduction of 30% in MMDs for CM after receiving treatment for a minimum of 3 months. Patient characteristics included age, gender, migraine diagnoses, migraine years, and the type of CGRP mAb from the EMR.

Statistical Analysis

Since this analysis was conducted retrospectively, the sample size was not based on any statistical consideration. The sample size was achieved depending on the number of cases fulfilling the inclusion criteria treated at ACPN. Continuous variables were summarized using mean ± standard deviation [SD] or median interquartile range [IQR], while categorical data were presented as numbers and percentages. The normality assumption was evaluated using the Shapiro–Wilk test. Given that the data did not follow a normal distribution, the Wilcoxon signed rank test was used to analyze the changes in quantitative variables before and after changes. A significance level of $p < 0.05$ was considered statistically significant for all variables. The statistical software SPSS version 26.0 (IBM Corp. SPSS Statistics, Armonk, NY, USA) was utilized for all data analyses.

3. Results

3.1. Demographics and Baseline Characteristics

The participant pool was composed of 53 individuals, all of whom had undergone a switch from one CGRP mAb to another; the descriptive statistics for this cohort are visualized in Table 2. Among the 53 participants, 42 (79.2%) of whom were female, 20 (37.7%) were diagnosed with CM, while the remaining 33 (62.3%) were diagnosed with EM. The mean age (SD) of participants in years was 39.2 (11.0). Furthermore, patients were categorized according to their switching profile and had the following distribution: CGRP/L to R mAb (n = 11; 20.7%), CGRP/R to L mAb (n = 24; 45.3%), and CGRP/L to L mAb (n = 18; 34.0%). All 53 patients were diagnosed with migraine headaches without aura.

Table 2. Patient demographics and clinical features at baseline. CGRP/L: CGRP ligand; CGRP/R: CGRP receptor.

	Total Cohort (n = 53)
Demographics	
Age (years), mean +/− SD.	39.2 +/− 11.0
Sex female, n (%)	42 (79.2%)
Migraine features	
Chronic migraine, n (%)	20 (37.7%)
Pain intensity, mild, n (%)	0 (0.0%)
Pain intensity, moderate, n (%)	48 (90.6%)
Pain intensity, severe, n (%)	5 (9.4%)
Patients with daily headaches, n (%)	10 (18.9%)
Age at migraine diagnosis, mean +/− SD	27.56 +/− 10.62
Migraine duration (years), mean +/− SD	11.6 +/− 11.3
Other features	
Positive family history of migraine, n (%)	16 (30%)
Received prior preventive treatment, n (%)	16 (30%)
Psychiatric comorbidity, n (%)	24 (45.0%)
First monoclonal antibody	
CGRP/L mAb, n (%)	29 (55.0%)
Galcanezumab, n (%)	28 (53)
Eptinezumab, n (%)	1 (2.0%)
CGRP/R mAb (erenumab), n (%)	24 (45.0%)
Second monoclonal antibody	
CGRP/L mAb, n	42
Galcanezumab, n	7
Eptinezumab, n	35
CGRP/R mAb (erenumab), n	11
Switching profile	
CGRP/L to CGRP/R, n	11
CGRP/L to another CGRP/L, n	18
CGRP/R to CGRP/L, n	24

Throughout the study, the frequency of participants' monthly migraine days (MMD) was assessed at three stages prior to and following their medication switch: at baseline, at a 3-month follow-up, and at a 6-month follow-up (this can be visualized in Figure 2). As exhibited in Table 3, the greatest mean (SD) MMD values were recorded at the baseline assessments; however, it is worth mentioning that the post-switch baseline mean of 10.21 (5.42) was lower than that of the pre-switch baseline mean of 12.92 (8.23). Following the pre-switch baseline assessment, the mean was reduced to 5.53 (5.73) by month 3; however, it rose slightly to 5.92 (6.69) by month 6. Following the post-switch baseline assessment, mean MMDs dropped to 5.74 (4.32) by month 3 and further decreased to 5.42 (4.98) by month 6. Patients began treatment on CGRP mAbs, as suggested by our local UAE guidelines, based on at least 4 MMDs, or fewer if the attacks were severe or disabling based on the Migraine Disability Assessment (MIDAS) or Headache Impact Test-6 (HIT-6) scores [22]. There was a minimum of a 3-month washout period prior to switching.

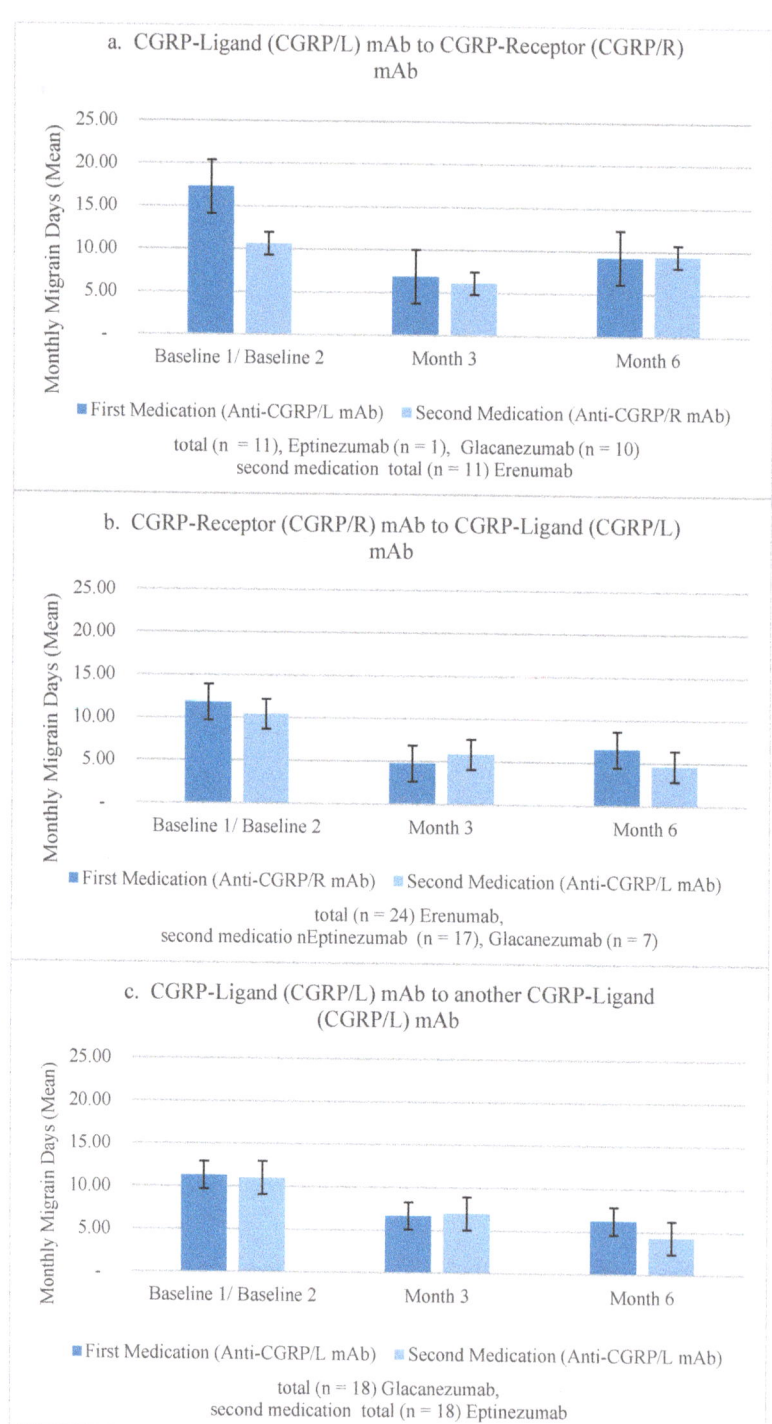

Figure 2. Mean MMDs of switchers. (**a**) MMDs of 11 patients who switched from CGRP/L to CGRP/R mAb. (**b**) MMDs of 24 patients who switched from CGRP/R to CGRP/L. (**c**) MMDs of 18 patients who switched from a CGRP/L to another CGRP/L mAb.

Table 3. MMD mean data before and after switching. Total number of patients (n = 53).

Drug	Mean	Minimum	Maximum	Standard Deviation
Pre-switch BL MMD	12.92	1.0	28.0	8.23
Pre-switch M3 MMD	5.53	0.0	28.0	5.73
Pre-switch M6 MMD	5.92	0.0	28.0	6.69
Post-switch BL MMD	10.21	2.0	28.0	5.42
Post-switch M3 MMD	5.74	0.0	15.0	4.32
Post-switch M6 MMD	5.42	0.0	28.0	4.98

3.2. First CGRP Monoclonal Antibody

A total of 29 patients were initiated on CGRP/L mAbs, while 24 patients were started on CGRP/R mAbs. Upon conducting a follow-up at month 3, it was observed that patients with CM exhibited a higher response rate compared to patients with EM. Specifically, 72% of CM patients responded positively to treatment with CGRP/L mAb, whereas 100% of CM patients responded to CGRP/R mAb. On the other hand, 61% and 63% of EM patients responded to CGRP/L mAb and CGRP/R mAb, respectively. However, it is worth noting that the CM group displayed higher rates of non-responsiveness when treated with CGRP/L mAb (27%) as opposed to CGRP/R mAb (0%). Upon analyzing the 6-month follow-up data, no significant improvement in response rates was observed. Notably, 8 EM patients remained non-responders to both classes of CGRP mAb. Further details regarding response rates during the initial observational period on the first medication are displayed in Figure 3.

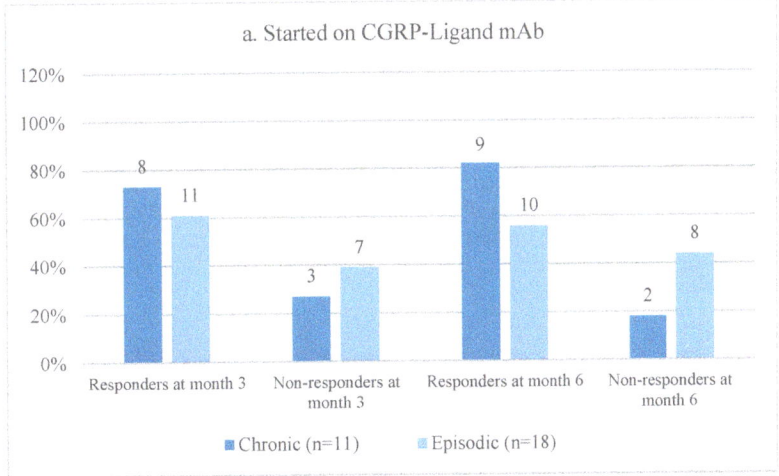

Figure 3. *Cont.*

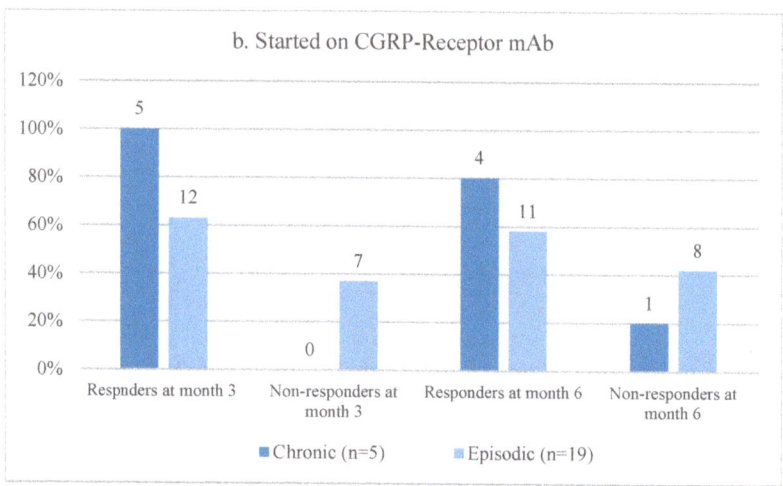

Figure 3. Responder and non-responder rates at month 3 and month 6 for patients with EM or CM on (**a**) CGRP/L mAb and (**b**) CGRP/R mAb during the first observational period.

3.3. Second CGRP Monoclonal Antibody

During the second observational period, the 24 patients who received CGRP/R mAb as their first CGRP mAb switched to anti-CGRP/L mAbs (7 galcanezumab and 17 eptinezumab), whereas out of the 29 patients who started on CGRP/L mAb (28 galcanezumab and 1 eptinezumab), 11 patients were switched to CGRP/R mAbs (erenumab) and 18 patients to another class of CGRP/L mAb (galcanezumab). All the patients in the latter group switched from galcanezumab to eptinezumab, while the one patient who initially received eptinezumab was switched to erenumab. Surprisingly, response rates during the second observational period at the month 3 follow-up dropped in the CM and EM patients who were switched from CGRP/R mAbs to CGRP/L mAbs, specifically from 100% and 63% to 71% and 41%, respectively (Figures 3b and 4a). On the other hand, CM patients who started on CGRP/L mAb had a higher response rate when they were switched to another anti-CGRP/L mAb (100%) rather than to an anti-CGRP/R mAb (87.5%) at month 3 (Figure 4b,c). Overall, CM had a better response rate than EM during the second observational period (Figure 4).

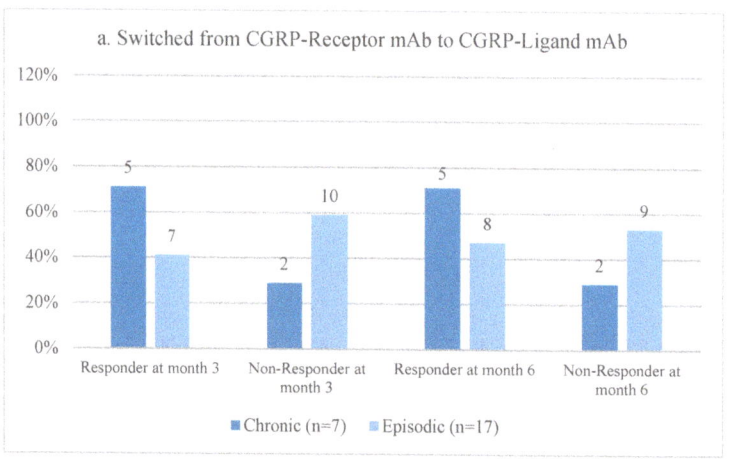

Figure 4. *Cont.*

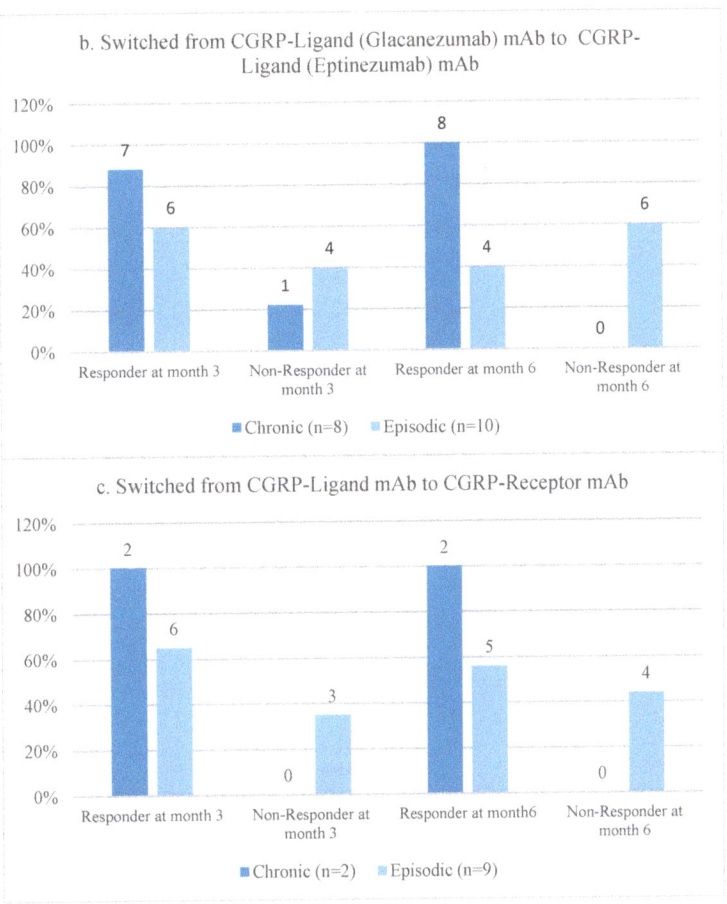

Figure 4. Responder and non-responder rates at month 3 and month 6 for patients with EM or CM (**a**) after switching from CGRP/R mAb to CGRP/L mAb, (**b**) from CGRP/L mAb to CGRP/L mAb, (**c**) or from CGRP/L mAb to CGRP/R mAb.

3.4. First versus Second CGRP Monoclonal Antibody

Tables 4 and 5 present the median differences in MMDs at 6 months compared to the baseline. These tables specifically focus on the first and second CGRP mAbs administered to different patient groups. Interestingly, the overall reduction in MMDs for all patients is precisely identical for both the first and second mAbs.

As shown in Table 6, patients were assessed on their reduction in MMDs from the 6-month follow-up before the switch to their 6-month follow-up after the switch as an additional evaluation of treatment efficacy following a medication switch. In line with the results of the Wilcoxon tests, among ligand–receptor switchers, only one (11.1%) participant experienced a greater than 50% reduction in MMDs, while the vast majority (66.7%) experienced less than a 25% reduction. Although a greater proportion of receptor–ligand switchers (19.1%) experienced a greater than 50% reduction in MMDs, an overwhelming majority (71.4%) experienced less than a 25% reduction. Interestingly, the ligand–ligand cohort exhibited the greatest proportion (33.4%) of participants experiencing a greater than 50% reduction, as well as the lowest proportion (44.4%) of those experiencing less than a 25% reduction. Tables 7 and 8 represent migraine pain severity and the overall improvement status after treatment respectively. Switching the route of administration from subcutaneous to intravenous could possibly influence treatment outcomes. This shift in administration route may impact pharmacokinetics and alter drug absorption, which may contribute to a better treatment response. It could also influence the patient's perception of treatment efficacy as a result of enhancing the placebo effect.

Table 4. Changes in MMDs during the first CGRP mAb from the first baseline.

	Median Difference (IQR) 6 Month	N
All patients	−5.1 (5.5)	53
p-value	<0.001	
Anti-CGRP/L before switching to anti-CGRP/R	−2.2 (7.0)	11
p-value	0.025	
Anti-CGRP/R before switching to anti-CGRP/L	−3.15 (4.5)	24
p-value	0.002	
Anti-CGRP/L before switching to another anti-CGRP/L	−3.21 (5.25)	18
p-value	0.001	

IQR, interquartile range.

Table 5. Changes in MMDs during the second CGRP mAb from the second baseline.

	Median Difference (IQR) 6 Month	N
All patients	−5.0 (5.0)	53
p-value	<0.001	
Anti-CGRP/R after anti-CGRP/L	−1.60 (9.0)	11
p-value	0.109	
Anti-CGRP/L after CGRP/R	−3.73 (3.75)	24
p-value	<0.001	
Anti-CGRP/L after another anti-CGRP/L	−3.47 (7.25)	18
p-value	0.001	

Table 6. M6–M6 percent reductions.

Switching Profile	Q1 Frequency (%)	Q2 Frequency (%)	Q3 Frequency (%)	Q4 Frequency (%)
Ligand–Receptor	6.0 (66.7)	2.0 (22.2)	0.0 (0.0)	1.0 (11.1)
Receptor–Ligand	15.0 (71.4)	2.0 (9.5)	1.0 (4.8)	3.0 (14.3)
Ligand–Ligand	8.0 (44.4)	4.0 (22.2)	3.0 (16.7)	3.0 (16.7)

Q1: <25% reduction in MMDs; Q2: 25% < x < 50% reduction in MMDs; Q3: 50% < x < 75% reduction in MMDs; Q4: >75% reduction in MMDs.

Table 7. Migraine pain severity.

Pain Severity	Initial n (%)	Final (%)
Severe	5 (9.4%)	3 (5.7%)
Moderate	48 (90.6%)	39 (73.6%)
Mild	0 (0.0%)	11 (20.8%)

Table 8. Overall improvement status after treatment.

Status	Number of Patients	Percentage
Improved	37	69.8%
No improvement	15	28.3%
Worsened	1	1.9%

3.5. Exposure and Safety

In this particular study, a total of 53 patients were included. Out of these patients, it was observed that four individuals had an adverse event (AE), three of which took place prior to the switch in treatment. However, it is important to mention that despite these AEs, these patients did not opt to discontinue the treatment, indicating that the AEs were of a minor nature. AEs included constipation, slight pain on injection site, and increased itchiness. The remaining patient reported an AE after the switch. This particular AE involved peri labial numbness and swelling, which occurred during the infusion. The patient was closely monitored and subsequently discharged safely. Treatment was well tolerated among the remaining 49 patients.

4. Discussion

Despite the recent growth in CGRP mAb use as a unique migraine treatment strategy, relatively little is known regarding how switching between CGRP mAb classes can impact the efficacy and tolerability of treatment. Therefore, this study represents another step in furthering our understanding of how CGRP mAb treatments can be safely and effectively applied in a clinical context. Moreover, to our knowledge, this is the first real-world study of its kind to be conducted in the United Arab Emirates and GCC region, thus including an underrepresented population in pivotal trials. Determined prior to data analysis, our primary endpoint was to determine the impact, if any, of switching between CGRP mAb medications on the effectiveness of MMD reduction. Furthermore, our secondary endpoint was to assess the safety and tolerability associated with that switching.

The 53 patients included in data analysis were classified according to their switching profile, including switching from receptor-targeted to ligand-targeted treatment (RL), from ligand-targeted to ligand-targeted (LL) treatment, and from ligand-targeted to receptor-targeted (LR) treatment. Using a Wilcoxon signed rank test, groups were compared at baseline (BL), month 3 (M3), and month 6 (M6) to assess if changes in MMDs were attributable to treatment. Although RL and LL patients experienced significant reductions in MMDs between BL and M6 after switching, this was not the case for LR patients. This incongruence between groups warrants further investigation with larger cohorts into the pathophysiology of CGRP mAb treatments in order to explain why switching in one direction produces starkly different outcomes than the other.

Indeed, prior to conducting the study, we expected switching between different classes of CGRP mAbs could yield improved results, especially for those switching from L to R or vice versa. However, to our surprise, our results showed that switching from ligand to ligand produced better outcomes. This unexpected finding underscores the importance of studying the mechanism of CGRP mAb treatments in greater detail. Conducting future studies with larger cohorts would provide a better insight into the pathophysiology of these treatments and may help further explain why switching from ligand to ligand produces a better outcome.

As part of our analysis, the Wilcoxon signed rank test included comparisons between M6 MMD data prior to and post switching. Across all switching profiles, there was no significant difference between M6 mean MMDs. There are two perspectives from which to interpret this outcome. On one hand, it is surprising that, even after switching medications, patients did not experience further significant improvements in their MMD reduction when compared to their previous medication. This could lead one to assume that if a patient is discontinuing a CGRP mAb treatment due to lack of effectiveness, it may not be significantly advantageous for them to consider switching to another CGRP mAb medication. However, it is simultaneously encouraging that the failure of a previous CGRP mAb medication due to side effects or poor tolerability may not necessarily suggest that future trial of another mAb would result in the same outcome.

Despite a lack of statistically significant differences between M6 values before and after switching, we found it valuable to quantify the percentage of MMD reduction according to switching profile. Notably, 33.4% of LL patients experienced at least a 50% reduction in MMDs 6 months post switch when compared to their 6-month data from their initial medication. Among LR and RL patients, less than 20% of each group experienced a similar degree of MMD reduction. These findings offer modest support to the notion that considering drug mechanism of action may lend itself to improved outcomes post switching. Unfortunately, as erenumab is the only drug included that targets CGRP receptors, there is no means of assessing a receptor–receptor switch for a similar phenomenon.

On the topic of safety, three of four documented AEs took place prior to switching, all of which were considered mild and did not impact patients' continuation of treatment. It is worth noting that despite experiencing AEs on their previous CGRP mAb treatment, the aforementioned three patients switching to another mAb did not result in worsening or new AEs. This is a promising development pointing to switching as a safe, tolerable, and, probably, effective process for those experiencing side effects with their first CGRP mAb prescription.

We have identified two retrospective studies examining lateral switching between CGRP mAb therapies [20,21] to serve as points of comparison with our findings relative to those in the existing literature. The study by Overeem et al. [20] conducted a real-world, multicenter analysis of 78 patients with PPTF on erenumab (receptor-targeted therapy) who switched to ligand-targeted therapies. Unlike the 50% meaningful response rate that was used in our study, their analysis yielded a >30% reduction in MMDs by month 3 after switching in 32% of patients and a >50% reduction in 12% of patients.

The study by Kaltseis et al. [20,21] conducted a larger retrospective assessment of 171 patients who received either one, two, or three different anti-CGRP mAbs. In contrast to the study by Overeem et al., non-response was set as a <50% reduction in MMDs in EM patients and a <30% reduction in CM patients. In total, 5.3% of participants discontinued treatment due to negative side effects. Compared to our study, that study was heavily focused on the quantity of PPTFs. Our study, however, carefully analyzed the impact of switching directionality on outcomes.

In addition, and in contrast to the study by Overeem et al. [20] where patients who switched from a CGRP/R mAb to any CGRP/L mAb experienced improved MMDs, our study did not observe similar outcomes, which could be due to the different characteristics of our cohorts compared to theirs.

When it comes to responding to treatment, it is important to consider that individuals respond differently. There are those who respond promptly, and there may also be individuals who respond later to treatment (late responders and ultra-late responders). A study by Barbanti et al. defined responders as patients with a ≥50% reduction in MMDs at weeks 9–12 from baseline and late responders as those who had a reduction in MMDs between weeks 13 and 16. Ultra-late responders displayed a reduction in MMD between weeks 21 and 24 [25]. This underscores the importance of carefully recognizing this possibility at the time we consider switching patients to a new class of mAbs if they fail their initial mAb therapy.

Our study had several limitations that must be acknowledged. Being retrospective in nature means that controlling certain variables that may have affected the results was not possible. Additionally, the sample size included was small, which limits the generalizability of our findings. As a result, it is worth noting that the data analyzed involved one patient who was initially on eptinezumab, and further studies may consequently be required to confirm our findings on ligand–ligand lateral switching interactions and to verify the generalizability of the data. Furthermore, we realize that in our study we allowed patients to consider switching to a new class of mAbs after a minimum of 3 months of treatment. We adopted this approach based on the EHF and our local UAE guidelines and following a thorough and shared decision process involving the patient and the treating physician. However, we acknowledge that there is a subset of patients who might be late responders and that a longer duration of initial treatment might have resulted in better response [25]. Furthermore, the effectiveness outcome was solely based on MMD reduction. Thus, it may not fully capture the impact of the intervention on other patient related outcomes.

Due to the relatively short observation period of six months for both the first and second medication, it is not possible to rule out the potential for further improvement that could have been attained if patients had prolonged their use of the initial medication before switching to an alternative one. Furthermore, we lack information regarding the potential occurrence of relapse after six months on the second medication following the switch. Lastly, our cohorts included 37 patients who had not previously tried other preventive therapies, representing, probably, less refractory patients than those previously studied in the literature. Out of the 53 patients, 16 individuals had previously attempted preventative treatment for migraine. One patient had tried two preventative therapies before switching to CGRPs mAbs, while the remaining 15 only had one preventative treatment failure prior to switching. Previous preventative treatments included propranolol, amitriptyline, flunarizine, topiramate, and onabotulinumtoxinA. It is important to acknowledge the prescriptions within this region in comparison to other regions across the globe. It is worth noting that currently there exists no prerequisite in this region for individuals to have undergone a specific number of unsuccessful preventative treatments prior to being administered a CGRP mAb.

5. Conclusions

This retrospective, real-world exploratory study examining the effectiveness and safety of switching between CGRP mAb treatments serves as an essential step into furthering our understanding of an under-researched topic. The findings of this study suggest that switching from a previous treatment does not significantly impact the new prescription's effectiveness nor safety.

Among 53 patients enrolled, none experienced significant changes in their MMDs when comparing their mean data for 6 months on the previous medication against 6 months on the new medication. Nevertheless, the data suggest that those switching from one ligand-targeted treatment to another ligand-targeted treatment were more likely to experience additional or compounded reductions in MMDs on top of improvements gained from their initial prescription.

Overall, the findings present in this study point to CGRP switching as a potentially safe and clinically viable practice that may have applications for those experiencing side effects on their current CGRP mAb. Further research is warranted to better understand the long-term implications of switching beyond a 6-month period, as well as if those switching to a CGRP mAb of the same mechanism are truly likely to experience greater improvements than their counterparts.

Author Contributions: I.A.Q., J.L.S., K.A. and V.S. helped collect data. A.A.F., B.A., H.A.B. and Y.B. helped analyze data and performed Medline searches. R.S. and T.A. helped with interpreting data, writing the manuscript, and overseeing the project. All authors have read and agreed to the published version of the manuscript.

Funding: This study received no funding.

Institutional Review Board Statement: This research was conducted in accordance with the Declaration of Helsinki and is consistent with GCP guidelines and the applicable regulatory requirements. The American Center for Psychiatry and Neurology (ACPN) Institutional Review Board has waived the need for informed consent for this study as it involved a retrospective analysis.

Informed Consent Statement: Patient consent was waived due to the study's retrospective design.

Data Availability Statement: All data generated or analyzed during this study are included in this published article. No data repository is available.

Conflicts of Interest: The authors declare no conflicts of interest.

References

1. Safiri, S.; Pourfathi, H.; Eagan, A.; Mansournia, M.A.; Khodayari, M.T.; Sullman, M.J.; Kaufman, J.; Collins, G.; Dai, H.; Bragazzi, N.L. Global, regional, and national burden of migraine in 204 countries and territories, 1990 to 2019. *Pain* **2022**, *163*, e293–e309. [CrossRef]
2. On behalf of Lifting the Burden: The Global Campaign against Headache; Steiner, T.J.; Stovner, L.J.; Jensen, R.; Uluduz, D.; Katsarava, Z. Migraine remains second among the world's causes of disability, and first among young women: Findings from GBD2019. *J. Headache Pain* **2020**, *21*, 137. [CrossRef]
3. Buse, D.C.; Scher, A.I.; Dodick, D.W.; Reed, M.L.; Fanning, K.M.; Adams, A.M.; Lipton, R.B. Impact of Migraine on the Family: Perspectives of People with Migraine and Their Spouse/Domestic Partner in the CaMEO Study. *Mayo Clin. Proc.* **2016**, *91*, 596–611. [CrossRef]
4. Wattiez, A.S.; Sowers, L.P.; Russo, A.F. Calcitonin gene-related peptide (CGRP): Role in migraine pathophysiology and therapeutic targeting. *Expert Opin Ther Targets* **2020**, *24*, 91–100. [CrossRef]
5. Shi, M.; Guo, J.; Li, Z.; Sun, H.; Yang, X.; Yang, D.; Zhao, H. Network meta-analysis on efficacy and safety of different anti-CGRP monoclonal antibody regimens for prophylaxis and treatment of episodic migraine. *Neurol. Res.* **2021**, *43*, 932–949. [CrossRef] [PubMed]
6. Edvinsson, L.; Haanes, K.A.; Warfvinge, K.; Krause, D.N. CGRP as the target of new migraine therapies—successful translation from bench to clinic. *Nat. Rev. Neurol.* **2018**, *14*, 338–350. [CrossRef]
7. Schuster, N.M.; Rapoport, A.M. New strategies for the treatment and prevention of primary headache disorders. *Nat. Rev. Neurol.* **2016**, *12*, 635–650. [CrossRef] [PubMed]
8. Raffaelli, B.; Reuter, U. The Biology of Monoclonal Antibodies: Focus on Calcitonin Gene-Related Peptide for Prophylactic Migraine Therapy. *Neurotherapeutics* **2018**, *15*, 324–335. [CrossRef] [PubMed]
9. Tepper, S.J.; Ashina, M.; Reuter, U.; Brandes, J.L.; Doležil, D.; Silberstein, S.D.; Winner, P.; Zhang, F.; Cheng, S.; Mikol, D.D.; et al. Long-term safety and efficacy of erenumab in patients with chronic migraine: Results from a 52-week, open-label extension study. *Cephalalgia* **2020**, *40*, 543–553. [CrossRef]
10. Kanaan, S.; Hettie, G.; Loder, E.; Burch, R. Real-world effectiveness and tolerability of erenumab: A retrospective cohort study. *Cephalalgia* **2020**, *40*, 1511–1522. [CrossRef]
11. Ruff, D.D.; Ford, J.H.; Tockhorn-Heidenreich, A.; Stauffer, V.L.; Govindan, S.; Aurora, S.K.; Terwindt, G.M.; Goadsby, P.J. Efficacy of galcanezumab in patients with episodic migraine and a history of preventive treatment failure: Results from two global randomized clinical trials. *Eur. J. Neurol.* **2020**, *27*, 609–618. [CrossRef]
12. Dhillon, S. Eptinezumab: First Approval. *Drugs* **2020**, *80*, 733–739. [CrossRef]
13. Winner, P.K.; McAllister, P.; Chakhava, G.; Ailani, J.; Ettrup, A.; Josiassen, M.K.; Lindsten, A.; Mehta, L.; Cady, R. Effects of Intravenous Eptinezumab vs Placebo on Headache Pain and Most Bothersome Symptom When Initiated During a Migraine Attack: A Randomized Clinical Trial. *JAMA* **2021**, *325*, 2348. [CrossRef] [PubMed]
14. Dodick, D.W.; Goadsby, P.J.; Silberstein, S.D.; Lipton, R.B.; Olesen, J.; Ashina, M.; Wilks, K.; Kudrow, D.; Kroll, R.; Kohrman, B.; et al. Safety and efficacy of ALD403, an antibody to calcitonin gene-related peptide, for the prevention of frequent episodic migraine: A randomised, double-blind, placebo-controlled, exploratory phase 2 trial. *Lancet Neurol.* **2014**, *13*, 1100–1107. [CrossRef]
15. Alex, A.; Vaughn, C.; Rayhill, M. Safety and Tolerability of 3 CGRP Monoclonal Antibodies in Practice: A Retrospective Cohort Study. *Headache J. Head Face Pain* **2020**, *60*, 2454–2462. [CrossRef]
16. López Moreno, Y.; Castro Sánchez, M.V.; García Trujillo, L.; Serrano Castro, P.J. Fracaso de un anticuerpo monoclonal anti-CGRP en el tratamiento de la migraña. ¿Tiene sentido probar otro? *Rev. Neurol.* **2022**, *75*, 87. [CrossRef] [PubMed]
17. Briceño-Casado, M.D.P.; Gil-Sierra, M.D.; De-La-Calle-Riaguas, B. Switching of monoclonal antibodies against calcitonin gene-related peptide in chronic migraine in clinical practice: A case series. *Eur. J. Hosp. Pharm.* **2021**, *30*, e19. [CrossRef]
18. Patier Ruiz, I.; Sánchez-Rubio Ferrández, J.; Cárcamo Fonfría, A.; Molina García, T. Early Experiences in Switching between Monoclonal Antibodies in Patients with Nonresponsive Migraine in Spain: A Case Series. *Eur. Neurol.* **2022**, *85*, 132–135. [CrossRef] [PubMed]
19. Ziegeler, C.; May, A. Non-Responders to Treatment with Antibodies to the CGRP-Receptor May Profit from a Switch of Antibody Class. *Headache J. Head Face Pain* **2020**, *60*, 469–470. [CrossRef]
20. Overeem, L.H.; Peikert, A.; Hofacker, M.D.; Kamm, K.; Ruscheweyh, R.; Gendolla, A.; Raffaelli, B.; Reuter, U.; Neeb, L. Effect of antibody switch in non-responders to a CGRP receptor antibody treatment in migraine: A multi-center retrospective cohort study. *Cephalalgia* **2022**, *42*, 291–301. [CrossRef]
21. Sacco, S.; Amin, F.M.; Ashina, M.; Bendtsen, L.; Deligianni, C.I.; Gil-Gouveia, R.; Katsarava, Z.; MaassenVanDenBrink, A.; Martelletti, P.; Mitsikostas, D.D.; et al. European Headache Federation guideline on the use of monoclonal antibodies targeting the calcitonin gene related peptide pathway for migraine prevention—2022 update. *J. Headache Pain* **2022**, *23*, 67. [CrossRef]
22. Alsaadi, T.; Kayed, D.M.; Al-Madani, A.; Hassan, A.M.; Krieger, D.; Riachi, N.; Sarathchandran, P.; Al-Rukn, S. Acute Treatment of Migraine: Expert Consensus Statements from the United Arab Emirates (UAE). *Neurol. Ther.* **2024**, 1–25. [CrossRef] [PubMed]
23. Headache Classification Committee of the International Headache Society (IHS). The International Classification of Headache Disorders, 3rd edition (beta version). *Cephalalgia* **2013**, *33*, 627–808.

24. Kaltseis, K.; Filippi, V.; Frank, F.; Eckhardt, C.; Schiefecker, A.; Broessner, G. Monoclonal antibodies against CGRP (R): Non-responders and switchers: Real world data from an austrian case series. *BMC Neurol.* **2023**, *23*, 174. [CrossRef] [PubMed]
25. Barbanti, P.; Aurilia, C.; Egeo, G.; Proietti, S.; D'Onofrio, F.; Torelli, P.; Aguggia, M.; Bertuzzo, D.; Finocchi, C.; Trimboli, M. Ultra-late response (>24 weeks) to anti-CGRP monoclonal antibodies in migraine: A multicenter, prospective, observational study. *J. Neurol.* **2024**. [CrossRef]

Disclaimer/Publisher's Note: The statements, opinions and data contained in all publications are solely those of the individual author(s) and contributor(s) and not of MDPI and/or the editor(s). MDPI and/or the editor(s) disclaim responsibility for any injury to people or property resulting from any ideas, methods, instructions or products referred to in the content.

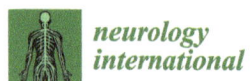 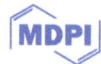

Case Report

Pulsed Radiofrequency for Auriculotemporal Neuralgia: A Case Report

Yan Tereshko [1], Enrico Belgrado [1], Christian Lettieri [1], Simone Dal Bello [1,*], Giovanni Merlino [1,2], Gian Luigi Gigli [2] and Mariarosaria Valente [1,2]

[1] Clinical Neurology Unit, Department of Head-Neck and Neurosciences, Udine University Hospital, Piazzale Santa Maria della Misericordia 15, 33100 Udine, Italy
[2] Department of Medicine (DMED), University of Udine, 33100, Udine, Italy
* Correspondence: simonedalbello@libero.it; Tel.: +39-043-255-9020; Fax: +39-043-255-2719

Abstract: Auriculotemporal neuralgia is a rare facial pain disorder with no therapeutic evidence for refractory cases. We described a male patient with right auriculotemporal neuralgia, refractory to anesthetic nerve blocks and botulinum toxin type A injections, who was successfully treated with pulsed radiofrequency without adverse events. Pulsed radiofrequency may be an effective and safe treatment for refractory auriculotemporal neuralgia.

Keywords: pulsed radiofrequency; pain; auriculotemporal neuralgia

Citation: Tereshko, Y.; Belgrado, E.; Lettieri, C.; Dal Bello, S.; Merlino, G.; Gigli, G.L.; Valente, M. Pulsed Radiofrequency for Auriculotemporal Neuralgia: A Case Report. *Neurol. Int.* **2024**, *16*, 349–355. https://doi.org/10.3390/neurolint16020025

Academic Editor: Yasushi Shibata

Received: 5 February 2024
Revised: 7 March 2024
Accepted: 8 March 2024
Published: 12 March 2024

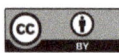

Copyright: © 2024 by the authors. Licensee MDPI, Basel, Switzerland. This article is an open access article distributed under the terms and conditions of the Creative Commons Attribution (CC BY) license (https://creativecommons.org/licenses/by/4.0/).

1. Introduction

The auriculotemporal nerve represents the terminal branch of the trigeminal nerve. Emerging from the foramen ovale outside the skull, the mandibular nerve, which is the third division of the trigeminal nerve, proceeds into the infratemporal fossa. Within this region, it bifurcates around the middle meningeal artery into two trunks: the anterior trunk and the posterior trunk. The latter further branches into the auriculotemporal nerve (ATn). The auriculotemporal nerve is responsible for providing cutaneous sensitivity to various areas, including the auriculotemporal region, external acoustic meatus, tragus, anterior portion of the ear, temporal scalp, posterior portion of the temple, tympanic membrane, temporomandibular joint capsule, and the parotid gland. Additionally, the auriculotemporal nerve carries parasympathetic fibers to the parotid gland [1].

Auriculotemporal neuralgia (ATN) is a rare disorder involving 0.23–0.4% of the patients in tertiary headache centers, characterized by unilateral side-locked pain localized in the territory of the auriculotemporal nerve [1–4]. The pain could be paroxysmal, moderate to severe in intensity, and variable in duration; however, continuous pain is often seen in this scenario. The pain can be spontaneous or can be triggered by pressure over the preauricular region, chewing, menses, gustatory stimuli, or facial tactile stimuli. The pain is usually throbbing (probably due to the temporal artery's proximity) but could also be stabbing, lancinating, or shock-like and can radiate to the occipital, retro-orbital, or temporal region [2]. Some authors have proposed different mechanisms that can cause this disorder: compression at the level of the fascia bands in the preauricular region, the wrapping around the superficial temporal artery, the entrapment at the level of the pterygoideus externus muscle or between the pterygoideus internus and externus muscles, and mandibular overclosure [5–9]. This disorder may be misdiagnosed since the temporal and pulsatile localization may resemble the clinical features of migraine; in the case of auriculotemporal neuralgia, the localization is side-locked, photo-phono-osmophobia is typically absent, and the pain is triggered or exacerbated only by applying pressure over the preauricular region involved [1,2]. The auriculotemporal nerve is a branch of the trigeminal nerve; however, the pain quality and the localization of the pain are completely different from trigeminal neuralgia, and the efficacy of carbamazepine is not established [1]. Since this is a very rare disorder with clinical characteristics that overlap with other more frequent facial pain conditions, diagnosis and therapy could be challenging.

Anesthetic auriculotemporal nerve blockade is considered therapeutic and diagnostic; sometimes, the response is transient, and multiple nerve blocks are required. In a recent case series and case report, botulinum toxin type A (BoNT/A) was a valid alternative therapy in refractory cases [2,10]. The treatment of refractory cases is challenging, and the literature needs to be more conclusive. Pulsed radiofrequency (PRF) is a common treatment modality for chronic pain [11]. Pulsed radiofrequency (PRF) is a technique that applies radiofrequency electrical current to a target nerve; the electrical current is of short duration (20 ms) and is followed by a resting phase (480 ms) that repeats for a specific time [12–14]. Pulsed radiofrequency (PRF) generates an electromagnetic field to modulate the transmission of nerve impulses; the changes induced by electric fields act selectively on small, non-myelinated nerve fibers, producing a motor-sparing effect. Research has highlighted that the analgesic effect of PRF is not linked to thermal effects or permanent neural damage, suggesting a potential neuromodulatory mechanism. This mechanism may alter synaptic transmission or the excitability of C fibers. PRF affects afferent pathways and may exhibit a local anti-inflammatory effect by involving the immune system in the nociceptive process. Histological evaluations indicate that PRF induces transient endoneural edema, persisting up to a week after treatment. Pain relief commonly observed after PRF treatment can last for several months. Currently, PRF is used in the treatment of conditions such as radicular pain, occipital and trigeminal neuralgia, as well as shoulder and knee pain. Still, it is also effective in migraine, tension-type headaches, and cluster headaches [11,15–19]. Radiofrequency energy used in this technique is not continuous but pulsed, allowing for sufficient cooling to maintain a target temperature below 42 °C and prevent nerve axonotmesis or neurotmesis [20,21]. In a 2009 study, however, microscopic alterations were found in mitochondria, microfilaments, microtubules and membranes of C-fibers, A-delta fibers, and A-beta fibers [22]. This technique was never described in auriculotemporal neuralgia; however, it has been used in other neuralgias with promising results [18,19].

2. Case Description

We present a case of right auriculotemporal neuralgia, refractory to multiple nerve blocks and BoNT/A injections, successfully treated with pulsed radiofrequency (PRF). The patient is a 49-year-old man who came in May 2022 to our tertiary headache center complaining of persistent throbbing pain in the right preauricular and temporal region with superimposed spontaneous painful stabbing paroxysmal pain.

Sometimes, the pain radiated to the occipital region. The background pain was mild (NRS 3/10), and the exacerbations were severe (NRS 8/10); the exacerbations lasted 20–40 min and occurred 3–4 times per day. The pain started in February 2021, a few weeks after a mild SARS-CoV-2 infection. Neurological examination highlighted tenderness in the right temporal preauricular region with allodynia, and the pressure over the preauricular region determined acute stabbing pain along the course of the auriculotemporal nerve. He denied nausea, vomiting, photophobia, phonophobia, and osmophobia. Anesthetic right auriculotemporal nerve blockade with 1 mL of bupivacaine abolished pain after 5 min, and the effect lasted for 20 days; the procedure was performed five other times with the same result. Brain Magnetic Resonance Imaging (MRI) reported mild vascular gliosis, and angio-CT was normal; echography of the right temporal region excluded temporal artery involvement, and the MRI of the temporomandibular articulation did not show any pathologic changes. The dental exam was normal.

Blood tests were unremarkable. Oxygen 100% 12 L/min for 15 min and verapamil 80 mg TID were ineffective. We excluded cervicogenic headache, atypical facial pain, hemicrania continua, myofascial pain, temporomandibular junction dysfunction, tooth pain, chronic migraine, temporal arteritis, and trigeminal neuralgia based on the clinical features, neurological examination, and diagnostic instrumental tools. The anesthetic block of the auriculotemporal nerve was effective in aborting pain. However, the effect was not long-lasting. A diagnosis of right auriculotemporal neuralgia was performed. Since the disturb was refractory to anesthetic blocks, botulinum toxin type A therapy was discussed with the patient, and he accepted. We performed onabotulinumtoxinA subcutaneous injections (85 U) in the right preauricular and temporal region regions along the course of the auriculotemporal nerve; the therapy improved pain from a baseline of NRS 8/10 to 4/10 at 1-month evaluation and to 5/10 at 3-month evaluation; the frequency of the exacerbations remained the same and the background pain remitted. The benefit lasted about three months, and then the background and exacerbating pain returned to the baseline; the procedure was repeated twice with the same result. The outcome of onabotulinumtoxinA was satisfactory; however, it could not remit pain completely, and the patient's quality of life was still impaired. We decided to perform pulsed radiofrequency with the patient's consent; the patient was informed of the off-label nature of the therapy and the lack of any evidence in the literature regarding its efficacy in this clinical condition; he gave written formal consent for the treatment with pulsed radiofrequency and for his images and clinical information to be published.

3. Methods

The procedure was performed using the Cosman G4™ RF generator device (Cosman Medical Inc., Marlborough, MA, USA) and kit EchoRF™. The patient was positioned in a prone position with the left aspect of the head lying on the bed, and disinfection with betadine was performed. We located the superficial temporal artery via palpation and inserted the RF needle (Cosman Medical Inc., Marlborough, MA, USA) (SCK 100 mm, 22G, curved, active tip 5 mm) 1 cm forward with the tip upward; when the needle was in position, the stylet was removed, and the RF probe was inserted (Figure 1). The correct position of the RF probe was confirmed using 50 Hz sensory stimulation at 0.3 V, which determined paresthesia in the territory of the right auriculotemporal nerve (the RF probe is at the target when the tingling sensation is evoked with a stimulation below 0.5 V). Then, a pulsed current was applied twice for 180 s (pulsed current for 20 ms at 2 Hz, followed by 480 ms of resting) with an 85 V output, an electrical current of 290 mA, and a 300 Ohm impedance. The temperature did not exceed 42 °C, preventing nerve damage.

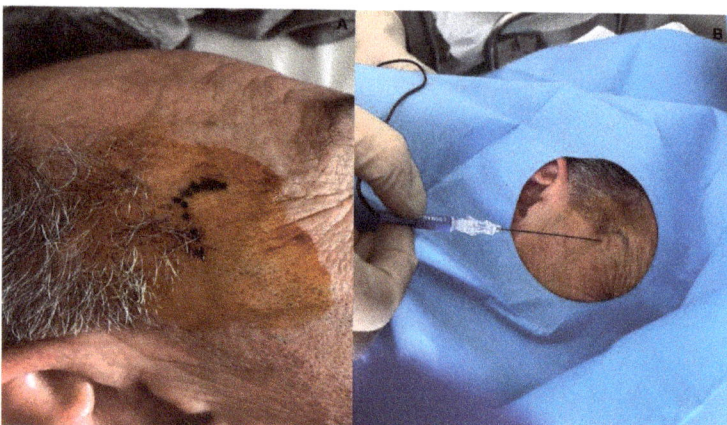

Figure 1. (**A**) shows the temporal area of the patient where the right superficial temporal artery was located with a landmark-guided technique. The auriculotemporal nerve was localized, drawing a line between the lateral cantus and the tragus; from the mid-point of this line, we proceeded upward, localizing the superficial temporal artery. The auriculotemporal nerve was about 0.5 cm anterior to the artery. (**B**) shows the RF needle inserted subcutaneously in the nearby of the right auriculotemporal nerve, anterior to the superficial temporal artery, with a cephalad direction and parallel to the auriculotemporal nerve. The 50 Hz sensory stimulation at 0.3 V determined the occurrence of paresthesia along the course of the auriculotemporal nerve and confirmed the correct stimulation site.

4. Results

The background and the exacerbating pain gradually improved during the four weeks after the procedure, and at 1-month follow-up, there was a complete paroxysmal and background pain remission (NRS 0). Allodynia was remitted shortly after a 3-month follow-up. The pain remission persisted during the 6-month and 12-month follow-up and is still ongoing. The patient denied any adverse events related to the procedure and was satisfied with the long-standing positive outcome.

5. Discussion

Auriculotemporal neuralgia is not specifically addressed in the third edition of the International Classification of Headache Disorders [23]. In the second edition (ICHD-II), the auriculotemporal neuralgia (ATN) was considered as a possible inclusion under epigraph 13.7, which encompasses "other terminal branch neuralgias" of the trigeminal nerve. Consequently, in the current context, ATN does not align accurately with any diagnostic categories outlined in the third edition of the International Classification of Headache Disorders (ICHD-III) [1,2].

The neuralgia of the auriculotemporal nerve may stem from nerve entrapment during its passage through the lateral pterygoid muscle or at the level of the roof of the infratemporal fossa, frequently due to a muscle spasm or other pathologic conditions. Other potential causes include the formation of synovial cysts, malformations, aneurysms of the middle meningeal artery, and fractures of the mandibular condyle. Perineural spread of tumors involving the auriculotemporal nerve has also been reported [1,2]. In this case report, there were no secondary causes of auriculotemporal nerve neuralgia; it is probable that the etiology could be traced to the entrapment of the nerve during its passage through the lateral pterygoid muscle or at the level of the roof of the infratemporal fossa, the compression at the level of the superficial temporal artery, or could be idiopathic since the MRI was negative. Since our patients reported the occurrence of this disorder weeks after a SARS-CoV-2 infection, it could have had a possible role in its pathology. There have been some cases of trigeminal neuralgia probably due to a SARS-CoV-2 infection; however, the link between COVID-19 and our case of auriculotemporal neuralgia is only determined by the time that occurred between the infection and the clinical presentation of this disorder. Therefore, a certain connection is not feasible [24].

Given the rarity of this condition, the availability of high-quality studies is limited. The literature contains only a few articles discussing therapeutic options for auriculotemporal neuralgia. The evidence supporting treatments is primarily based on case series documenting positive responses to applying local anesthetic blocks of the auriculotemporal nerve, with or without steroids. Other mentioned therapeutic options include the use of medications such as carbamazepine and gabapentin or the use of botulinum toxin with controversial results [2,10,25]. Other treatment options may include cryoneuroablation and peripheral nerve stimulation, the latter used on male patients with chronic migraine pain in the distribution auriculotemporal nerve region [26,27]; however, these therapies were described only in single case reports and not on a large population of patients. To date, the most effective and reliable therapy is the anesthetic nerve blockade, while the other therapeutic options are still inconclusive. The treatments involving local anesthetic blocks of the auriculotemporal nerve and botulinum toxin injections yielded results for our patient that were not entirely satisfactory. Consequently, we decided to apply pulsed radiofrequency as a last resort since this approach successfully treats neuropathic pain conditions, and the short-term and long-term adverse events are very low [11,15–19].

Pulsed radiofrequency was never described in auriculotemporal neuralgia. However, this procedure has already been utilized in similar conditions such as occipital and trigeminal neuralgia [11]. Therefore, its application in other types of neuralgia, such as auriculotemporal nerve neuralgia, should be encouraged. This mini-invasive technique uses a pulsed current and maintains a target temperature below 42 °C, preventing nerve axonotmesis or neurotmesis [20,21]. The nerve stimulation affects pain by inducing long-term depression (LDT), inhibiting the C-fibers, and reducing pain signaling from the periphery to the central nervous system [28,29]. Moreover, it has been demonstrated that PRF enhances the descending inhibitory pathway [30]. On a molecular level, PFR exerts action on pain, decreasing dorsal horn microglia release of inflammatory cytokines and therefore reduces the facilitation in nociceptive signaling and sensitization [31–33]; moreover, it exerts its analgesic effect by the increase in mRNA expression of endogenous opioid precursors and related opioid peptides in the central nervous system [34].

Our patient improved after one PRF procedure and is still pain-free after twelve months, without any adverse events or nerve damage. No other cases reported in the literature were treated with PRF, and we hope our report may prompt others to use this therapy in this rare neuralgia and even in refractory cases. Moreover, it is unknown if the therapy may determine a complete remission of pain or may provide only temporary long-standing pain relief. In occipital neuralgia and trigeminal neuralgia, the literature reports temporary benefit; in the case of trigeminal neuralgia, a recent study applied PRF, CRF, and CCPRF to the Gasserian ganglion in a cohort of TN patients; the results in the PRF group were less satisfactory when compared to the other two groups, with pain relief of 82%, 9.1%, and 0% at 6-month, 12-month, and 24-month follow-up [35]. In most studies, the benefit lasted at least 3 months in occipital neuralgia [36].

Additional studies will be required to confirm the effectiveness of pulsed radiofrequency in managing auriculotemporal neuralgia, even though the rarity of this condition complicates the implementation of in-depth research.

Author Contributions: Y.T.: Conceptualization, Investigation, Data Curation, Visualization, Writing—Original Draft, Project Administration; E.B.: Conceptualization, Supervision, Writing—Review and Editing, Resources, Project Administration, supervision; C.L.: Writing—Review and Editing, Visualization; S.D.B.: Investigation, Data Curation, Writing—Original Draft G.M.: Supervision; G.L.G.: Writing—Review and Editing, Visualization; M.V.: Writing—Review and Editing, Project Administration, Supervision. All authors have read and agreed to the published version of the manuscript.

Funding: This research received no external funding.

Institutional Review Board Statement: All procedures contributing to this work comply with the ethical standards of the relevant national and institutional committees on human experimentation and with the declaration of Helsinki. The patient gave formal written consent for the treatment with BoNT/A and for his data and images to be used for research. Friuli Venezia Giulia (CEUR)'s ethics committee waived the need for this study's approval since the responsibility of case reports is entirely in the hands of the authors, and they describe something that has already been carried out (statement of the 3 December 2021).

Informed Consent Statement: Informed consent was obtained from all subjects involved in the study.

Data Availability Statement: The original contributions presented in the study are included in the article, further inquiries can be directed to the corresponding author.

Conflicts of Interest: The authors declare no conflicts of interest.

Abbreviations

ATN	auriculotemporal neuralgia
BoNT/A	botulinum toxin type A
CT	computerized tomography
AEs	adverse events
NRS	numeric rating scale
MRI	magnetic resonance imaging

References

1. Ruiz, M.; Porta-Etessam, J.; Garcia-Ptacek, S.; de la Cruz, C.; Cuadrado, M.L.; Guerrero, A.L. Auriculotemporal Neuralgia: Eight New Cases Report. *Pain Med.* **2016**, *17*, 1744–1748. [CrossRef]
2. Tereshko, Y.; Belgrado, E.; Lettieri, C.; Gigli, G.L.; Valente, M. Botulinum Toxin Type A for the Treatment of Auriculotemporal Neuralgia—A Case Series. *Toxins* **2023**, *15*, 274. [CrossRef]
3. Damarjian, E. Auriculo-temporal neuralgia—An original diagnostic and therapeutic approach. *R. I. Med. J.* **1970**, *53*, 100–101.
4. Kosminsky, M.; Nascimento, M.G.D. Primary auriculotemporal neuralgia. Case report. *Rev. Dor* **2015**, *16*, 312–315. [CrossRef]
5. Janis, J.E.; Hatef, D.A.; Thakar, H.; Reece, E.M.; McCluskey, P.D.; Schaub, T.A.; Theivagt, C.; Guyuron, B. The zygomaticotemporal branch of the trigeminal nerve: Part II. Anatomical variations. *Plast. Reconstr. Surg.* **2010**, *126*, 435–442. [CrossRef]
6. Chim, H.; Okada, H.C.; Brown, M.S.; Alleyne, B.; Liu, M.T.; Zwiebel, S.; Guyuron, B. The auriculotemporal nerve in etiology of migraine headaches: Compression points and anatomical variations. *Plast. Reconstr. Surg.* **2012**, *130*, 336–341. [CrossRef] [PubMed]
7. Loughner, B.A.; Larkin, L.H.; Mahan, P.E. Nerve entrapment in the lateral pterygoid muscle. *Oral Surg. Oral Med. Oral Pathol.* **1990**, *69*, 299–306. [CrossRef] [PubMed]
8. Anil, A.; Peker, T.; Turgut, H.B.; Gülekon, I.N.; Liman, F. Variations in the anatomy of the inferior alveolar nerve. *Br. J. Oral Maxillofac. Surg.* **2003**, *41*, 236–239. [CrossRef]
9. Fernandes, P.R.B.; de Vasconsellos, H.A.; Okeson, J.P.; Bastos, R.L.; Maia, M.L.T. The anatomical relationship between the position of the auriculotemporal nerve and mandibular condyle. *Cranio* **2003**, *21*, 165–171. [CrossRef] [PubMed]
10. Pinto, M.J.; Guerrero, A.L.; Costa, A. Botulinum toxin as a novel therapeutic approach for auriculotemporal neuralgia. *Headache* **2021**, *61*, 392–395. [CrossRef]
11. Jorge, D.D.M.F.; Huber, S.C.; Rodrigues, B.L.; Da Fonseca, L.F.; Azzini, G.O.M.; Parada, C.A.; Paulus-Romero, C.; Lana, J.F.S.D. The Mechanism of Action between Pulsed Radiofrequency and Orthobiologics: Is There a Synergistic Effect? *Int. J. Mol. Sci.* **2022**, *23*, 11726. [CrossRef]
12. Podhajsky, R.J.; Sekiguchi, Y.; Kikuchi, S.; Myers, R.R. The histologic effects of pulsed and continuous radiofrequency lesions at 42 degrees C to rat dorsal root ganglion and sciatic nerve. *Spine* **2005**, *30*, 1008–1013. [CrossRef]
13. Vallejo, R.; Benyamin, R.M.; Kramer, J.; Stanton, G.; Joseph, N.J. Pulsed radiofrequency denervation for the treatment of sacroiliac joint syndrome. *Pain Med.* **2006**, *7*, 429–434. [CrossRef]
14. West, M.; Wu, H. Pulsed radiofrequency ablation for residual and phantom limb pain: A case series. *Pain Pract.* **2010**, *10*, 485–491. [CrossRef] [PubMed]
15. Batistaki, C.; Madi, A.I.; Karakosta, A.; Kostopanagiotou, G.; Arvaniti, C. Pulsed Radiofrequency of the Occipital Nerves: Results of a Standardized Protocol on Chronic Headache Management. *Anesthesiol. Pain Med.* **2021**, *11*, e112235. [CrossRef] [PubMed]
16. Chua, N.H.L.; Vissers, K.C.; Sluijter, M.E. Pulsed radiofrequency treatment in interventional pain management: Mechanisms and potential indications—A review. *Acta Neurochir.* **2011**, *153*, 763–771. [CrossRef]
17. Bogduk, N. Pulsed radiofrequency. *Pain Med.* **2006**, *7*, 396–407. [CrossRef] [PubMed]
18. Fang, L.; Tao, W.; Jingjing, L.; Nan, J. Comparison of High-voltage- with Standard-voltage Pulsed Radiofrequency of Gasserian Ganglion in the Treatment of Idiopathic Trigeminal Neuralgia. *Pain Pract.* **2015**, *15*, 595–603. [CrossRef]
19. Lan, M.; Zipu, J.; Ying, S.; Hao, R.; Fang, L. Efficacy and safety of CT-guided percutaneous pulsed radiofrequency treatment of the Gasserian ganglion in patients with medically intractable idiopathic trigeminal neuralgia. *J. Pain Res.* **2018**, *11*, 2877–2885. [CrossRef]
20. Park, D.; Chang, M.C. The mechanism of action of pulsed radiofrequency in reducing pain: A narrative review. *J. Yeungnam Med. Sci.* **2022**, *39*, 200–205. [CrossRef]
21. Chang, M.C. Efficacy of Pulsed Radiofrequency Stimulation in Patients with Peripheral Neuropathic Pain: A Narrative Review. *Pain Physician* **2018**, *21*, E225–E234. [CrossRef]
22. Erdine, S.; Bilir, A.; Cosman, E.R.; Cosman, E.R.J. Ultrastructural changes in axons following exposure to pulsed radiofrequency fields. *Pain Pract.* **2009**, *9*, 407–417. [CrossRef]
23. Arnold, M. Headache Classification Committee of the International Headache Society (IHS) The International Classification of Headache Disorders, 3rd edition. *Cephalalgia* **2018**, *38*, 1–211. [CrossRef]
24. Molina-Gil, J.; González-Fernández, L.; García-Cabo, C. Trigeminal neuralgia as the sole neurological manifestation of COVID-19: A case report. *Headache* **2021**, *61*, 560–562. [CrossRef]
25. O'Neill, F.; Nurmikko, T.; Sommer, C. Other facial neuralgias. *Cephalalgia* **2017**, *37*, 658–669. [CrossRef] [PubMed]
26. Trescot, A.M. Headache management in an interventional pain practice. *Pain Physician* **2000**, *3*, 197–200. [CrossRef] [PubMed]
27. Simopoulos, T.; Bajwa, Z.; Lantz, G.; Lee, S.; Burstein, R. Implanted auriculotemporal nerve stimulator for the treatment of refractory chronic migraine. *Headache* **2010**, *50*, 1064–1069. [CrossRef] [PubMed]
28. Sluijter, M.E.; van Kleef, M. Pulsed radiofrequency. *Pain Med.* **2007**, *8*, 381–388. [CrossRef] [PubMed]
29. Huang, R.-Y.; Liao, C.-C.; Tsai, S.-Y.; Yen, C.-T.; Lin, C.-W.; Chen, T.-C.; Lin, W.-T.; Chang, C.-H.; Wen, Y.-R. Rapid and Delayed Effects of Pulsed Radiofrequency on Neuropathic Pain: Electrophysiological, Molecular, and Behavioral Evidence Supporting Long-Term Depression. *Pain Physician* **2017**, *20*, E269–E283. [PubMed]

30. Hagiwara, S.; Iwasaka, H.; Takeshima, N.; Noguchi, T. Mechanisms of analgesic action of pulsed radiofrequency on adjuvant-induced pain in the rat: Roles of descending adrenergic and serotonergic systems. *Eur. J. Pain* **2009**, *13*, 249–252. [CrossRef] [PubMed]
31. Cho, H.K.; Cho, Y.W.; Kim, E.H.; Sluijter, M.E.; Hwang, S.J.; Ahn, S.H. Changes in pain behavior and glial activation in the spinal dorsal horn after pulsed radiofrequency current administration to the dorsal root ganglion in a rat model of lumbar disc herniation: Laboratory investigation. *J. Neurosurg. Spine* **2013**, *19*, 256–263. [CrossRef]
32. Cho, H.K.; Kang, J.H.; Kim, S.-Y.; Choi, M.-J.; Hwang, S.J.; Cho, Y.-W.; Ahn, S.-H. Changes in Neuroglial Activity in Multiple Spinal Segments after Caudal Epidural Pulsed Radiofrequency in a Rat Model of Lumbar Disc Herniation. *Pain Physician* **2016**, *19*, E1197–E1209.
33. Jiang, R.; Li, P.; Yao, Y.-X.; Li, H.; Liu, R.; Huang, L.-E.; Ling, S.; Peng, Z.; Yang, J.; Zha, L.; et al. Pulsed radiofrequency to the dorsal root ganglion or the sciatic nerve reduces neuropathic pain behavior, decreases peripheral pro-inflammatory cytokines and spinal β-catenin in chronic constriction injury rats. *Reg. Anesth. Pain Med.* **2019**, *44*, 742–746. [CrossRef] [PubMed]
34. Moffett, J.; Fray, L.M.; Kubat, N.J. Activation of endogenous opioid gene expression in human keratinocytes and fibroblasts by pulsed radiofrequency energy fields. *J. Pain Res.* **2012**, *5*, 347–357. [CrossRef] [PubMed]
35. Elawamy, A.; Abdalla, E.E.M.; Shehata, G.A. Effects of Pulsed Versus Conventional Versus Combined Radiofrequency for the Treatment of Trigeminal Neuralgia: A Prospective Study. *Pain Physician* **2017**, *20*, E873–E881. [PubMed]
36. Manolitsis, N.; Elahi, F. Pulsed radiofrequency for occipital neuralgia. *Pain Physician* **2014**, *17*, E709–E717. [CrossRef]

Disclaimer/Publisher's Note: The statements, opinions and data contained in all publications are solely those of the individual author(s) and contributor(s) and not of MDPI and/or the editor(s). MDPI and/or the editor(s) disclaim responsibility for any injury to people or property resulting from any ideas, methods, instructions or products referred to in the content.

MDPI AG
Grosspeteranlage 5
4052 Basel
Switzerland
Tel.: +41 61 683 77 34

Neurology International Editorial Office
E-mail: neurolint@mdpi.com
www.mdpi.com/journal/neurolint

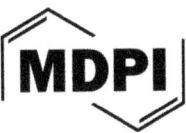

Disclaimer/Publisher's Note: The statements, opinions and data contained in all publications are solely those of the individual author(s) and contributor(s) and not of MDPI and/or the editor(s). MDPI and/or the editor(s) disclaim responsibility for any injury to people or property resulting from any ideas, methods, instructions or products referred to in the content.

www.ingramcontent.com/pod-product-compliance
Lightning Source LLC
LaVergne TN
LVHW070723100526
838202LV00013B/1157